CONTEMPORARY TOPICS
IN IMMUNOBIOLOGY
VOLUME 3

CONTEMPORARY TOPICS IN IMMUNOBIOLOGY

A Continuation Order Plan is available for this series. A continuation order will bring delivery of each new volume immediately upon publication. Volumes are billed only upon actual shipment. For further information please contact the publisher.

CONTEMPORARY TOPICS IN IMMUNOBIOLOGY

VOLUME 3

EDITED BY

MAX D. COOPER
University of Alabama
Birmingham, Alabama

and

NOEL L. WARNER
The Walter and Eliza Hall Institute
Victoria, Australia

PLENUM PRESS • NEW YORK – LONDON

Library of Congress Catalog Card Number 68-26769

ISBN-13: 978-1-4684-3047-9   e-ISBN-13: 978-1-4684-3045-5

DOI: 10.1007/978-1-4684-3045-5

Contributors

A. C. Allison   *Clinical Research Centre, Harrow, Middlesex, England*

Max D. Cooper   *Spain Immunology Research Laboratories, Departments of Pediatrics and Microbiology, University of Alabama in Birmingham, Birmingham, Alabama*

Joseph M. Davie   *Departments of Pathology and Microbiology, Washington University School of Medicine, St. Louis, Missouri*

Richard K. Gershon   *Department of Pathology, Yale University School of Medicine, New Haven, Connecticut*

Leonard A. Herzenberg   *Department of Genetics, Stanford University School of Medicine, Stanford, California*

Leonore A. Herzenberg   *Department of Genetics, Stanford University School of Medicine, Stanford, California*

Alexander R. Lawton, III   *Spain Immunology Research Laboratories, Departments of Pediatrics and Microbiology, University of Alabama in Birmingham, Birmingham, Alabama*

Rose Lieberman   *Laboratory of Immunology, National Institutes of Allergy and Infectious Diseases, National Institutes of Health, Bethesda, Maryland*

Graham F. Mitchell   *Basel Institute for Immunology, Grenzacherstrasse 487, CH-4058, Basel, Switzerland*

Peter J. Morris   *Reader in Surgery and Director, Tissue Transplantation Laboratories, Department of Surgery, University of Melbourne, Royal Melbourne Hospital, Australia*

William E. Paul   *Laboratory of Immunology, National Institutes of Allergy and Infectious Diseases, National Institutes of Health, Bethesda, Maryland*

Hans Wigzell   *Department of Tumor Biology, Karolinska Institutet, Stockholm, Sweden*

Henry H. Wortis   *Department of Pathology, Tufts University School of Medicine, Boston, Massachusetts*

Preface

Contemporary immunobiology is an ever-diversifying field that embraces many aspects of cellular and humoral immune responsiveness. This includes the phylogeny, ontogeny, induction, regulation, expression, and differentiation of the immune-cell series, as well as the relationship of these to the pathogenesis of many disease processes. It is clearly beyond the limitations of each volume in this series to comprehensively cover progress in each of these fields. Three general areas of contemporary investigations are discussed in the current issue: cellular events of B cell differentiation, including antigen recognition and responsiveness of B lymphocytes; regulation of the immune response by T cells, and the roles of this regulatory system in allotype suppression and in autoimmunity; and the genetic control of immune responses and its possible relation to disease pathogenesis.

Analysis of responsiveness of B lymphocytes has been greatly aided by the availability of athymic nude mice. The immunological responsiveness of these mice to a wide range of stimuli has been reviewed and analyzed by H.H. Wortis. This article concludes with the provocative thesis that in the future "nudes will supply new rather than confirmatory data . . . (especially regarding) the development of neoplasia." In contrast to the studies on the congenitally athymic mice, G.F. Mitchell considers many of the problems inherent in studies of T cell deficient animals in relation to T cell modification of B cell responses, and considers an hypothesis relating "T cell independence," antigen persistence, and low-affinity antibody production. The recognition of antigen by B cells is considered in some depth first by J.M. Davie and W.E. Paul and then by H. Wigzell. The former authors consider current techniques for the demonstration of antigen-binding cells, and the presence and significance of these cells in nonimmune animals, in immunity and in tolerance. The relationship of the cell-surface-bound immunoglobulin to humoral antibody is discussed by H. Wigzell in terms of immunoglobulin class, affinity for antigen, and specificity for antigen. Analysis of B cell differentiation has been approached in a different manner by A.R. Lawton and M.D. Cooper, who use class-specific antibodies to immunoglobulins to modify subsequent B cell expression of immunoglobulin production. In considering the available data from avian and mammalian studies, these authors present a compelling thesis of antigen-independent B cell differentiation that involves sequential switching of heavy-chain genes in the fetal/neonatal period.

In the past seven years, evidence of T cell involvement in the complete differentiation of the B cell pathway has continued to mount. However, more recently, another function of T cells has become increasingly recognized, namely, a regulatory or suppressive role. The current data in this field are comprehensively detailed and analyzed by R.K. Gershon, who concludes that "the antigen-reactive T cell can be thought of as the conductor of the immunological orchestra . . . in that this T cell decides on the basis of the energetics of the binding of its receptor(s) whether to turn other cells on or off." In summarizing their studies on allotype suppression in mice, L.A. Herzenberg and L.A. Herzenberg also present relevant data toward the thesis that suppressive or regulatory T cells may be involved and operate to inhibit expression of immunoglobulin by B cells. These general concepts of T and B cell involvement in regulation of the immune responses are then extended by A.C. Allison to the self-tolerance situation, and a thesis on the failure of suppressive T cells to control autoimmune expression is developed.

Much recent interest has developed in the genetic controls of the induction of antibody responses, and R. Lieberman and W.E. Paul describe a striking example of this in the response of mice to immunoglobulin allotypic and idiotypic antigens. Through the use of congenic and recombinant strains, they clearly demonstrate the existence of several gene loci involved in this control. The relationship of these genes to the major histocompatibility loci is discussed. This topic is further extended to man in the comprehensive review of histocompatibility antigens and disease by P.J. Morris. In this chapter, the current data on HL-A antigens and disease association are considered, and compared to genetic controls of disease susceptibility in animals and to immune-response gene action in animals. It is noted that, while a parallel argument could be made for mouse and man in linking immune-response genes with histocompatibility genes, there is as yet relatively little direct information available in man, and other possible mechanisms of HL-A association with disease should be considered.

In compiling this issue of the series, it is our hope that these chapters, representing some of the challenging areas of contemporary immunobiology, will act as stimuli to "contemporary investigators" in their own researches in these areas, and will serve as well to update other interested investigators, teachers, and students in the ever-expanding horizons of contemporary immunobiology.

M.D. COOPER

December, 1973   N.L. WARNER

Contents

Chapter 3. On the Relationship Between Cellular and Humoral Antibodies
Hans Wigzell

Chapter 4. T Cell Modification of B Cell Responses to Antigen in Mice
    Graham F. Mitchell

**Chapter 5. Genetic Control of Antibody Responses to Myeloma Proteins
    of Mice**
    Rose Lieberman and William E. Paul

Chapter 6. Histocompatibility Systems, Immune Response, and Disease in Man
Peter J. Morris

Chapter 7. Antigen-Binding Receptors on Lymphocytes
Joseph M. Davie and William E. Paul

Chapter 8. Modification of B Lymphocyte Differentiation by Anti-Immunoglobulins
Alexander R. Lawton, III, and Max D. Cooper

Chapter 9. The Roles of T and B Lymphocytes in Self-Tolerance and Autoimmunity
A. C. Allison

Chapter 10. Immunological Studies of Nude Mice
Henry H. Wortis

Chapter 1

T Cell Control of Antibody Production

Richard K. Gershon

Department of Pathology
Yale University School of Medicine
New Haven, Connecticut

INTRODUCTION

The discovery that the thymus was involved in the development of the immune system (Miller, 1961; Archer *et al.*, 1962; Jankovic *et al.*, 1962) ushered in the "golden age of 'thymology' " (Miller, 1967). A second golden age (Miller, 1967) began with the discovery that thymus-derived lymphocytes [soon to be christened T cells (Roitt *et al.*, 1969)] did not themselves make circulating antibodies, but rather assisted other nonthymus-derived lymphocytes to do so (Miller and Mitchell, 1969; Davies, 1969; Claman and Chaperon, 1969). This second class of lymphocytes was christened B cells (Roitt *et al.*, 1969), a term with sufficient ambiguity to gain the acceptance of those who thought these cells differentiated to a functional state in mammalian bone marrow and those who thought a mammalian equivalent of the bursa of Fabricius played a role in their differentiation.

The importance of the cooperative interactions between these 2 cell types was best dramatized in the hapten-carrier cell transfer studies of Mitchison (1971*a-c*), Boak *et al.* (1971), and Britton *et al.* (1971). He demonstrated that events which followed carrier recognition by the T cell led to antihapten antibody production by the B cell. His observations have been confirmed and extended by Paul (1970) and Katz and Benacerraf (1972). On the basis of these discoveries T cells came to be known by another name—"helper" cells.

Recently, however, evidence has accumulated which suggests that helper cells may also be "harmer" cells, in that they may act to suppress the response of other cells as well as to assist them in carrying out their immune functions. This discovery, along with the realization that there are at least two subclasses of

1

T cells (Asofsky *et al.*, 1971), may serve to usher in a third golden age of thymology. We can only hope that, with these new elements to build on, this will not be an age of "fool's gold," as it has been said that with 2 variables one can create an elephant, with three the universe. In any case, the use of the term "regulator cells" (Katz and Benacerraf, 1972) for T cells seems an appropriate one for this age. In this article I would like to discuss some of the evidence establishing a "suppressor" role for T cells and some of the implications this function may have on current immunologic theory.

Both specific and nonspecific T cell mediated suppressor effects have been reported, and in some cases, the specificity of the suppression is unclear. It is important to distinguish between these two types of effects, as the mechanisms controlling them must clearly be different, although not necessarily unrelated. Thus, I will discuss the evidence for each type of effect separately.

EVIDENCE FOR A SUPPRESSOR EFFECT OF T CELLS

Specific Effects

Tolerance Induction

Perhaps the first direct suggestion that T cells might have immunosuppressive effects was made during thymology's first golden age, and thus, its true significance was not fully appreciated at the time. Horiuichi and Waksman (1968) performed a series of experiments demonstrating that the thymus was a place where the induction of tolerance transpired. In one of these experiments they injected BGG[1], both in an aggregated and soluble form, directly into various lymphoid tissues of the rat. Their most striking finding, to my mind, was that almost immediately after injection of antigen into the thymus, the rats exhibited a significant and specifically suppressed immune response to BGG administered in complete Freunds adjuvant. Similar, although less striking, suppressive effects were produced by intrasplenic and intralymph node injection. The latter two cases can be explained by tolerance induction in circulating lymphocytes present in the injected organs, which would result in a diminished pool of BGG reactive immunocompetent cells. Such an explanation cannot account, however, for the results produced by intrathymic injection. The thymus is not a path of cell recirculation, and the induction of tolerance in thymic cells should not significantly affect the immune response of peripheral tissues, at least not acutely. Indeed, even adult thymectomy does not diminish immunologic responsiveness for quite some time. Thus, these experiments suggest that the thymus, or more likely the lymphocytes within it, can suppress the response

---

[1] For complete listing of abbreviations, see end of chapter.

of the peripheral competent lymphocytes. The controls the authors performed made it seem highly unlikely that tolerogenic amounts of free antigen escaped from the thymus. However, the possibility that the intrathymic injections had disrupted the blood thymus barrier, resulting in tolerance induction in circulating cells, was not formally excluded.

More recently, Ha and Waksman (1973) have begun to reinvestigate these findings, looking for immunosuppressive T cell dependent effects directly. They have shown that thymocytes from BGG inoculated rats can, upon adoptive transfer to normal rats, specifically suppress both cell-mediated and antibody responses to BGG.

Our own interest in the possible existence of suppressor cells stemmed from some observations we made on the behavior of an unusual hamster tumor, originally described by Dr. H. S. N. Greene (Greene and Harvey, 1960). We noted that hamsters bearing transplanted tumors developed a strong cell-mediated immune response against the tumor (concomitant immunity) (Gershon et al., 1967). This immunity could be rapidly and specifically abrogated by surgical resection of the tumor (Gershon et al., 1968b; Gershon and Carter, 1969; Gershon and Kondo, 1969). The rapidity with which the immunity disappeared after resection suggested to us that some active immunosuppressive agent was responsible. These observations reminded us of earlier work which had shown that the administration of large amounts of antigen to animals which exhibited a state of "pure" delayed hypersensitivity could lead to a rapid loss of 24-hr skin test reactivity (Uhr and Pappenheimer, 1958; Leskowitz and Waksman, 1960). Thus, when Davies and his colleagues (1967) published their exciting findings showing that T cells participated in the immune response to sheep red cells (SRBC), but that they did not actually produce antibodies, we felt that this cell was a prime candidate as a suppressor cell in our tumor system.

To investigate possible suppressor effects of T cells we performed some experiments to test whether immunological tolerance of a B cell function was dependent on the presence of T cells (Gershon and Kondo, 1970). Since we knew that B cells were unable to make significant amounts of anti-SRBC antibody without T cell help we wanted to know if in the absence of T cell help they would become paralyzed when confronted with large amounts of SRBC. We therefore deprived adult CBA mice of T cells by thymectomy and lethal irradiation, protected them with a syngeneic bone marrow graft, and, over the course of the next 4 weeks, gave them a very large amount of SRBC (2.5×10^{10} cells). Four days after the last SRBC injection the mice were reconstituted with thymocytes and immunized with SRBC, and their sera were titrated for hemagglutinating antibodies at various intervals. We found that the pretreatment with SRBC in the absence of T cells had no significant effect on the ability of thymocytes to reconstitute the mercaptoethanol resistant (MER) fraction of the anti-SRBC response (cf. nonpretreated controls). Except for one interesting effect which I will discuss below, the mercaptoethanol sensitive (MES) anti-bodies were also little affected by the pretreatment with antigen. Thus, the major fraction of the B cell population seemed to be totally insensitive to the vast amount of antigen they were presented with in the absence of T cells. On the other hand, in parallel experiments, mice which had been reconstituted with a small number of thymocytes at the time of bone marrow reconstitution (prior to the "tolerizing" antigen injections) were markedly impaired in their ability to make anti-SRBC antibodies, even after the addition of normal thymocytes. Since we were able to show that the first injection of thymocytes had not pre-empted space in the lymphoid tissues preventing functional localization of the second inoculum, these experiments showed that the interaction of the SRBC with the thymocytes during tolerance induction had resulted in a turning off of the B cells so they could no longer cooperate with the added T cells, or a turning off of the added T cells, or both. It was clear that residual antigen was not turning off the added cells since these cells functioned quite well in B mice which had gotten the same amount of antigen.

Subsequent experiments (Gershon and Kondo, 1972c) showed that the unresponsive mice contained significant numbers of B cells capable of making anti-SRBC antibody. The B cells could not be activated, however, unless we added normal thymocytes and then activated these cells with an antigen other than SRBC. Thus, in order to get the mice which had been pretreated with SRBC in the presence of T cells to make anti-SRBC antibody, we had to give them both normal thymocytes and another antigen. Neither inoculum was effective when given alone. We used horse RBC(HRBC) as the second antigen, but the anti-SRBC antibodies made had no demonstrable binding affinity for the HRBC. We did not try other antigens and do not know if the second antigen acted totally nonspecifically or had its effect due to its close relationship to the SRBC. We interpret these experiments in the following manner: The interaction of the SRBC with thymocytes during the period of tolerance induction had resulted in the production of a substance which could specifically suppress the cooperative functions of normal thymocytes. The nonspecific effects of stimu-lating the normal thymocytes with another antigen, HRBC, inhibited the sup-pression. As a result, the added thymocytes could utilize the stimulatory capacity of the SRBC which remained from the tolerizing injections and induce B cells to make anti-SRBC antibodies. The importance of a two step mechanism (i.e., HRBC doing one thing and SRBC doing another) was emphasized by two other experiments: (1) adding SRBC to the HRBC increased the anti-SRBC response, and (2) removal of the cells from the SRBC depot created by the tolerizing injections, by transferring cells to irradiated secondary hosts, pre-vented the HRBC from producing an anti-SRBC response (Gershon and Kondo, 1971c).

The interpretation that a T cell dependent factor was specifically suppressing the normal thymocytes injected into the tolerant recipients was supported by the transfer studies cited above (Gershon and Kondo, 1971c). In these experiments adoptively transferred spleen cells of SRBC unresponsive mice were able to specifically suppress cooperation between normal T and B cells in secondary host. They did not interfere with the cooperative interaction between these cells in response to HRBC.

To summarize, these experiments showed (1) the ability of SRBC reactive B cells to cooperate with T cells could not be abrogated by treating B mice with large doses of SRBC; (2) if B mice were reconstituted with small numbers of thymocytes, the same SRBC dose schedule that failed to affect cooperation in mice lacking T cells specifically abrogated B and T cooperation to this antigen; and (3) the lack of cooperation was most likely due to the production of a factor with "infectious" qualities, in that it rendered other T cells specifically unresponsive.

These experiments support the notion of a specific T cell dependent immunosuppressive factor. They do not, however, show that this factor is directly made by T cells. The factor almost certainly is not normal antibody for a number of reasons previously discussed (Gershon and Kondo, 1971c), not the least of which is that it is made by spleen cells of mice selected by the absence of detectable antibody and not made by mice selected by the presence of antibody.

McCullagh (1970a–b) has also presented data supporting the notion of the production of a factor during tolerance induction with the capacity to specifically render normal cells unresponsive. He rendered rats tolerant to SRBC by repeated injections of antigen from birth. Normal syngeneic thoracic duct cells transferred to these rats failed to overcome the tolerant state. The failure of the transferred cells to abrogate tolerance could not be attributed to their failure to colonize lymphoid tissue, as McCullagh demonstrated their localization in the spleen and also showed that they retained the ability to respond to SRBC if they were recovered before three days residence in the tolerant host. Although these experiments did not incriminate the T cell as the source of the factor which rendered the inoculated cells nonresponsive, its specificity and disassociation from conventional antibody make his results similar enough to ours for us to suspect the T cell responsible. Another interesting feature of McCullagh's work was the demonstration that allogeneic thoracic duct cells could cause the tolerant host's own B cells to make antibody. This was true both when the allogeneic cells were reactive (but not if they were tolerant) to the host (parent→F_1) or when the host was reactive to the injected cells (F_1→ parent). The first instance is compatible with the nonspecific activation of B cells by allogeneic T cells (Katz and Osborne, 1972) [the so-called allogeneic effect (Katz et al., 1971a)] but the second case is not. The second case may be similar to our work, in that nonspecific T cell activation prevented "infectious tolerance." The allogeneic effect appears to be different, however, since even SRBC tolerant parental cells were able to break the tolerance to SRBC in F_1 mice. Thus, this may be a totally nonspecific effect and have nothing to do with escaping from tolerance infection. On the other hand, the allogeneic effect may actually cause tolerant cells to escape from their suppressed state. In any case, both McCullagh's work and our experiments cited above point up very clearly that the failure to break tolerance with adoptively transferred cells is not sufficient evidence to prove the presence of tolerant B cells in recipient mice.

There are several other reports showing that normal cells cannot break a tolerant state (Chase, 1963; Crowle and Hu, 1969; Tong and Boose, 1970), although none of these reports demonstrates functional localization of the inoculated cells. In addition, there are several recent reports in which the adoptive transfer of cells from tolerant or partially tolerant mice was able to confer specific nonreactivity on immunocompetent mice (Asherson et al., 1971; Terman et al., 1971; Elkins, 1972a).

Perhaps the most direct demonstration of specific suppressive factors released by T cells is Feldmann's recent demonstration that supernatants from cultures of carrier "educated" T cells (thymus cells inoculated into lethally irradiated mice, primed with antigen and harvested from the spleen) cultured with the priming carrier complexed to a hapten, specifically suppressed the *in vitro* antihapten antibody response of B cells depleted of macrophages (Feldmann, 1973).

Increased Responsiveness to "Thymus Independent" Antigens

Another place where specific T cell dependent immunosuppressive factors may affect the immune response is illustrated by the heightened antibody response made by T cell depleted mice to "thymus independent" antigens [such as pneumococcal polysaccharide type III (S-III) (Baker et al., 1970a–b; Barthold et al., 1973), polyvinylpyrrolidone (PVP) (Kerbel and Eidinger, 1971a, 1972), and bacterial lipopolysaccharide (endotoxin) (Möller and Michael, 1971; Andersson and Blomgren, 1971)]. Although there is little direct information that the diminished B cell response made by mice with more T cells is due to the production of specific factors, there is good reason to believe that it is not due to the production of nonspecific factors such as those that cause antigenic competition (see Antigenic Competition). In addition, some recent results from Baker's laboratory indicate that the suppression is specific; therefore, I will discuss these effects under the heading of specificity.

Baker and his colleagues showed that inoculation of many different strains of mice with a single dose of antilymphocyte serum (ALS) at the time of immunization with S-III produced a marked increase in the anti-S-III antibody response (Baker et al., 1970a–b; Barthold et al., 1973). They suggested that this increase might be due to the inactivation, by the ALS, of a thymus-derived suppressor cell, since ALS is known to act primarily, in the dose range they studied, on T cells (Leuchars *et al.*, 1968; Bert *et al.*, 1971). This view was supported by their ability to suppress the enhanced response by reinoculating the treated mice with syngeneic normal thymocytes. It is important to emphasize that S-III is an antigen that has not been demonstrated to elicit any of cooperative T cell dependent effects such as heavy IgG production (Baker and Stashak, 1969; Baker *et al.*, 1971*b;* Howard *et al.*, 1971), heightened secondary responses (Baker *et al.*, 1971*c*), or delayed hypersensitivity (Gerety *et al.*, 1970), and, indeed, does not appear to stimulate T cells to synthesize significant amounts of DNA (Davies *et al.*, 1970; Krüger and Gershon, 1972). Other antigens which lack the ability to utilize T cell cooperation have also been shown to produce increased antibody responses after adult thymectomy, ALS treatment, and the two combined (Kerbel and Eidinger, 1971*a,* 1972). In some studies on the thymus dependency of these antigens the data showed that the addition of thymocytes to rigorously thymus-deprived mice suppressed their response (Möller and Michael, 1971; Andersson and Blomgren, 1971). Thus, at least some, and maybe all, nonprotein polymeric antigens do not elicit T cell help but, rather, cause these cells to produce suppressor factors.

Baker has recently extended his work by showing that low zone tolerance to S-III (Baker *et al.*, 1971*a*) can be overcome by treatment with ALS (Baker, personal communication). Mice given 0.005 µg. of S-III (a dose which hardly yields a detectable plaque forming cell response) 48 hr prior to immunization with an optimal dose of antigen (0.5 µg.), have a markedly depressed antibody response. However, if these mice are given an injection of ALS at the time of immunization, their response returns to normal. Since pretreatment with the same dose of S-I does not affect the S-III response, some form of specificity is suggested.

Baker has also extended his studies to congenitally athymic "nude" (nu/nu) mice (Baker, personal communication). He has shown that the antibody response of nu/nu mice is significantly greater than that produced by nu/+ or +/+ controls. In addition, only the controls show enhancement following treatment with ALS. He therefore suggests nu/nu mice lack a population of T cells that normally exert a negative influence on the antibody response to S-III. The absence of such suppressor cells permits nu/nu mice to give a greater response to S-III than do controls. The lack of suppressor cells *per se* however, does not enable nu/nu mice to respond to S-III in a manner comparable to that observed for control mice treated with ALS. Consequently, he postulates that nu/nu mice also lack amplifier T cells.

Suppression of Antibody Subclasses

A particularly intriguing specific suppressor effect of T cells has been demonstrated by Tada and his associates (1971; Okumura and Tada, 1971*a,* 1971*b;* Taniguchi and Tada, 1971). They reported that the homocytotrophic antidinitrophenyl (DNP) antibody response of rats immunized with DNP-Ascaris could be increased by a number of maneuvers which deplete T cells. This enhanced response could be rapidly abrogated by the inoculation of thymocytes from syngeneic rats hyperimmunized to either Ascaris or DNP-Ascaris, whereas cells from rats hyperimmunized to DNP-bovine serum albumin (BSA) were without effect (Okumura and Tada, 1971b). Their experiments virtually rule out antibody as a causative agent, as the carrier (ascaris) immune cells were suppressive while anticarrier antibody was not. In addition, they show the same carrier specificity for T cell suppression as has previously been shown for T cell helpers.

Subclasses of Suppressor T Cells

Droege's demonstration of suppressor effects produced by thymocytes is also potentially quite interesting (Droege, 1971). He showed that thymocytes from 6-week old normal chickens could markedly depress the antibody of 6-week normal syngeneic recipients. Thymocytes from neonatally bursectomized animals were nonsuppressive but could be shown in other experiments to contain helper cells. He also showed that neonatally bursectomized chickens lacked a population of cells, defined by electrophoretic mobility, in their thymuses (Droege et al., 1972). The electrophoretic mobility of the missing population was distinct from plasma cells. These experiments suggest suppressor T cells may be separatable from helper cells. The bursal dependence of the suppressor T cell might suggest to some that this T cell is, in fact, a B cell. However, Droege showed that his chicken thymus cells were totally unable to reconstitute the antibody response of bursectomized recipients, indicating an absence of B cells. They boosted the response of a 10-day-old nonbursectomized control, however, indicating the presence of helper cells. It would seem worthwhile to keep an open mind to the possibility that these bursa dependent thymocytes represent a special population similar to the rodent T cells which disappear so rapidly after adult thymectomy (Bach et al., 1970, 1971). Kerbel and Eidinger (1972) have shown that adult thymectomy can lead to increased antibody responses, and Mosier and Cantor (1971) have shown that cells from adult thymectomized mice have increased reactivity in mixed lymphocyte reactions (see Interactions Between T Cell Subpopulations). In addition, Simpson and Cantor (personal communication) have recently shown markedly improved killing of allogeneic target cells by immunized cells from adult thymectomized mice.

Nonspecific Effects

The specific suppressive events I have discussed were all measured either by antibody production or in situations where antibody could, at least theoretically, be produced. Since antibody itself has been shown to be immunosuppressive, it is liminally possible, as skeptics might argue, that these effects were B cell-mediated. However, another type of T cell suppressor effect seems to be totally nonspecific, in contradistinction to B cell products. Thus, these are even less likely to be B cell dependent.

Antigenic Competition

The induction of an immune response to one antigen may significantly interfere with the response to another, totally unrelated, antigen (Adler, 1964). The mechanism by which this interference is brought about remained obscure until Radovich and Talmage (1967) showed that the more spleen cells they transferred to irradiated recipients the more antigenic competition they produced. They concluded on this basis that the production of an immunosuppressive substance was the most likely explanation for their results. The concept of a nonspecific immunosuppressant as the cause of antigenic competition was supported by demonstrations that adoptively transferred syngeneic lymphoid cells are unable to function in a milieu of antigenic competition even after lethal irradiation of the recipient animals (Waterston, 1970; Gershon and Kondo, 1971a; Möller, 1971). We have recently extended this finding to show that even allogeneic cells are suppressed in a lethally irradiated host stimulated 2 days previously with SRBC (Menkes et al., 1972). The thymic dependence of this effect was emphasized by experiments showing that thymus-deprived mice failed to exhibit antigenic competition, even after immunization with adjuvant material that boosted their antibody response to respectable levels (Gershon and Kondo, 1971a). Reconstitution of these mice with graded doses of thymocytes, however, progressively increased the competition. Thus, in the absence of prestimulation with SRBC, mice with increased numbers of thymocytes made progressively more antibody to HRBC. On the other hand, they made progressively less anti-HRBC antibody if they were given SRBC on day minus 4. The degree of depression of the HRBC response was totally unrelated to the amount of anti-SRBC antibody produced (Gershon and Kondo, 1971a–b).

Further proof for the thymus dependency of antigenic competition was adduced by Möller (1971), who showed that antigens which did not have a thymus dependent component to their immune response were relatively poor at initiating antigenic competition. In addition, he showed that nonspecific T cell stimulators could produce antigenic competitionlike effects (Sjöberg et al., 1973).

Whereas the thymic dependency of antigenic competition seems well established, the idea that it is due to an actively inhibiting substance is not. Several workers have suggested that it is due to a saturation of macrophage sites by specific T cell dependent cooperating factors (Taylor and Iverson, 1971; Taussig and Lachmann, 1972; Feldmann, 1972a). I find this explanation unattractive because (1) antigens which give no evidence of stimulating T cell cooperating factors can produce competition (Möller, 1971; Ben-Efraim and Liacopoulos, 1967; Eidinger and Baines, 1971); (2) these same antigens which require no such factors to elicit a normal immune response can be interfered with (Möller, 1971; Ben-Efraim and Liacopoulos, 1967; Eidinger and Baines, 1971; Sjöberg, 1973); (3) spleen cells from mice undergoing antigenic competition may respond quite well when removed from the local environment and placed in tissue culture (Waterston, 1970). The tissue culture response is macrophage dependent (Feldmann and Palmer; 1971); (4) competition is completely nonspecific in that it does not spare the specific response (O'Toole and Davies, 1971; Gershon, unpublished observations). Thus, macrophages clogged with specific T cell cooperating factors should be able to help the immune response to the antigen which stimulated their production. They do not (Gershon, unpublished observations); and (5) most directly, Veit and Michael (1972) have demonstrated an increase in a factor which can directly and nonspecifically inhibit T cell responses in mouse serum, during the period when antigenic competition would be most pronounced. This factor is most likely an alphaglobulin (Veit and Michael, 1973) and similar to other immunosuppressive alphaglobulins (Kamrin, 1955; Mowbray, 1963; Cooperband et al., 1968; Carpenter et al., 1971; Riggio et al., 1969), which have been shown to be concentrated in thymic tissue (Carpenter et al., 1971) and to be increased in the serum during graft rejection (Riggio et al., 1969). It may also be related to proliferation inhibition factor (Green et al., 1970), the release of which is produced by T cell stimulators.

It should be emphasized that there is little evidence that the suppressive agent in antigenic competition is made directly by T cells. Sjöberg (1972) has recently suggested that T cell activated macrophages may be the cellular source (see Suppressor Macrophages).

Desensitization

Another form of infectious nonspecific immunosuppression is produced during desensitization of guinea pigs. Dwyer and Kantor (1973) have immunized guinea pigs to a variety of antigens in complete Freunds adjuvant and then desensitized them with a soluble form of one of these antigens. They found that the desensitized pigs were acutely anergic in that they did not have delayed skin reactions to the desensitizing antigen or to the other antigens to which they had been immunized but not desensitized. The anergy was infectious in that adding normal or even preimmunized cells could not overcome it, although the immunized cells transferred skin reactivity to nondesensitized, nonimmune pigs. Interestingly, similar to Waterston's (1970) finding with antigenic competition, cells removed from the anergic pigs were quite capable of responding to antigen *in vitro* or on adoptive transfer. Further, the anergic state was short-lived in the desensitized hosts, even if desensitization with the specific antigen was continued. However, continuation of the desensitization procedure maintained the specific effect while the nonspecific one disappeared. These findings are reminiscent of some studies reported by Liacopoulos (Liacopoulos and Neven, 1964; Liacopoulos and Herlem, 1968). He showed that tolerizing doses of BGG produced significant antigenic competition even though no anti-BGG antibody was made. However, continuation with the tolerizing regimen caused the nonspecific suppression to disappear. Thus, it seems that specifically stimulated T cells may release or cause to be released substances with nonspecific immunosuppressive effects even during tolerance induction, but that fully tolerant T cells do not. (Evidence that the same holds true for the specific suppressor is given under Meaning in Life.) Moreover, the ease with which new cells, introduced into an environment where these events are transpiring, are shut off, and the difficulty in transferring this infectious characteristic to syngeneic recipients or tissue culture [the Field phenomenon is another example of this (Field and Gibbs, 1966; Field et al., 1967)], suggests that local environmental or architectural influences play an important role in these events.

Effects in the Absence of Viable B Cells

To rule out what we considered to be the extremely unlikely possibility that these nonspecific events were being mediated by B cell products, we investigated T cell suppressor effects in lethally irradiated mice reconstituted only with weanling thymocytes. Such mice have no detectable antibody forming capacity (Miller and Mitchell, 1969; Claman and Chaperon, 1969). However, their lymphoid organs have the capacity to support DNA synthesis of the inoculated T cells, but only if these cells are stimulated with antigen (Gershon and Hencin, 1971). We found the DNA synthetic T cell response in such mice to be precisely the same, at least qualitatively, as the response of chromosomally marked T cells in B cell reconstituted mice (Krüger and Gershon, 1972; Carter et al., 1969). In both cases (with one interesting exception which I will discuss below), there is a 1—3 day latent period, a 1—2 day burst of activity, and a subsequent sharp decline. This holds true even in situations where the antigen is the host tissue (i.e., GVH reactions) (Gershon and Liebhaber, 1972). We attributed the decline in DNA synthesis to suppressor activity for a number of reasons (Gershon and Liebhaber, 1972), not the least of which was that cells removed from the original host and re-exposed to antigen went through another similar cycle of DNA synthesis, although with a shortened latent period (Mills and Gershon, in prep.). This shows that potentially reactive cells were present in the lymphoid tissues, but were incapable of reacting unless transferred out of the suppressive environment. It was a simple matter to show that the fall in DNA synthesis was not due to loss of antigen, as the reintroduction of antigen just prior to the fall only made the fall more precipitous (Gershon and Hencin, in prep.). It is intriguing that increasing the responding number of cells hastened the shutoff and that the shutoff occurred at the time when antigenic competition is at its maximum, supporting the notion that the two phenomena are similarly caused. Using this assay system we were able to show antergistic reactions between immune and normal syngeneic T cells as well as between parental and F_1 cells in F_1 mice (Gershon *et al.*, 1972). We coined the term antergy (Liebhaber *et al.*, 1972) to mean that the sum of the reactions of the combined cell populations was less than one of the cell populations operating alone. This is a more proper antonym for synergy than is antagonism, and it avoids the implication that one cell acts in opposition to the other; a more complex series of interactions is possible. Illustrative of the possible complexity is Haskill's recent finding that small numbers of a lymphocyte subpopulation markedly inhibit the response of other cells, but that increasing their number decreases the inhibition (Haskill and Axelrod, 1972).

Thus, T cells seem to be quite capable of shutting each other off in the absence of significant numbers of viable B cells. The mechanism by which they do so is not clear, but the information available to date suggests that their products have some of the characteristics of the chalones (Maugh, 1972) released by a wide variety of tissues. An important question yet to be answered is their target organ specificity. Are they T cell specific, lymphocyte specific, leukocyte specific, etc.? The preliminary association made between T cell shutoff and alphaglobulin production (Veit and Michael, 1973) suggests they may have less target organ specificity than the chalones heretofore reported.

SUPPRESSOR MACROPHAGES

Although B cells seem to be an unlikely source of nonspecific T cell dependent suppressor factors, macrophages as a source remain a distinct possibility. It is generally assumed the immunosuppressive effects of reticuloendothelial (R.E.) blockade are due to direct stoppage of macrophage function by the injected material. Friedman's work, however, suggests a number of analogies between R.E. blockade and antigenic competition (Friedman and Sabet, 1970). There are a large number of reports of inhibition of *in vitro* immune responses by excess numbers of macrophages (Chen and Hirsch, 1972). Macrophage released factors have been implicated in this suppressor effect (Hoffmann and Dutton, 1971; Gery *et al.*, 1972; Gery and Waksman, 1972) and the release of the factors has been shown to be controlled, to a degree, by T cells (Gery *et al.*, 1972; Gery and Waksman, 1972; Yoshinaga *et al.*, 1972). T cell control of other macrophage functions is well established (Mackaness, 1969). Thus, it is possible that some, or even all, of the suppressive T cell effects discussed above are mediated indirectly through macrophages. Indeed, Sjöberg (1972) has reported that the infectious suppressive effect that spleen cells from mice undergoing a GVH reaction have on normal spleen cells *in vitro* can be abolished by treatment with iron powder but not with an antitheta antiserum. He interpreted these findings to suggest a T cell dependent macrophage mediated suppressor mechanism. However, recent evidence indicates that stimulated T cells may be resistant to killing with antitheta antibodies and complement (Kerbel and Eidinger, 1971*b;* Rich *et al.,* 1973). Further, Howard *et al.* (1966) have noted the transformation of chromosomally marked thoracic duct cells into liver macrophages during a GVH reaction, indicating that T cells may acquire macrophage-like characteristics. Thus, the cellular source of the inhibitor remains to be established. It must be remembered that macrophage factors can activate T cells (Gery *et al.,* 1972) and, therefore, the macrophage activated T cells might just as well be responsible for the apparent macrophage mediated suppression as the macrophage is for T cell dependent suppression. It seems that products from purified cell populations must be isolated and characterized before we will be able to tell who is doing what and to whom.

SUPPRESSOR ANIMALS

At present we know that the products of all three of the cell types involved in immune responses (B cell, T cell, and macrophage) may act either directly or in cooperation with one or more of the other cell types, in a suppressor role. It is possible that these suppressor effects account for the poor performance of immunologically competent cells inoculated into intact syngeneic adult animals, in comparison to their ability to perform after inoculation into irradiated hosts (Celada, 1966; Elkins, 1972*b*). The irradiation may serve to inactivate host suppressor cells. It does not seem to function by increasing space for the lodgment of the inoculated cells (Lance and Taub, 1969). The possibility that host T cells may be active in shutting off the inoculated cells is suggested by the observation that adding back F_1 thymocytes to F_1 hosts after irradiation can suppress the activity of inocula of parental thymocytes (Gershon *et al.,* 1972). It is also known that parental thymocytes are more active in producing GVH reactions in newborn F_1 mice, which are relatively T cell deficient, than they are in adults (Elkins, 1972*b*). One last suggestive piece of evidence stems from a recent observation from our laboratory: T cells, educated against tumor cell antigens, were shown to kill tumor cells more efficiently in syngeneic hosts that were lethally irradiated than in intact animals (Frank *et al.,* in prep.). Their increased killing ability could be diminished by reinoculating the irradiated hosts with normal thymocytes.

INTERACTIONS BETWEEN T CELL SUBPOPULATIONS

Recent discoveries have indicated that two types of T cells may cooperate with each other in certain immune responses (Asofsky *et al.,* 1971). I will discuss this subject only insofar as it may apply to suppressor effects. Basically, preliminary evidence points very strongly toward the cell referred to as T_1 by Raff and Cantor (1971) as the principal cell involved in suppressor effects. This is the short-lived cell which disappears rapidly after adult thymectomy and has a predilection for splenic localization. Thus, adult thymectomy has been noted by several workers to lead to a rapid rise in immune responsiveness to a number of antigens (Kerbel and Eidinger, 1972; Mosier and Cantor, 1971; Simpson and Cantor, personal communication). Similarly, Baker *et al.* (1970*b*) found thymus cells (which are rich in T_1) suppressed the antibody response to S-III while peripheral blood cells (which are rich in T_2) increased it. Splenectomy has been commonly noted to increase tumor immunity (Gershon and Carter, 1969; Gershon and Kondo, 1969), and we have found that removal of spleen seeking thymocytes from an inoculum of unfractionated parental thymocytes can markedly increase the DNA synthetic response of lymph node seeking cells in lethally irradiated F_1 mice (Gershon *et al.*, in press). Consequently, it might seem attractive to ascribe suppressor function to T_1 type cells and helper function to T_2. It would also be attractive to relate these findings to Droege's work (see Subclasses of Suppressor T Cells) in that T_1 cells of mice might be analogous to the bursal dependent suppressor T cells he has described, particularly if the charge differential of these cells is a factor in their binding to a highly charged substance such as histamine. A recent report from Sela's laboratory suggests that a subpopulation of cells which bind to histamine coated beads plays an important suppressor role in antibody responses (Shearer *et al.*, 1972). I doubt that this simplified scheme will prove to be correct. For example, a number of workers have shown that ALS, which acts principally on T_2 type cells (Raff and Cantor, 1971), can cause enhanced antibody responses (Baker *et al.*, 1970*a–b*; Barthold *et al.*, 1973; Kerbel and Eidinger, 1971*a*; Okumura and Tada, 1971*b*; Anderson *et al.*, 1972). Although it has not been unequivocally demonstrated that this ability of ALS is due to removal of T cells, since it does not have this effect in T-deprived mice (Baker, personal communication), this seems to be its most likely mode of action. Further, although splenectomy usually increases tumor immunity and DNA synthesis of lymph node seeking T cells, as noted above, it also can have, under certain conditions, the opposite effect and decrease these responses (Gershon and Carter, 1969; Gershon and Kondo, 1969; Gershon *et al.*, in press). We have analyzed these circumstances in some detail and think that suppressor effects, as well as helper effects, are mediated through T_2 type cells but that the T_1 cells act to moderate or indirectly regulate the T_2 cell. Space does not permit the detailed analysis of these experiments, but I hope they will be published soon. I mention them here simply to sound a cautionary note against the natural tendency to simplify a highly complex system.

Finally, one should consider the "experiment of nature" presented us by the NZB mouse. I have avoided, up to now, any discussion of a possible suppressor T cell role in autoimmune phenomena, or in allotype suppression, as these subjects are being specifically covered in this volume (Allison, this volume; Herzenberg and Herzenberg, this volume). However, some recent data of ours concerning the behavior of NZB thymocytes may have some bearing on T-T suppressor interactions. In essence, we found that thymocytes from NZB mice, as early as 5 weeks after birth, were highly deficient in the ability to respond to H-2 antigens in the lymph nodes of lethally irradiated recipient mice, but responded excessively in their spleens (Gershon, unpublished observations). In addition, the spleen seeking cells lacked the auto-shutoff tendency seen in other mouse strains (Gershon and Liebhaber, 1972). If these two observations (the deficiency of nodal responses and lack of splenic shutoff) are causally related, the T_2 nature (lymph node seeking) of the suppressor cell is supported. Thus, the lack of T_2 cells could help to explain the tendency NZB mice have to make autoantibodies (Mellors, 1967; Howie and Helyer, 1968) and their resistance to tolerance induction (Weir et al., 1968; Staples and Talal, 1969) [particularly in their T cells (Playfair, 1971a)] , while they also lack the GVH amplifying cells (Cantor et al., 1970) discussed above and the other cellular functions ascribed to T_2 cells (Waksman et al., 1972). Our studies mentioned above also indicate a lack of amplifying cells, as well as suppressor cells, in the NZB thymuses, as the dose dependent latent period which occurs before spleen seeking cells start to react to antigen (Gershon and Liebhaber, 1972), was significantly prolonged.

SUBCLASSES OF B CELLS

The evidence for subclasses of T cells seems quite strong, while such evidence for different classes of B cells is not only more limited but also more indirect. Nonetheless, I would like to speculate a bit on certain possibilities that might make some seemingly paradoxical T cell effects seem more comprehensible.

As I mentioned earlier, in discussing the thymus dependency of tolerance to SRBC (Tolerance Induction), the MER antibody response was unaffected by pretreating B mice with large doses of SRBC prior to reconstituting them with thymocytes (Gershon and Kondo, 1970). The late appearing (day 10 and after) MES antibodies were likewise unaffected. The early appearing (days 4 and 7) MES antibody response was, however, significantly depressed. The depression did not depend on the amount of time allowed to elapse between termination of the antigen pretreatment and thymocyte reconstitution. This result suggests that a class of B cells, responsible for the earliest MES antibody response to SRBC, was made unresponsive to SRBC by antigen pretreatment in the absence of T cells and that its nonparticipation in the immune response was inconsequential to the response of the B cells which were unaffected by the antigen pretreatment. It is interesting that the sum of the antibody response made by nonpretreated B mice (thymic independent response, (a) and the response made by pretreated B mice subsequently reconstituted with thymocytes (thymus dependent response, (b) equalled the response of control B mice reconstituted with thymocytes (a and b). Thus, we put forth the following notion. Two classes of B cells exist; one (B_1) requires no help from the thymus to be triggered to antibody production and similarly requires no help to be made unresponsive. Its product is IgM. A second class of B cells (B_2) will not respond to antigen in any fashion without T cell help; it will neither become tolerant nor will it make antibody. This B cell also makes IgM but is the precursor of the cell which undergoes the switch to IgG and IgA production (Lawton *et al.*, 1972; Pierce *et al.*, 1972*a–b*) (and also possible to IgE). Playfair (1971*b*) has also put forth evidence for a subclass of B_1 cells which do not cooperate with T cells.

To develop this notion further, we suggest that B_1 cells are phylogenetically primitive (see Table I for B_1 and B_2 characteristics); they are the descendants of the first antibody making cells, which appeared prior to the development of thymic function. Subsequent thymic development allowed the development of B_2 cells which could make more specialized products which would include antibody molecules with a high free energy of binding (high affinity antibodies). This concept is consistent with our present state of knowledge of the phylogenetics of immunology in that sharks seem only to have B_1 type antibody responses (Grey, 1969; Voss and Sigel, 1971; Sigel *et al.*, 1972), and a recent, very thorough search for a thymus in these beasts has been fruitless (Simic, personal communication), although some lymphoid tissue in a thymic location has been noted by others in younger animals (Good and Papermaster, 1964; Sigel, personal communication). The eventual discovery of a thymuslike organ, such as the structure found in lampreys (Good and Papermaster, 1964), in

Table I. Characteristics of B_1 and B_2 Type Antibody
Responses

	B_1	B_2
Immunoglobulin class	IgM	IgM, G, A, E
Heterogeneity	$\pm - +$	$+ + - ++++$
Energy of interaction with antigen	$+$	$+ + - ++++$
Heightened secondary	$\pm$	$+ + - ++++$
Cross reactions [degeneracy Little and Eisen, 1969)]	$\pm$	$+ +$
Ease of tolerance induction	Easy	Hard
Dose range of immunization	Narrow	Wide
Phylogenetic appearance	Early	Late

animals with only B_1 type antibody responses will not discredit the hypothesis, however. It is assumed that thymic function has also progressed during evolution. For example, such phylogenetically advanced creatures as reptiles clearly have thymuses and B_2 type antibody responses (Grey, 1969). Nonetheless, they still are deficient in their production of high affinity antibody subsets (Grey, 1969), a B_2 function which is highly thymus dependent in mice (Gershon and Paul, 1971; Gershon and Kondo, 1972a-b). Further evidence for the lack of a thymic function in sharks consists of the inability of their lymphoid cells to respond to PHA, or histocompatibility antigens (Simic, personal communication; Sigel et al., personal communication) under conditions which allow them to respond to nonthymus dependent stimulators.

Thus, we suggest an antigen responsive antibody making cell evolved during the course of evolution. Its product was a monomeric molecule homologous to mammalian IgM. Subsequent to this, evolutionary pressure selected for cells that could make products which were more efficacious at eliminating noxious foreign material. The initial result was a polymerization of the IgM. The precise association of this development with the development of thymic functions is unclear. At or about this time helper cell thymic function started to develop and allowed the emergence of a new type of B cell which could make more specialized products. This hypothetical historical sequence predicts that T cells should have B_1 cell type receptors (i.e., monomeric IgM) which appears to be the case (Feldmann, 1972a; Marchalonis et al., 1972; Feldmann et al., 1973). The B_1 response has persisted through evolution, at least as far as the mouse. Therefore, we would expect that the antibody response of a B mouse and a shark to be very similar. Known similarities are predominant IgM production, lack of memory, and deficiency in maturation to high affinity type antibodies.

The fact that development of those immune responses which are classically associated with thymic function, such as graft rejection, seem to have preceded antibody production in evolution, does not affect the hypothesis I have put forth. Graft rejection in primitive animals, including sharks, is indeed rather poor (Simic, personal communication; Good and Papermaster, 1964; Sigel et al., personal communication) and there is no need to attribute it to T cells.

MEANING OF "THYMUS INDEPENDENCY"

The immunological literature is replete with references to "thymus independent antigens." I would like to put forth the notion that there is no such thing as a thymus independent antigen but only a "thymus independent antibody." To my mind, this differentiation is not semantic nitpicking but has important theoretical and conceptual implications. It also is intrinsically related to the B_1, B_2 concept that I have put forth above.

The idea that there are "thymus independent antigens" probably stems from some early observations of Humphrey *et al.* (1964) who noted that neonatally thymectomized mice generally had a depressed antibody response to SRBC but were not significantly impaired in their antibody response to Keyhole limpet hemocyanin (KLH) or to S-III. At that time (Golden Age 1; see Introduction) it was widely thought that the thymus was little concerned with antibody production but rather with cell-mediated immunological events. As work progressed and thymus deprivation mechanisms became more efficient, the antibody responses to more and more antigens were noted to be deficient in thymus-deprived mice, and a classification of thymus dependent and independent antigens began to appear.

We have found a great distinction between two classes of antigens which were classified as thymus independent as late as 1972. One class is an exceptionally good stimulator of DNA synthesis in T cells [this includes Brucella organisms and the polymerized flagella antigen of *Salmonella adelaide* (POL)] while the other (S-III, PVP, endotoxin) is extremely poor (Krüger and Gershon, 1972; Gery *et al.*, 1972). [Interestingly KLH, which only recently became a "thymus dependent antigen" (Unanue, 1970; Krüger and Gershon, 1971), is in the first category.] On this basis we suggested that the antibody response to the good T cell stimulators was not thymus independent at all, but rather that these antigens produced exceptionally good thymus independent antibody responses (B_1 type response—see Subclasses of B Cells) which, in the absence of T cell directed feedback, obscured the lack of a thymus dependent component (Krüger and Gershon, 1972). This prediction has recently been confirmed by Warner, who has shown thymusless "nude" mice are quite deficient in their IgG response to the first 2 antigens (Warner, personal communication). Interestingly, the second class of antigens fails to elicit much of an IgG response even in normal mice (Kerbel and Eidinger, 1971a; Andersson and Blomgren, 1971; Baker and Stashak, 1969; Britton and Möller, 1968). Thus, if one talks of an IgG response, there appears to be no such thing as a thymus independent antigen. If one talks of IgM responses, the situation is less clear. It would appear that certain polymeric nonprotein antigens are extremely poor at eliciting a helper T cell effect and, therefore, the immune responses they elicit are not diminished by removal of cells which are of no help to them. Thus, the immune response of normal mice to these antigens is qualitatively similar to the response of sharks and B mice to any antigen. However, I do not think that we can yet completely rule out the possibility that T cells can help the response to these antigens. Baker's work suggests that some helper cells exist but that suppressor cells may obscure the help (Baker *et al.*, 1971c; Baker, personal communication). This point requires further clarification, but it is fair to say that T cell help is at best quite limited.

Therefore, when examining the antibody response to an antigen it is important to characterize the nature of the response as to whether it has B_1 or B_2 type characteristics. A known "thymus dependent antigen," SRBC, still produces a thymus independent antibody response (Playfair, 1971b; Kindred, 1971; Pantelouris and Flisch, 1972), but this response is clearly of B_1 character. Certain maneuvers, such as coupling the SRBC to endotoxin which is a good B_1 stimulator, markedly enhanced the IgM response (Möller *et al.*, 1972). This has been interpreted to mean that endotoxin can replace T cell function. However, since no investigation of the IgG response was made in that study, such an interpretation is invalid. It is possible (I think, likely) that rather than performing a T cell function the endotoxin was acting as a "thymus independent carrier" with the SRBC as the hapten and simply boosting the thymus independent (B_1) IgM antibody response. These results then are probably more related to the studies which showed that DNP coupled to the homopolymer levan (polyfruc tose), a nonstimulator of T cells, could elicit only an IgM anti-DNP antibody response, which was of similar magnitude in normal and in B mice (Del Guerico and Leuchars, 1972). It would appear that whatever the physical characteristics are that are required to trigger B_1 cells, they can be imparted to an antigen by coupling it to another which has those characteristics. It is an open question whether this enhanced immunogenicity results from B-B interaction, similar to the carrier-hapten, T-B interaction reported by Mitchison (1971a–c; Boak *et al.*, 1971; Britton *et al.*, 1971), or if the addition of the carrier acts simply to allow the antigen to directly trigger the precursor cell in the way that the addition of an extra lysine group to a homolysine polymer gives the polymer the ability to trigger T cells (Schlossman and Levin, 1971). I personally lean toward the latter interpretation and feel that distinguishing between the two is extremely important to understanding the nature of B cell triggering.

Another antigen has been shown to act as good carrier in B mice (Feldmann and Basten, 1971; Feldmann, 1972a). This antigen, POL, however, is in the other class of so-called "thymus independent antigens," as it not only is a good direct stimulator of B cells but it also is an excellent stimulator of T cells (Krüger and Gershon, 1972). Thus, one would predict that the anti-DNP antibodies made by B mice after stimulation with DNP-POL would be similar to the antibodies made by mice to DNP-levan but different from those made by normal mice stimulated with DNP-POL, in that they would be deficient in an IgG component. This point has not been investigated. If it is true that some large antigens with repeating determinants elicit qualitatively distinct antibody responses in the presence or absence of T cells, it becomes quickly obvious that T cell help is more than simple alteration of antigen to allow it to be presented to the B cell in a form which mimics a "thymus independent antigen" (Feldmann and Basten, 1971; Feldmann, 1972a–c).

The key question in regard to thymus dependency, as I see it, is why some antigens can stimulate T cells to perform a helper function and others cannot.

Theories based solely on repeating determinants are inadequate as POL and S-III, used as examples of antigens of this class, are wildly different in their T cell stimulatory capacity. Perhaps this attribute helps them to stimulate B_1 cells, but this is only half the story.

T CELL DISCRIMINATION OF SIGNALS

The easiest explanation for the apparent differences between T and B cell recognition of antigen is that they have receptors of different specificity. This explanation is not as simple as it might seem, however, as it requires evolution to generate two different types of highly specialized molecules which appear to serve similar functions. Such biological ineconomy is most unusual. Generally speaking, B cell products appear to have greater discriminatory power than do T cell receptors. However, it must be pointed out that the tests for discrimination are highly biased in favor of the B cell. Demonstration of antibody binding to antigen is the usual test for B cell recognition, while tests for T cell recognition require not only a recognition event to occur but for this to lead to a measurable cellular event. More recently, antigen binding assays have become a popular way to demonstrate receptors on immunologically competent cells (see Möller, 1970). In this assay too, B cells have a selective advantage by virtue of mechanisms other than receptor specificity and which may have something to do with the relationship of the receptor to the cell membrane (Marchalonis *et al.,* 1972).

Another selective advantage for the B cell is that it often has the T cell to help it produce its product. Thus, it is possible that the end product of B cell differentiation, under T cell influence or help, does not have precisely the same specificity as the receptor on the originally stimulated cell. It is widely assumed that the progression of a B cell response from low to high affinity is due to competitive selective stimulation of high affinity precursors by antigen (Siskind and Benacerraf, 1969). This assumption requires that there be more low than high affinity precursors, otherwise it should not take time for the competitive selection to occur. It also requires that there be some advantage to the organism to have relatively more low affinity precursors. In light of recent demonstrations that low affinity molecules will not react with more antigenic determinants but probably with less than antibodies of higher affinity (Gershon and Kondo, 1972*a*; Little and Eisen, 1969; Underdown and Eisen, 1971), I can see no such advantage. One must consider the possibility that T cell products, in conjunction with antigen, assist in the emergence of molecules with new specificities either by differentiational or mutational mechanisms. This could explain why high affinity molecules are so thymus dependent (Gershon and Paul, 1971; Gershon and Kondo, 1972*b*). If cells bearing high affinity receptors existed prior to T cell action one would expect them to be expressed preferentially under the adverse conditions that exist in T deprived mice, and they appear not to be. Also, the fact that B cells are more mitotically active than are T cells (Davies, 1969;

Gershon *et al.*, 1971) makes them a better equipped cell population for undergoing changes.

The importance of distinguishing between a lack of recognition and a lack of response is emphasized by the recent demonstrations of suppressor T cell effects produced by antigens that elicit none of the commonly used responses that measure T cell recognition (see Increased Responsiveness to "Thymus Independent" Antigens). Some form of recognition event between the antigen and the T cell must have occurred for this to have happened.

Therefore, at the present time it would seem unwise to assume differences in antigen recognition between T & B cells. Indeed, evidence for T cell recognition of haptens is accumulating (Mitchison, 1971*c;* Katz and Benacerraf, 1972; Leskowitz *et al.*, 1966; Paul, 1970; Alkan *et al.*, 1971; Alkan *et al.*, 1972; Walters *et al.*, 1972; Roelants, personal communication).

Role in Genetically Controlled Responsiveness to Antigen

Another possible example of T cell recognition without T cell response occurs in mice which are genetically incapable of making antibody to a synthetic amino acid polymer, GAT. The gene(s) controlling responsiveness to this antigen seem to be inextricably linked to those which code for the major histocompatibility antigens (Merryman and Maurer, 1972). Nonresponder mice have potentially responsive B cells as they make significant amounts of anti-GAT antibody when immunized with the polymer complexed to an immunogenic carrier (Gershon *et al.*, 1973). Thus, this situation seems quite similar to previously reported cases of genetically controlled histocompatibility-linked unresponsiveness (McDevitt and Benacerraf, 1969; Benacerraf and McDevitt, 1972). Due to the inability of these antigens to elicit T cell responses in nonresponder animals and also on the basis that maneuvers which elicit T cell help [the allogeneic effect (Katz and Osborne, 1972; Katz *et al.*, 1971*a*), for example] can turn nonresponders into responders (Ordal and Grumet, 1972), it has been suggested that nonresponder T cells may lack receptors for the antigen. We have recently presented evidence that such is not the case (Gershon *et al.*, 1973). Thymocytes from nonresponder mice will synthesize significant amounts of DNA when they confront the antigen in the spleens of lethally irradiated syngeneic mice. They differ significantly from responder thymocytes, however, in that they will not respond to the antigen upon a second confrontation, while the responders make a heightened secondary response. We suggest that the antigen-induced T cell DNA synthesis indicates that a recognition event transpired and the lack of a second response indicates that this event did not lead to memory, as it did in the case of the responder mice, but probably led to tolerance. We have been able to show the occurrence of significant amounts of DNA synthesis during tolerance induction in T cell populations to other antigens (see Do Tolerant Cells Exist?).

We have recently accumulated further evidence for T cell recognition of

GAT by nonresponder animals. We have found a negative form of memory, in that a secondary response to this antigen in intact nonresponder mice produces antigenic competition while a primary response does not (Gershon *et al.*, in prep.). Similarly, the PHA response of spleen cells from GAT immunized nonresponder mice is significantly diminished by inclusion of the antigen in the culture medium (Gershon *et al.*, in prep.). We have also shown that pretreatment of nonresponder mice with free polymer can impair the response of these mice to GAT conjugated to an immunogenic carrier (Gershon *et al.*, 1973) but does not do this if the mice are thymus-deprived during the pretreatment period (Gershon *et al.*, in prep.).

Thus, in many ways, GAT in nonresponder mice behaves the way an antigen like S-III does in all mice. [Other workers have shown nonresponder mice make only a primary IgM response to other synthetic antigens (Grumet, 1972).] Another similarity is that S-III can elicit a striking secondary response if it is conjugated to an immunogenic carrier (Paul *et al.*, 1971). In light of these parallels, I suggest a parallel mechanism: that the T cell receptor can discriminate between various types of signals and on this basis decide whether to release or cause to be released factors which may be immunosuppressive or immuno-enhancing. Some possible models of how this might be governed appear under Possible Models.

Based on the interesting experiments of Parish (1971*a*), confirming and extending earlier studies of Benacerraf and Gell (1959), it would seem that the energetics of the binding would be of crucial importance. Parish showed that acetoacetylated flagellin had reduced affinity for antiflagellin antibodies and could render adult rats tolerant (in terms of antibody formation) to a subsequent challenge of flagellin (1971*a*). These rats, however, had heightened delayed hypersensitivity reactions to the antigen (Parish, 1971*b*). He found the same reciprocity between these two responses using other means of chemical modification of the antigen. On the other hand, the acetoacetylated antigen induced tolerance to both responses in neonatal rats. Parish has recently extended these findings to other antigens (1972). He interpreted his findings to indicate that the affinity of antigen for receptors on cells appears to be of crucial importance in determining whether antibody formation or antibody suppression occurs. I find this interpretation quite reasonable and, in light of the rapidly accumulating evidence for T cell regulatory effects discussed above, suggest that this discriminatory event takes place at the T cell level. [Entia non multiplicanda praeter necessitatem—William of Ockham (see Tornay, 1938)].

The way such regulation could explain the linkage between immunological unresponsiveness and genes that control cell surface antigens is to postulate that these antigens contribute, by virtue of their proximity, to the binding energy of receptor and antigen. This could be done through steric or electrochemical forces. A recent paper has emphasized the importance of the relationship between the charge of the antigen and the charge of the cell with which it binds (Phie and Sehon, 1972). Thus, a nonresponder animal would be one whose surface antigens happened to be either particularly complementary or anti-complementary to a given antigen and, consequently, made it bind either too tightly or too loosely to the receptor. This hypothesis could also explain why all F_1 animals in a responder:nonresponder cross are responders (McDevitt and Benacerraf, 1969; Benacerraf and McDevitt, 1972). The dilution of the antigens of the cell surface would dilute their effects on the receptor. However, covering the responder antigens on F_1 cells with a specific antiserum would then return them to a nonresponder status, as has been demonstrated (Shevach et al., 1972), by leaving only those receptors which are affected by nonresponder histo-compatibility antigens available for interaction with the antigen.

Role of Physical Characteristics of Antigen

A number of other procedures that might change the physical characteristics of an antigen and, thus, affect the energy with which it binds to its receptor have been shown to change immunogens into tolerogens. Deaggregation of gamma globulin by ultracentrifugation is a particularly good example (Dresser, 1962). Substances which are either nonimmunogenic or very weakly immunogenic such as d-amino-acid polymers (Schechter et al., 1964), isogenic serum (Walters et al., 1972; Golan and Borel, 1971), polymers which are nonimmunogenic by virtue of the histocompatibility antigens of the immunized host (Katz et al., 1971b), and S-III (Mitchell and Humphrey, 1973) have been shown to act as tolerogenic carriers. That is to say, hapten specific tolerance can be induced by treating animals with the hapten conjugated to these substances. Some of these substances have also been shown to act as haptens, and in this case hapten specific tolerance can be induced by treatment with the nonconjugated substance (Gershon et al., 1973; Schecter et al., 1964). One possible interpretation of these findings is that these substances act directly on B cells, and, thus, B cell tolerance is induced by the direct presentation of the hapten to the B cell. However, since many of these substances can produce antigenic competition (Ben-Efraim and Liacopoulos, 1967; Gershon et al., in prep.) and/or stimulate other suppressor T cell functions (Baker et al., 1970a–b; Baker, personal communication), it is possible that the mechanism by which the tolerance is produced is via a negative helper effect.

Role of Antibody

Another possible example where T cell signal discrimination might be important is in the regulation of the immune response by antibody and in particular antigen-antibody complexes. It is well established that antibody can be an immunosuppressive agent (Uhr and Möller, 1968), and there have been a number of demonstrations that it also might act in an adjuvantlike fashion (Terres and Wolins, 1959; Möller and Wigzell, 1965), particularly the IgM fraction (Henry and Jerne, 1968; Dennert, 1971). Recent evidence has suggested that antigen-antibody complexes can not only block some T cell-mediated immunological effects (Sjögren *et al.,* 1971), but that immune complexes can produce immunological tolerance (Feldmann and Diener, 1970; Hellström *et al.,* 1971; Wegmann *et al.,* 1971; Voisin, 1971). It is possible that the antibody complexed to the antigen alters the energetics of the interaction of the antigen with T cell receptor in such a fashion as to cause a maximum production of suppressor effects and/or a minimum amount of helper effects. It has been established that antibody can produce significant conformational changes in antigen, and such conformational changes can markedly affect the antigens' ability to stimulate an immune response (Conway-Jacobs *et al.,* 1970). Interestingly, soluble antigens tend to be tolerogenic, antigen-antibody complexes in antigen excess are soluble and lose solubility as the ratio of antibody to antigen is increased, and tumor enhancement can be affected with very small doses of antibody but not with larger doses (Hutchin *et al.,* 1967; Kaliss, 1969; Skurzak *et al.,* 1972). The possible relationship of these observations to each other and to the alterations they may have on binding of antigen and T cell receptor are intriguing to me.

There is some evidence that antibody can differentially affect T cell helper and suppressor functions. For example, we found a dose of anti-SRBC antibody that would not affect or perhaps even increase the suppressive effect SRBC immunization has on a subsequent HRBC response (Antigenic Competition) while it prevented a detectable antibody response to the SRBC (Gershon and Kondo, 1971*b*). Whether the antibody altered the T cell response or simply neutralized the helper effect could not be decided on the basis of these experiments, however. Increased amounts of antibody neutralized both effects (helper and suppressor) pointing up again the importance of molar ratios of antigen to antibody in determining the effect the complexes will have.

Evidence that antigen-antibody complexes may work at the T cell level can be found in the work of Pearlman (1967) and also McBride and Schierman (1970), based on the fact that the T cell is the cell which regulates carrier effects (Mitchison, 1971*a-c*; Boak *et al.,* 1971; Britton *et al.,* 1971). These authors found that passive immunization with anticarrier antibody, in a proper dose, could increase antihapten responses. Interestingly, the passive antibody suppressed the antibody response to the carrier indicating, perhaps, a different effect of antibody at the T and B cell levels. (Parish's antigen alteration techniques have the same differential effect; see Role in Genetically Controlled Responsiveness to Antigen.)

Thus, it is possible that S-III, acetoacetylated POL, deaggregated gammaglobulin, synthetic polypeptides in nonresponder mice, d-amino acids, and antigen-antibody complexes in certain molar ratios all act in a similar way: they have characteristics apart from their antigenic determinants which affect their binding with T cell receptors in a manner that causes this cell to act in a suppressor fashion without eliciting a helper effect.

Role in Antigen Dose Effects

Immunological tolerance is known to occur in two antigen dose levels (Mitchison, 1964). This, too, can be explained in terms of T cell discrimination of signals. Thus, a high antigen dose, by virtue of the number of receptors it hits or by mass action effects at a single receptor level, could trigger an excess amount of suppressor. Low zone tolerance would be explained not by excess suppressor production but by the absence of triggering of helper material. Both cases would yield a preferential suppressor effect, but by 2 different mechanisms. This concept predicts a quantitative difference in the 2 forms of tolerance; that produced in the high zone should be stronger, broader, and harder to break. Available evidence indicates that such is the case (Mitchison, 1971a; Paul et al., 1969). Liacopoulos et al. (1972) have shown that less antigenic competition occurs during tolerance induction in a low zone than in a high zone, supporting the notion that less suppressor is produced in low zone tolerance induction. We have shown that a dose of SRBC that produces a good antibody response in B mice reconstituted with a given number of thymocytes induces a high degree of tolerance in the same number of thymocytes if they are immunized in mice that have no B cells (so called tabla rasae mice) (Spiesel and Gershon, 1972). In this case, it would appear that the production of helper material was wasted in the mice without B cells and concomitant immunization which might obscure or alter tolerance induction was avoided. The relevance of this observation to the model for low zone tolerance is that it shows that avoidance of helper activity can facilitate tolerance induction without requiring an increase in tolerance inducing factors.

DO TOLERANT CELLS EXIST?

The question of whether immunological tolerance results from the deletion of cells with specificity for antigen or to their inactivation has been a poser to immunologists ever since the discovery of the phenomenon. With the advent of thymology's second golden age (Miller, 1967) and the knowledge that two cells participated in the immune response, evidence that bore on this question which was acquired in the first golden age [reviewed by Dresser and Mitchison (1968)] required re-evaluation. The concept of suppressor T cells offers a mechanism by which cells can be made nonresponsive to antigen without requiring clonal deletion. Indeed, recent reports of undiminished or even increased numbers of antigen binding cells in tolerant animals (Naor and Sulitzeanu, 1969; Howard *et al.*, 1969; Ada, 1970, Sjöberg, 1971) indicate that clonal deletion is not required. It could be argued that the antigen binding cells in those studies were B cells and that the relevant T cells were lacking but their absence was not picked up by the binding assay. It is known that tolerant animals can have antigen responsive B cells (Gershon and Kondo, 1972*c*; McCullagh, 1970*a,b*). However, these studies were done with antigens which elicit significant amounts of antibody in B mice (Howard *et al.*, 1969; Ada, 1970; Sjöberg, 1971) so an alternate explanation must be sought. Active suppression by T cells is a possible mechanism. Such a mechanism could also explain the observation that mice tolerant to S-III and without detectable antibody in their serum have large numbers of cells which can form plaques when incubated with S-III tagged red cells in agar (Howard *et al.*, 1969). It has been theorized that the PFC are operative *in vivo* but that their product, antibody, is neutralized by the antigen which remains from tolerance induction, and, thus, is not found in the serum (Howard, 1972). The fact that this antigen is poorly catabolized, and goes in and out of macrophages where it can be stripped of its antibody burden, makes this hypothesis attractive. I find it hard, however, to conceive of microgram amounts of antigen doing such a thing, particularly since we know that removal of antibody is a great stimulus for the production of more antibody (Graf and Uhr, 1969). It seems more likely that these potential PFC are being actively suppressed *in vivo* and escape from the suppressor influence when removed from the animal. Parallels for such a mechanism have been found in antigenic competition (Waterston, 1970), desensitization (Dwyer and Kantor, 1973), tolerance to SRBC (McGregor *et al.*, 1967), tolerance to endotoxin (Möller and Sjöberg, 1972) and tumor immunity (Ortiz de Landazuri and Herberman, 1972), and even in the ordinary DNA synthetic T cell response to antigen (Gershon and Liebhaber, 1972; Mills and Gershon, in prep.). These results imply that actively suppressed B cells can exist.

We have presented evidence that actively suppressed T cells may exist also (Spiesel and Gershon, 1972). We immunized thymocytes to SRBC in the spleens of lethally irradiated recipient mice and determined the amount of DNA synthesis that resulted, by measuring the uptake of ^{125}I-5-iodo-2-deoxyuridine. We found that, with a constant dose of thymocytes, increasing the antigen dose increased the amount of DNA synthesis (Gershon and Hencin, 1971). This was also true if the adjuvant, pertussis vaccine, was incorporated with the SRBC (Spiesel and Gershon, 1972). The use of pertussis, however, increased the stimulatory capacity of the SRBC. We had previously shown that the action of pertussis was to increase antigen dependent recruitment of T cells into responding lymphoid tissue, thus making more cells available to react with antigen (Taub and Gershon, 1972). We then harvested the T cells which had been immunized in the spleens of the lethally irradiated mice and tested their ability to boost the antibody response of B mice. Interestingly, we found an inversion of the dose hierarchy seen in the DNA synthesis experiments. That is to say, the lowest antigen dose studied produced the least DNA synthesis and the most help. The highest dose led to the most DNA synthesis and the least help. In fact, the cells immunized with the highest dose gave no help at all. An intermediate dose was intermediate in both assays. These results suggested to us that the higher antigen doses were rendering the thymocytes tolerant. The role the DNA synthesis was playing in this process was not clear, but since we knew that DNA synthesis could generate memory cells (Gershon *et al.*, 1971) we considered the possibility that memory T cells were being generated and then shut off, perhaps by suppressor factors. To test this possibility, we incubated the immunized T cells in B mice for various periods of time to see if tolerance might wane. It did indeed, and after 6 weeks of rest the T cells immunized with the largest antigen dose were super helpers. Interestingly, those cells immunized with the lowest dose lost helping activity with time. Thus, the antigen dependent DNA synthesis we observed during the immunization was correlated with long-term memory. The expression of this memory was temporarily blocked and its expression was correlated with the demise of the cells mediating the short-term memory. It is possible that the blocking of the expression of the long-term memory cells was mediated by a suppressor T cell with a life span similar to that of those cells mediating the short term memory. We showed that the long term memory could not be produced by antigen carryover and that the increased DNA synthesis at the time of original exposure to the antigen seemed to be the responsible factor. We did not, however, do a pertussis carryover control, and, thus, as has been pointed out to us (Mitchison, personal communication), it is possible that a carryover of antigen and pertussis immunized a few cells that had escaped tolerance induction in the original host, and these cells proliferated to form memory cells in the second host. We consider this possibility extremely unlikely for a number of reasons, but we have no direct experiments to disprove it. These are now in progress. However, we had similar findings some years ago in another system in which we were able to rule out post tolerance, antigen induced T cell proliferation as a cause of passage from tolerance to memory (Gershon, 1970; Gershon *et al.*, unpublished observations). These experiments were pilot studies, and we are presently repeating some of this work. However, they illustrate the particular point in question quite well, so I will present some of the preliminary data here.

We gave standardly prepared (Davies, 1969) B mice a histocompatible thymus graft with chromosomally (T6) marked cells. Over the course of the next 30 days we gave these mice large doses of SRBC. We used the 30-day period because we knew that after 30 days the mitotic cells in the thymus graft switch from T_6 to host type and that from this time on there would no longer be seeding of T_6 thymocytes to peripheral tissues (Davies, 1969). At the termination of the pretreatment schedule we removed the thymus grafts of half the mice and these animals had no further source of any T cells. At intervals thereafter we immunized the mice with SRBC or with HRBC and measured the mitotic response of T_6 cells as well as the antibody response. Some of the mice were immunized directly and some had their spleen cells transferred to lethally irradiated recipients.

SRBC pretreatment severely depressed both the T_6 mitotic response and the antibody response to SRBC. The specificity of the suppression of T_6 mitoses was poor, as has previously been noted (Gershon *et al.*, 1968), in that the mitotic response to HRBC was also diminished, although not as severely as the specific suppression. The mitotic response to a totally unrelated antigen, oxzazolone, was normal. The antibody response to HRBC, however, was not significantly different from controls. With time the anti-SRBC antibody response recovered and actually acquired secondary response type characteristics, as it was predominately IgG in both mice with and without intact thymus grafts. The findings of a hyperimmune state when tolerance wanes has previously been noted, but the question of whether the memory was acquired before or after the tolerance induction could not be decided (Dresser and Mitchison, 1968). In this case, however, the nature of the T_6 mitotic response, after the waning of tolerance, gave some added clues, as no source of new T_6 cells was present in these animals after the period of tolerance induction. However, one group of mice, those with intact thymus grafts, had a source of new T cells without T_6 chromosomes. The mitotic response of cells transferred from both groups of mice to lethally irradiated recipients, 11–12 weeks after the termination of tolerance induction, is given in Table II. In mice with intact thymus grafts, 65% of the cells in mitosis were of T_6 genotype 3 days after stimulation with SRBC and only 40% were T_6 in mice stimulated with HRBC. The mitotic response of

Table II. Percentage of Cells in Mitosis with T_6 Chromosomes Three Days after Stimulation with Various Materials

Mitotic stimulus	Experimental group	
	Thymus graft excised	Thymus graft intact
SRBC	91	65
HRBC	86	40
PHA	87	49

their peripheral blood cultured with PHA was 49%. In mice whose thymus grafts were removed at the termination of the tolerance induction the T_6 response was about 90% in both groups, as was the response of their peripheral blood cells to PHA. Since the cells which respond mitotically to PHA are essentially all T cells (Doenhoff *et al.*, 1970), these results suggest that the peripheral T cell pool had been diluted about 50% in mice with intact thymus grafts. However, the T_6 cells responded preferentially to the non-T_6 cells when stimulated with SRBC, indicating a form of memory. We have shown that memory is reflected in T cell mitosis (Davies, 1969; Gershon *et al.*, 1971). We suggest these memory cells were formed during the tolerance induction, and the reason they did not respond earlier was that they had been suppressed. If the memory was generated by antigen remaining after the termination of tolerance induction it should have affected the non-T_6 cells coming from the thymus and we should not have seen a preferential T_6 effect on stimulation with SRBC. Thus, these studies support the notion that memory cells can be functionally suppressed without deletion. They also raise the important question of whether the waning is due to the loss of a cell which is actively suppressing the response or to a waning of the suppressor material produced during the tolerance induction. The answer to this question has important practical applications.

These results are also, at first glance, contradictory to those studies which showed that thymectomy prevented the recovery from tolerance (Taylor, 1964; Claman and Talmage, 1963; Aisenberg and Davis, 1968). The differences in results between our experiments and these, as well as between experiments which have demonstrated memory after the waning of tolerance and those which have not (Dresser and Mitchison, 1968), can all be explained by the mode and efficiency of tolerance induction. The production of memory cells is certainly not a necessary occurrence in tolerance induction. Thus, studies with poor immunogens and good tolerogens, like soluble heterologous globulins, would be highly unlikely to generate memory cells during tolerance induction. Similarly, the use of cytotoxic drugs also would help prevent immunization during induction (Aisenberg and Davis, 1968). Our use of a good immunogen like SRBC clearly is a poor way to produce tolerance, as it has a low yield of tolerant mice (50%) and many of those which we are calling tolerant were not rigorously so. However, this inefficiency has allowed us to make some observations that might otherwise be obscured.

MEANING IN LIFE

The experiments discussed above emphasize a particular problem in assessing much of the work I have presented, that of overall significance. Does the demonstration of temporarily suppressed cells in partially tolerant mice mean that such cells also exist in fully tolerant animals? Does the demonstration of T cell dependent suppressor mechanisms, in certain experimental situations, mean that such mechanisms are of general importance in immunoregulation? At present the observations discussed herein stand only as models which must be experimentally tested in multiple situations before their general validity can be assessed. Consideration of their existence is important, however, in the evaluation of experimental results. For example, when a particular experimental maneuver leads to an increased immune response it is not sufficient to assume that this result was brought about through a plethora of positive factors. The alternative of a paucity of negative ones must be considered. Of course, similar considerations apply to the reverse situation.

A similar problem exists in assessing the significance of the immunosuppressive factors, most likely antigen-antibody complexes, found in putatively tolerant animals (Wegmann *et al.,* 1971). Recently, it has been demonstrated that rigorously tolerant animals lack these factors (Beverley *et al.,* 1973). Does this mean that these factors are unrelated to the tolerance inducing mechanism? This is another question which is unanswerable at present. However, a recent observation by Elkins (1972*a*) suggests an answer. He found that lymphocytes from rat strain A, tolerant to the transplantation antigens of rat strain B, had no capacity to interfere with the ability of normal A lymphocytes to mount a GVH reaction against rats with B strain antigen. If, however, he broke the tolerance of A strain rats by the adoptive transfer of large numbers of normal cells, the cells from these rats could then specifically suppress the response of normal A cells against B antigens. Thus, it seems full tolerance abrogates the ability to demonstrate active suppression, probably because fully tolerant cells are also unreactive to the tolerogenic stimuli and, thus, not making much of their product (see Desensitization). Only during the period of tolerance induction, or in a case where tolerance is incomplete, will active suppression be readily demonstrable.

Space does not permit a detailed analysis of Ramseir's and Lindenmann's (1972) extremely interesting recent findings. Their relationship to some of the mechanisms considered above are not clear at present. However, on the basis of available data, it seems to me that suppressor T cell-mediation of the effects they have described is a distinct possibility.

POSSIBLE MODELS

At present, we know of 3 distinct cell types—T cells, B cells, and macrophages—which interact with one another in the generation of an antibody response. It is highly likely that these 3 main classes of cells have important functional subdivisions. There are 4 net effects of their interaction: specific and nonspecific helper effects as well as specific and nonspecific suppressor effects. Is it possible to build a cellular model which could reasonably account for all the known interactions? I cannot, but I would like to offer some simplified versions which might illustrate some of the problems facing theory building in light of the rapidly accumulating, somewhat bewildering, new information (Fig. 1). For the sake of simplification, the models start post T cell recognition and, thus, avoid all the possible ways, such as macrophage prehandling, receptor cross-linkage, etc., that the T cells' decision to start or stop an antibody response is made. I have also confined them, for the sake of simplicity, to deal only with specific effects.

Model A. This is the simplest model: one receptor class, one T cell class, and one product. In this model, after the signal is given to the T cell, its only decision is how much product (IgT) to make. The B cell is influenced then, as to whether or not to "fire," by the amount of product. In Model A_1 this is a direct effect, too much IgT, no response. In model A_2 this is a semidirect effect [this is Feldmann's (1972a) model]. IgT on a macrophage is stimulatory, and suppression occurs in IgT excess due to spillover and a direct action on the B cell. In model A_3 (indirect effect) the amount of IgT on the macrophage influences this cell as to whether to give the B cell a go or stop signal. The way the macrophage could do this could also be direct or indirect, as above, and, in addition, other classes of T cells can be thrown in at any point for a super cascade effect (dotted lines). All these models, however, have the same serious flaw: they do not account for the suppression produced by poor T cell stimulators.

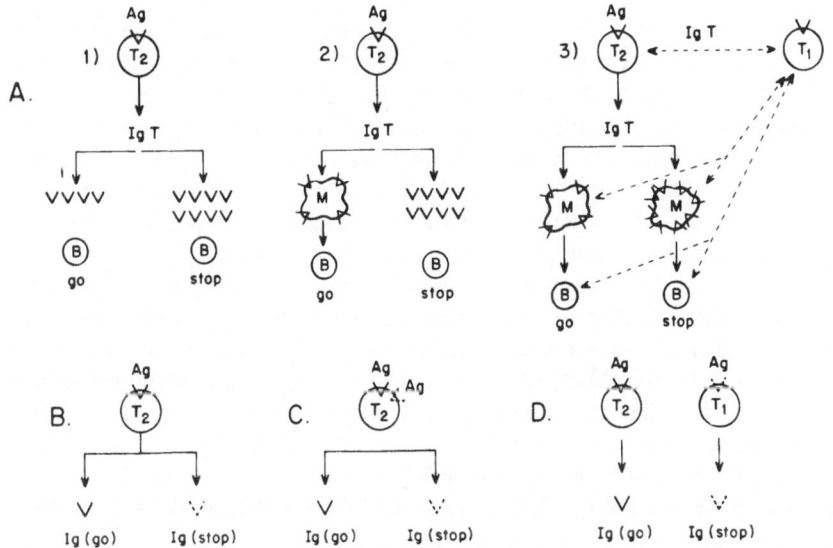

Figure 1. Schematic presentation of the possible models for T cell control of B cell functions discussed under Possible Methods. Ag = antigen, V = T cell receptor (symbol is also used for T cell product), T = T cell, M = macrophage, and B = B cell.

To account for this, one then moves to model B; one receptor class, one T cell class, and two products, Ig(go) and Ig(stop). In this case the T cell must discriminate between signals, as in model A, but instead of deciding how much to put out it must decide which product. How the products produce their effects could be direct, semidirect, or indirect, through macrophages or other T cells, as in model A. The advantage of this model is that it could have stop (suppressor) made in the absence of go (helper) and vice versa. The difficulty with it is to find a mechanism by which a single receptor can discriminate between signals to produce two different substances.

Model C overcomes this difficulty. This is two receptor classes, one T cell class, two products. Again direct, semidirect, and indirect variations of this model may obtain. This model allows the T cell to have a discriminatory effect by virtue of having different receptors which can be differentially triggered. It seems to be the simplest one which can account for the known duality of T cell function. Its major flaw is that it does not account for the differential effect on the two modes (suppression and help) produced by removal of one T cell subpopulation (i.e., increased antibody production after adult thymectomy).

Model D, two receptor classes, two T cell classes, two products, can do this. The problem with this model is that it does not account for those experimental results which indicate that suppressor effects are mediated by the same T cell subpopulation that produces helper effects (see Interactions Between T Cell Subpopulations).

Thus, as far as I can determine, no simple model is adequate to account for the presently known complexities involved in the bidirectional regulatory role T cells play in their interactions with B cells. The problem of model building becomes even more complex if one insists that it take into account T cell control of cells other than B cells: i.e., macrophages (Mackaness, 1969), eosinophiles (Basten and Beeson, 1970), basophils (Dvorak *et al.,* 1970), and other T cells (Asofsky *et al.,* 1971; Raff and Cantor, 1971), and the possible controlling influences on the T cell of the feedback products of their target cells. The possible effects of interactions between specific and nonspecific products is another variable adding to the complexity. Thus, the amplification, specialization, specificity, and attendant control mechanisms required by the system suggest that the complexity of the cellular interactions in the immune response will not be less than those found in complement activation, blood clotting, or vision (Wald, 1965).

At the inception of thymology's "second golden age" (Miller, 1967) a leading article in *Lancet* (1968) noted: "Endocrinologists speak of an endocrine orchestra, implying an interaction between the various components of the system which determines overall endocrine function. This idea might well be adopted by immunologists." The evidence accumulated since then suggests that the T cell is the leader of the band.

SUMMARY

A synthesis of the evidence and ideas I have discussed in this article is as follows. A T cell with attributes such as recirculating capacity and long life, which make it especially well equipped for this function, serves as an overseer of the immune response. Without its action no major aspect of the immune response which developed in the evolutionary period subsequent to the appearance of sharks, either occurs or is made tolerant. This T cell decides on the basis of the energetics of the binding of its receptor(s) with antigen whether to turn other cells on or off. The degree to which it does either or both also is dependent on the nature of the receptor: antigen bond as well as on its sensitivity to feedback signals from target cells (B cells, macrophages, eosinophiles, basophils, and probably other classes of T cells). Specific feedback signals include antigen-antibody complexes which, in the proper molar ratio, act to cause the T cell to turn off the response. Macrophages serve as an important source of nonspecific signals. A phylogenetically primitive B cell functions in the absence of T cell action but is quickly shut off when T cells are stimulated. Thus, the antigen reactive T cell can be thought of as the conductor of the immunological orchestra.

ABBREVIATIONS

Antigens

BGG .... bovine gamma globulin
BSA .... bovine serum albumin
DNP .... dinitrophenyl
GAT .... a linear amino acid copolymer of glutamic acid, alanine, and tyrosine
HRBC .... horse red blood cells
POL .... polymerized flagellar antigen of *Salmonella adelaide*
PVP .... polyvinylpyrrolidone
SIII .... the purified polysaccharide antigen from type III pneumococcus
SRBC .... sheep red blood cells
ALS .... antilymphocyte serum
GVH .... graft versus host disease
MER .... mercaptoethanol resistant
MES .... mercaptoethanol sensitive
PFC .... plaque forming cells
PHA .... phytohemagglutinin
R.E. .... reticuloendothelial

T cell .... thymus processed lymphocytes
B cells .... nonthymus processed lymphocytes which are the
                                          precursors of antibody forming cells
B mice .... mice which lack significant numbers of T cells

ACKNOWLEDGMENTS

The author's research was supported by Public Health Service grants from the NIH CA 08597 and AI 10,497 and his subsistence by a research career development award CA10316. He is also indebted to his technical assistants, students, and colleagues who collaborated in the studies reported, and in particular to Kazunari Kondo who did the work.

NOTE ADDED IN PROOF

Since this review was written, a spate of new demonstrations of suppressor T cell activity have been reported, not all of which are as yet published. It is not possible to review and interpret all these findings here, but just listing them would probably be of some value to those interested in the subject:

Thymus dependence of tolerance induction (Phillips-Quagliata *et al.*, 1973; Waldmann and Munro, in press).

Adoptive transfer of specific immunologic unresponsiveness with T cells (Basten *et al.*, personal communication; Claman, personal communication; Huchet and Feldmann, in press; Mosier, personal communication; Okumura and Tada, 1973; Weber and Kölsch, in press; Zan-Bar, *et al.*, in preparation; Zembala and Asherson, 1973).

Activation of suppressor T cells with mitogens (Dutton, 1972; Rich and Pierce, 1973).

Deficiency of suppressor T cell activity in mice with autoimmune disease (Hardin *et al.*, 1973; Morse, personal communication).

Immunosuppression by spleen-seeking T cells (Folch and Waksman, 1973; Wu and Lance, submitted).

Enhancement of tumor growth by immunized T cells (Kirkwood and Gershon, in press).

In addition, it should be noted that nonspecific suppressor activity of a T cell function has been noted in a B cell population (Gorczynski, submitted) and that tolerance to SRBC can be induced in B cells of nude mice (Mitchell, in press). The first observation may be a case of antigen-antibody complexes activating suppressor T cells (see T Cell Discrimination of Signals – Role of Antibody). In the latter case it may be that the nude mouse has a preponderance of B_1 type B cells (see subclasses of B cells) due to lack of thymic influence.

REFERENCES

Ada, G. L., 1970. *Transpl. Rev.* **5**:105.

Adler, F. L., 1964. *Progr. Allergy* **8**:41.

Aisenberg, A. C., and Davis, C., 1968. *J. Exp. Med.* **128**:1327.

Alkan, S. C., Williams, E. B., Nitecki, D. E., and Goodman, J. W., 1972. *J. Exp. Med.* **135**:1228.

Alkan, S. C., Nitecki, D. E., and Goodman, J. W., 1971. *J. Immunol.* **107**:353.

Allison, A. C., The role of T and B lymphocytes in self tolerance and autoimmunity. In this volume.

Anderson, H. R., Dresser, D. W., Iverson, G. M., Lance, E. M., Wortis, H. H., and Zebra, J., 1972. *Immunol.* **22**:277.

Andersson, B., and Blomgren, H., 1971. *Cell. Immunol.* **2**:411.

Archer, O. K., Pierce, J. C., Papermaster, B. W., and Good, R. A., 1962. *Nature* **195**:191.

Asherson, G. L., Zembala, M., and Barnes, R. M., 1971. *Clin. Exp. Immunol.* **9**:109.

Asofsky, R., Cantor, H., and Tigelaar, R. E., 1971. In *Progress in Immunology*, B. Amos, ed., Academic Press, New York, p. 369.

Bach, J. F., Dardenne, M., and Davies, A. J. S., 1971. *Nature* **231**:110.

Bach, J. F., Muller, J. Y., and Dardenne, M., 1970. *Nature* **227**:1251.

Baker, P. J., personal communication.

Baker, P. J., and Stashak, P. W., 1969. *J. Immunol.* **103**:1342.

Baker, P. J., Prescott, B., Barth, R. F., Stashak, P. W., and Amsbaugh, D. F., 1971a. *Ann. N.Y. Acad. Sci.* **181**:34.

Baker, P. J., Stashak, P. W., Amsbaugh, D. F., and Prescott, B., 1971b. *Immunology* **20**:469.

Baker, P. J., Prescott, B., Stashak, P. W., and Amsbaugh, D. F., 1971c. *J. Immunol.* **107**:719.

Baker, P. J., Barth, R. F., Stashak, P. W., and Amsbaugh, D. F., 1970a. *J. Immunol.* **104**:1313.

Baker, P. J., Stashak, P. W., Amsbaugh, D. F., Prescott, B., and Barth, R. F., 1970b. *J. Immunol.* **105**:1581.

Barthold, D. R., Stashak, P. W., Amsbaugh, D. F., Prescott, B., and Baker, P. J., 1973. *Cell. Immunol.* **6**:315.

Basten, A., and Beeson, P. B., 1970. *J. Exp. Med.* **131**:1288.

Basten, A., Sprent, J., and Miller, J.F.A.P., personal communication.

Benacerraf, B., and Gell, P. G. H., 1959. *Immunology* **2**:53.

Benacerraf, B., and McDevitt, H. O., 1972. *Science* **175**:273.

Ben-Efraim, S., and Liacopoulos, P., 1967. *Immunology* **12**:517.

Bert, G., Forrester, J. A., and Davies, A. J. S., 1971. *Nature New Biol.* **234**:87.

Beverley, P. C. L., Brent, L., Brooks, C., Medawar, P., and Simpson, E., 1973. *Transpl. Proc.*

Boak, J. L., Mitchison, N. A., and Pattison, P. H., 1971. *Eur. J. Immunol.* **1**:63.

Britton, S., and Möller, G., 1968. *J. Immunol.* **100**:1326.

Britton, S., Mitchison, N. A., and Rajewsky, K., 1971. *Eur. J. Immunol.* **1**:65.

Cantor, H., Asofsky, R., and Talal, N., 1970. *J. Exp. Med.* **131**:223.

Carpenter, C. B., Boylston, A. W., II, and Merrill, J. P., 1971. *Cell. Immunol.* **2**:425.

Carter, R. L., Davies, A. J. S., Leuchars, E., Wallis, V., and Gershon, R. K., 1969. *Lymphatic Tissue and Germinal Centers in Immune Response*, Plenum Press, New York, p. 143.

Celada, F., 1966. *J. Exp. Med.* **124**:1.

Chase, M. W., 1963. In A. Bussard (ed.), *La Tolerance Acquise et la Tolerance Naturelle a l'egard de substances angigeniques definies*, Centre National de la Recherche Scientifique, Paris VIIe, p. 139.

Chen, C., and Hirsch, J. G., 1972. *J. Exp. Med.* **136**:604.

Claman, H., personal communication.

Claman, H. N., and Chaperon, E. A., 1969. *Transpl. Rev.* **1**:92.

Claman, H. N., and Talmage, D. W., 1963. *Science* **141**:1193.

Conway-Jacobs, A., Schechter, B., and Sela, M., 1970. *Biochem.* **9**:4870.

Cooperband, S. R., Bondwik, H., Schmid, K., and Mannick, J. A., 1968. *Science* 159:1243.
Crowle, A. J., and Hu, C. C., 1969. *J. Immunol.* 103:1242.
Davies, A. J. S., 1969. *Transpl. Rev.* 1:43.
Davies, A. J. S., Carter, R. L., Leuchars, E., Wallis, V. W., and Dietrich, F. M., 1970. *Immunology* 19:945.
Davies, A. J. S., Leuchars, E., Wallis, V., and Koller, P. C., 1967. *Transplantation* 5:222.
Del Guercio, P., and Leuchars, E., 1972. *J. Immunol.* 109:951.
Dennert, G., 1971. *J. Immunol.* 106:951.
Doenhoff, M. J., Davies, A. J. S., Leuchars, E., and Wallis, V., 1970. *Proc. Roy. Soc. B.* 176:69.
Dresser, D. W., 1962. *Immunology* 6:378.
Dresser, D. W., and Mitchison, N. A., 1968. *Adv. Immunol.* 8:129.
Droege, W., 1971. *Nature* 234:549.
Droege, W., Malchow, D., and Strominger, J. L., 1972. *Eur. J. Immunol.* 2:156.
Dutton, R.W., 1972. *J. Exp. Med.* 136:1445.
Dvorak, H. F., Dvorak, A. M., Simpson, B. A., Richerson, H. B., Leskowitz, S., and Karnovsky, M. J., 1970. *J. Exp. Med.* 132:558.
Dwyer, J. M., and Kantor, F. S., 1973. *J. Exp. Med.*
Eidinger, D., and Baines, M., 1971. *Can. J. Microbiol.* 17:857.
Elkins, W. L., 1972a. *Cell Immunol.* 4:192.
Elkins, W. L., 1972b. *Progr. Allergy* 15:78.
Feldmann, M., 1973. *Nature, New Biol.,* 242:84.
Feldmann, M., 1972a. *J. Exp. Med.* 136:737.
Feldmann, M., 1972b. *Eur. J. Immunol.* 2:130.
Feldmann, M., 1972c. *J. Exp. Med.* 135:735.
Feldmann, M., and Basten, A., 1971. *J. Exp. Med.* 134:103.
Feldmann, M., and Diener, E., 1970. *J. Exp. Med.* 131:247.
Feldmann, M., and Palmer, J., 1971. *Immunology* 21:695.
Feldmann, M., Cone, R. E., and Marchalonis, J. J., 1973, *Cell Immunol.* 9:1.
Field, E. O., and Gibbs, J. E., 1966. *Clin. Exp. Immunol.* 1:195.
Field, E. O., Cauchi, M. N., and Gibbs, J. E., 1967. *Transplantation* 5:241.
Folch, H., and Waksman, B. H., 1973. *Cell Immunol.* 9:12.
Frank, G., Freedman, L., and Gershon, R. K., in preparation.
Friedman, H., and Sabet, T. Y., 1970. *Immunology* 18:883.
Gerety, R. J., Ferraresi, R. W., and Raffel, S., 1970. *J. Exp. Med.* 131:189.
Gershon, R. K., unpublished observations.
Gershon, R. K., 1970. *Fed. Proc.* 29:626.
Gershon, R. K., and Carter, R. L., 1969. *J. Nat. Cancer Inst.* 43:533.
Gershon, R. K., and Hencin, R., in preparation.
Gershon, R. K., and Hencin, R., 1971. *J. Immunol.* 107:1723.
Gershon, R. K., and Kondo, K., 1972a. *Immunology* 23:321.
Gershon, R. K., and Kondo, K., 1972b. *Immunology* 23:335.
Gershon, R. K., and Kondo, K., 1972c. *Science* 175:996.
Gershon, R. K., and Kondo, K., 1971a. *J. Immunol.* 106:1524.
Gershon, R. K., and Kondo, K., 1971b. *J. Immunol.* 106:1532.
Gershon, R. K., and Kondo, K., 1971c. *Immunology* 21:903.
Gershon, R. K., and Kondo, K., 1971d. *J. Nat. Cancer Inst.* 46:1169.
Gershon, R. K., and Kondo, K., 1970. *Immunology* 18:723.
Gershon, R. K., and Kondo, K., 1969. *J. Nat. Cancer Inst.* 43:545.
Gershon, R. K., and Liebhaber, S. A., 1972. *J. Exp. Med.* 136:112.
Gershon, R. K., and Paul, W. E., 1971. *J. Immunol.* 106:872.
Gershon, R. K., Maurer, P. H., and Merryman, C. F., in preparation.
Gershon, R. K., Lance, E. M., and Kondo, K., *J. Immunol.* (In press).
Gershon, R. K., Maurer, P. H., and Merryman, C. F., 1973. *Proc. Nat. Acad. Sci.* 70:250.
Gershon, R. K., Cohen, P., Hencin, R., and Liebhaber, S. A., 1972. *J. Immunol.* 108:586.
Gershon, R. K., Krüger, J., Naysmith, J. D., and Waksman, B. H., 1971. *Nature* 232:639.

Gershon, R. K., Wallis, V., Davies, A. J. S., and Leuchars, E., 1968a. *Nature* 218:280.
Gershon, R. K., Carter, R. L., and Kondo, K., 1968b. *Science* 159:646.
Gershon, R. K., Carter, R. L., and Kondo, K., 1967. *Nature* 213:674.
Gershon, R. K., Wallis, V., Davies, A. J. S., and Leuchars, E., unpublished observations.
Gery, I., and Waksman, B. H., 1972. *J. Exp. Med.* 136:143.
Gery, I., Gershon, R. K., and Waksman, B. H., 1972. *J. Exp. Med.* 136:128.
Golan, D. T., and Borel, Y., 1971. *J. Exp. Med.* 134:1046.
Good, R. A., and Papermaster, B. W., 1964. *Adv. Immunol.* 4:1.
Graf, M. W., and Uhr, J. W., 1969. *J. Exp. Med.* 130:1175.
Green, J. A., Cooperband, S. R., Rutstein, J. A., and Kibrick, S., 1970. *J. Immunol.* 105:48.
Greene, H. S. N., and Harvey, E. K., 1960. *Cancer Res.* 20:1094.
Grey, H. M., 1969. *Adv. Immunol.* 10:51.
Grumet, F. C., 1972. *J. Exp. Med.* 135:110.
Ha, T. Y., and Waksman, B. H., 1973, *J. Immunol.* 110:1290.
Hardin, J., A., Chused, T. M., and Steinberg, A. D., 1973. *J. Immunol.* 111:650.
Haskill, S. J., and Axelrod, M. A., 1972. *Nature New Biol.* 237:251.
Hellström, I., Hellström, K. E., and Allison, A. C., 1971. *Nature* 230:49.
Henry, C., and Jerne, N. K., 1968. *J. Exp. Med.* 128:133.
Herzenberg, L. A., and Herzenberg, L. A., Short-term and chronic allotype suppression in mice. In this volume.
Hoffmann, M., and Dutton, R. W., 1971. *Science* 172:1047.
Horiuichi, A., and Waksman, B. H., 1968. *J. Immunol.* 101:1322.
Howard, J. G., 1972. *Transpl. Rev.* 8:50.
Howard, J. G., Christie, G. H., and Courtenay, B., 1971. *Proc. Roy. Soc. B.* 178:417.
Howard, J. G., Elson, J., Christie, G. H., and Kinsby, R. G., 1969. *Clin. Exp. Immunol.* 4:41.
Howard, J. G., Boak, J. L., and Christie, G. H ., 1966. *Ann. N.Y. Acad. Sci.* 129:327.
Howie, J. B., and Helyer, B. J., 1968. *Adv. Immunol.* 9:215.
Huchet, R., and Feldmann, M., *Eur. J. Immunol.*, in press.
Humphrey, J. H., Parrott, D. M. V., and East, J., 1964. *J Immunol.* 7:419.
Hutchin, P., Amos, D. B., and Prioleau, W. E., Jr., 1967. *Transplantation* 5:68.
Jankovic, B. D., Waksman, B. H., and Arnason, B. G., 1962. *J. Exp. Med.* 116:159.
Kaliss, N., 1969. *Intern. Rev. Exp. Pathol.* 8:241.
Kamrin, B. B., 1955. *Ann. N.Y. Acad. Sci.* 73:848.
Katz, D. H., and Benacerraf, B., 1972. *Adv. Immunol.* 15:1.
Katz, D. H., and Osborne, D. P., Jr., 1972. *J. Exp. Med.* 136:455.
Katz, D. H., Paul, W. E., Goidl, E. A., and Benacerraf, B., 1971a. *J. Exp. Med.* 133:169.
Katz, D. H., Davie, J. M., Paul, W. E., and Benacerraf, B., 1971b. *J. Exp. Med.* 134:201.
Kerbel, R. S., and Eidinger, D., 1972. *Eur. J. Immunol.* 2:114.
Kerbel, R. S., and Eidinger, D., 1971a. *J. Immunol.* 106:917.
Kerbel, R. S., and Eidinger, D., 1971b. *J. Exp. Med.* 133:1043.
Kindred, B., 1971. *Eur. J. Immunol.* 1:59.
Kirkwood, J., and Gershon, R. K. *Oncology,* in press.
Krüger, J., and Gershon, R. K., 1972. *J. Immunol.* 108:581.
Krüger, J., and Gershon, R. K., 1971. *J. Immunol.* 106:1065.
Lance, E. M., and Taub, R. N., 1969. *Nature* 221:841.
Lancet 1:185 (1968)
Lawton, A. R., III, Asofsky, P., Hylton, M. B., and Cooper, M. D., 1972. *J. Exp. Med.* 135:277.
Leskowitz, S. W., and Waksman, B. H., 1960. *J. Immunol.* 84:58.
Leskowitz, S., Jones, V., and Zak, S., 1966. *J. Exp. Med.* 123:229.
Leuchars, E., Wallis, V. J., and Davies, A. J. S., 1968. *Nature* 219:1325.
Liacopoulos, P., and Herlem, S. G., 1968. *Intern. Arch. Allergy* 34:95.
Liacopoulos, P., and Neven, T., 1964. *Immunology* 7:26.
Liacopoulos, P., Couderc, J., and Gille, M. F., 1972. *Eur. J. Immunol.* 2:359.
Liebhaber, S. A., Barchilon, J., and Gershon, R. K., 1972. *J. Immunol.* 109:238.

Little, J. R., and Eisen, H. N., 1969. *J. Exp. Med.* **129**:247.
Mackaness, G. B., 1969. *J. Exp. Med.* **129**:973.
Marchalonis, J. J., Cone, R. E., and Atwell, J. L., 1972. *J. Exp. Med.* **135**:956.
Maugh, T. H., II, 1972. *Science* **176**:1407.
McBride, R. A., and Schierman, L. W., 1970. *J. Exp. Med.* **131**:377.
McCullagh, P. J., 1970a. *Aust. J. Exp. Biol. Med. Sci.* **48**:369.
McCullagh, P. J., 1970b. *J. Exp. Med.* **132**:916.
McDevitt, H. O., and Benacerraf, B., 1969. *Adv. Immunol.* **11**:31.
McGregor, D. D., McCullagh, P. J., and Gowans, J. L., 1967. *Proc. Roy. Soc. B.* **168**:229.
Mellors, R. C., 1967. *Intern. Rev. Exp. Pathol.* **5**:217.
Menkes, J. S., Hencin, R. S., and Gershon, R. K., 1972. *J. Immunol.* **109**:1052.
Merryman, C, F., and Maurer, P. H., 1972. *J. Immunol.* **108**:135.
Miller, J. F. A. P., 1967. *Lancet* **2**:1299.
Miller, J. F. A. P., 1961. *Lancet* **2**:748.
Miller, J. F. A. P., and Mitchell, G. F., 1969. *Transpl. Rev.* **1**:3.
Mills, V., and Gershon, R. K. In preparation.
Mitchell, G. F., *The Lymphocyte: Structure and Function.* Marchalonis, J. J. (ed.) M. Decker Inc., New York, in press.
Mitchell, G. F., and Humphrey, J. H., 1973. In *IV Conference of Germinal Centers and Lymphatic Tissue in the Immune Response,* Plenum Press, New York.
Mitchison, N. A., personal communication.
Mitchison, N. A., 1971a. In O. Makela, A. Cross, and T. V. Kosumen (eds.), *Cell Interactions and Receptor Antibodies in Immune Responses,* Academic Press, New York, p. 249.
Mitchison, N. A., 1971b. *Eur. J. Immunol.* **1**:10.
Mitchison, N. A., 1971c. *Eur. J. Immunol.* **1**:18.
Mitchison, N. A., 1971d. *Eur. J. Immunol.* **1**:68.
Mitchison, N. A., 1964. *Proc. Roy. Soc. B.* **161**:275.
Möller, G., 1971. *J. Immunol.* **106**:1566.
Möller, G. (ed.), 1970. *Transpl. Rev.* **5**. Munksgaard, Copenhagen.
Möller, G., and Michael, J. G., 1971. *Cell, Immunol.* **2**:309.
Möller, E., and Sjöberg, O., 1972. *Transpl. Rev.* **8**:26.
Möller, G., and Wigzell, H., 1965. *J. Exp. Med.* **121**:969.
Möller, G., Andersson, J., and Sjöberg, O., 1972. *Cell. Immunol.* **4**:416.
Morse, S., personal communication.
Mosier, D., personal communication.
Mosier, D., and Cantor, H., 1971. *Eur. J. Immunol.* **1**:459.
Mowbray, J. F., 1963. *Immunology* **6**:217.
Naor, D., and Sulitzeanu, D., 1969. *Intern. Arch. Allergy Appl. Immunol.* **36**:112.
Okumura, L., and Tada, T., 1971a. *J. Immunol.* **106**:1019.
Okumura, L., and Tada, T., 1971b. *J. Immunol.* **107**:1682.
Okumura, K., and Tada, T., 1973. *Nature New Biol.* **245**:180.
Ordal, J. C., and Grumet, F. C., 1972. *J. Exp. Med.* **136**:1195.
Ortiz de Landazuri, M., and Herberman, R. B., 1972. *J. Exp. Med.* **136**:969.
O'Toole, C. M., and Davies, A. J. S., 1971. *Nature* **230**:187.
Pantelouris, E. M., and Flisch, P. A., 1972. *Eur. J. Immunol.* **2**:236.
Parish, C. R., 1972. *Eur. J. Immunol.* **2**:151.
Parish, C. R., 1971a. *J. Exp. Med.* **134**:1.
Parish, C. R., 1971b. *J. Exp. Med.* **134**:21.
Paul, W. E., 1970. *Transpl. Rev.* **5**:130.
Paul, W. E., Katz, D. H., and Benacerraf, B., 1971. *J. Immunol.* **107**:685.
Paul, W. E., Thorbecke, G. J., Siskind, G. W., and Benacerraf, B., 1969. *Immunology* **17**:85.
Pearlman, D. S., 1967. *J. Exp. Med.* **126**:127.
Phie, J. O., and Sehon, A. H., 1972. *Nature New Biol.* **235**:156.
Phillips—Quagliata, J. M., Bensinger, D. O., and Quagliata, F., 1973. *J. Immunol.* **111**: in press.

Pierce, C. W., Solliday, S. M., and Asofsky, R., 1972*a. J. Exp. Med.* 135:675.
Pierce, C. W., Solliday, S. M., and Asofsky, R., 1972*b. J. Exp. Med.* 135:698.
Playfair, J. H. L., 1971*a. Immunology* 21:1037.
Playfair, J. H. L., 1971*b. Nature New Biol.* 231:149.
Radovich, J., and Talmage, D. W., 1967. *Science* 158:512.
Raff, M. C., and Cantor, H., 1971. In B. Amos (ed.), *Progress in Immunology,* Academic Press, New York, p. 83.
Ramsier, H., and Lindenmann, J., 1972. *Transpl. Rev.* 10:57.
Rich, R. R., Mosier, D. D., and Pierce, C. W., 1973. In *7th Leukocyte Culture Conference,* Academic Press, New York.
Rich, R. R., and Pierce, C. W., 1973. *J. Exp. Med.* 137:649.
Riggio, R. R., Schwartz, G. H., Bull, F. G., Stenzel, K. H., and Rubin, A. L., 1969. *Transplantation* 8:689.
Roelants, G., personal communication.
Roitt, I. M., Greaves, M. F., Torrigiani, G., Brostoff, J., and Playfair, J. H. L., 1969. *Lancet* 2:367.
Schechter, I., Bauminger, S., and Sela, N., 1964. *Biochem. Biophys. Acta* 93:686.
Schlossman, S. F., and Levin, H. A., 1971. In S. Cohen, G. Cudkowicz, and R. T. McCluskey (eds.), *Cellular Interactions in the Immune Response,* S. Karger, Basel, p. 153.
Shearer, G. M., Melmon, K. L., Weinstein, Y., and Sela, M., 1972. *J. Exp. Med.* 136:1302.
Shevach, E. M., Paul, W. E., and Green, I., 1972. *J. Exp. Med.* 136:1207.
Sigel, M. M., personal communication.
Sigel, M. M., Voss, E. W., Jr., and Rudikoff, S., 1972. *Comp. Biochem. Physiol.* 42A:249.
Sigel, M. M., Ortiniz-Muniz, G., Lee, J. C., and Lopez, D. M., personal communication.
Simic, M. M., personal communication.
Simpson, E., and Cantor, H., personal communication.
Siskind, G. W., and Benacerraf, B., 1969. *Adv. Immunol.* 10:1.
Sjöberg, O., 1972. *Clin. Exp. Immunol.* 12:365.
Sjöberg, O., 1971. *J. Exp. Med.* 133:1015.
Sjöberg, O., Möller, G., and Andersson, J., 1973. *Eur. J. Immunol.,* in press.
Sjögren, H. O., Hellström, I., Bansal, S. C., and Hellström, K. E., 1971. *Proc. Nat. Acad. Sci.* 68:1372.
Skurzak, H. M., Klein, E., Yoshida, T. O., and Lamon, E. W., 1972. *J. Exp. Med.* 135:997.
Spiesel, S. Z., and Gershon, R. K., 1972. *Nature New Biol.* 238:271.
Staples, P. J., and Talal, N., 1969. *J. Exp. Med.* 129:123.
Tada, T., Taniguchi, M., and Okumura, K., 1971. *J. Immunol.* 106:1012.
Taniguchi, T., and Tada, T., 1971. *J. Immunol.* 107:579.
Taub, R. H., and Gershon, R. K., 1972. *J. Immunol.* 108:377.
Taussig, M. J., and Lachmann, P. J., 1972. *Immunology* 22:185.
Taylor, R. B., 1964. *Immunology* 7:595.
Taylor, R. B., and Iverson, G. M., 1971. *Proc. Roy. Soc. B.* 176:393.
Terman, D. S., Minden, P., and Crowle, A. J., 1971. *Fed. Proc.* 30:650.
Terres, G., and Wolins, W., 1959. *Proc. Soc. Exp. Biol. Med.* 102:632.
Tong, J. L., and Boose, D., 1970. *J. Immunol.* 105:426.
Tornay, S. (ed.), 1938. *Ockham: Studies and Selections,* Open Court Publishing Co. LaSalle.
Uhr, J. W., and Möller, G., 1968. *Adv. Immunol.* 8:81.
Uhr, J. W., and Pappenheimer, A. M., Jr., 1958. *J. Exp. Med.* 108:891.
Unanue, E., 1970. *J. Immunol.* 105:1339.
Underdown, B. J., and Eisen, H. N., 1971. *J. Immunol.* 106:1431.
Veit, B. C., and Michael, J. G., 1973. *J. Immunol.* 111:341.
Veit, B. C., and Michael, J. G., 1972. *Nature New Biol.* 235:238.
Voisin, G. A., 1971. *Progr. Allergy* 15:328.
Voss, E. W., Jr., Sigel, M. M., 1971. *J. Immunol.* 106:1232.
Waksman, B. H., Raff, M. C., and East, J., 1972. *Clin. Exp. Immunol.* 11:1.
Wald, G., 1965. *Science* 150:1028.

Waldmann, H., and Munro, A. J., *Eur. J. Immunol.*, in press.
Walters, C. S., Moorhead, J. W., and Claman, H. N., 1972. *J. Exp. Med.* **136**:546.
Warner, N., personal communication.
Weber, G., and Kölsch, E., *Eur. J. Immunol.*, in press.
Weir, D. M., McBride, W., and Naysmith, J. D., 1968. *Nature* **219**:1276.
Wegmann, T. G., Hellström, I., and Hellström, K. E., 1971. *Proc. Nat. Acad. Sci.* **88**:1644.
Waterston, R. H., 1970. *Science* **170**:1108.
Wu, C-Y and Lance, E. M., *Cell Immunol.*, submitted.
Yoshinaga, M., Yoshinaga, A., and Waksman, B. H., 1972. *J. Exp. Med.* **136**:956.
Zan-Bar, I., Nachtigal, D., and Feldman, M., in preparation.
Zembala, M., and Asherson, G. L., 1973. *Nature* **244**:227.

Chapter 2

Short-Term and Chronic Allotype Suppression in Mice

Leonore A. Herzenberg and Leonard A. Herzenberg

Department of Genetics
Stanford University School of Medicine
Stanford, California

INTRODUCTION

The phenomenon called allotype suppression, in which exposure of the neonate to antibody against its own immunoglobulins suppresses production of those immunoglobulins, offers fertile ground for studying the mechanisms of differentiation and regulation of the immune system. Frequently the suppression is short-lived, and is measurable in weeks post exposure rather than months. In other cases, however, the short exposure of the young animal to antibody to an allotypic antigen on immunoglobulins appears to permanently modify the immune system of the treated animal so that it never regains its normal capacity for immunoglobulin production. Studies on the mechanisms of these short- and long-term suppressions may therefore be expected to provide useful information about some of the sensitive regulation points which keep the entire immune system in balance.

Allotype Suppression in Rabbits

Allotype suppression was originally described in the rabbit. Dray *et al.* immunized female rabbits to allotypic antigens carried on immunoglobulin molecules (i.e., allotypes). Mating these females with homozygous males of the immunizing allotype resulted in heterozygous progeny which were suppressed for production of the paternal type immunoglobulins. It was subsequently

This work is supported by N.I.H. Grants # CA 04681-14, AI 08917-09, and HD 01287-10.

shown that the suppression is due to exposure to maternal antiallotype antibody since progeny from normal mothers injected with the antibody also become suppressed (Mage and Dray, 1965).

Most of the rabbits suppressed by perinatal exposure to antiallotype antibody eventually do produce some immunoglobulins of the suppressed allotype; however, decreased production of the allotype is generally evident well into adulthood if not throughout the life of the animal. To compensate for the decrease in total immune globulins, which is considerable in the rabbit since the suppressed allotypes occur on the Fd portion of the immunoglobulin molecule and hence in several different immunoglobulin classes, suppressed rabbits either produce more immunoglobulins carrying the nonsuppressed allelic allotype (Mage, 1967) or, in the case of suppressed homozygotes, more of other classes of immunoglobulins (Dubiski, 1967; David and Todd, 1969) coded for by genes of other loci (Appella et al., 1968; Kim and Dray, 1973).

To date, it has been difficult to make progress elucidating the mechanism(s) of allotype suppression in the rabbit, perhaps due to the logistics of rabbit work, or perhaps due to the problems of studying cellular interactions with noninbred animals. Nonetheless, it has been established (among other things) that decrease in circulating allotype reflects a decrease in the number of plasma cells producing that allotype (Lummus et al., 1967) and that suppression decreases the amount of allotype in the antibody produced in response to a particular antigen as well as the amount of allotype in the general immunoglobulins in circulation (Mage, 1967). Rose Mage and co-workers have recently shown that suppressed rabbits also lack antibody-forming-precursor-type cells bearing the suppressed allotype on the cell membrane (Harrison et al., 1973a) and these begin to appear as suppression is ending (Harrison et al., 1973b).

Allotype Suppression in Mice

Our studies on allotype suppression in the mouse, with which we will largely concern ourselves for the remainder of this review, were stimulated originally by the demonstration of suppression in the rabbit. Following a similar protocol, we immunized female mice of one strain with an allotypic antigen from a second strain, mated males of the second strain to the immune female, and followed the development of the paternal type immunoglobulin in the heterozygous progeny. With the strains used in our first studies we found that the onset of production of paternal type immunoglobulin in the mouse was considerably delayed in progeny of immune mothers, although all suppressed progeny recovered from suppression and showed essentially normal levels of immunoglobulin by about 15 weeks of age (Herzenberg et al., 1967). In later studies we showed that by using a paternal strain which has severe immunoglobulin abnormalities (i.e., SJL/J), we could produce progeny with a long-term or "chronic" suppression (Jacobson and Herzenberg, 1972; Jacobson et al., 1972). In these hybrids (SJL

X BALB/c) the chronic suppression is due to the generation of a transferable population of thymus-derived (T-cells) which actively suppresses production of the allotype (Herzenberg *et al.*, 1971; Herzenberg, 1972; Herzenberg *et al.*, 1973 and see below).

In order to describe and discuss the studies which led to these conclusions, it is perhaps useful at this point to digress slightly for a brief review of the normal production of immunoglobulins in the mouse and some relevant information about mouse allotypy.

Immunoglobulin Allotypes in Mice

Distinct allotypic antigens have been found on heavy chains of four classes of mouse immunoglobulins (Herzenberg *et al.*, 1968). Antigens of two of these classes, Ig-1 on IgG_{2a} heavy chains and Ig-4 on IgG_1 heavy chains, have been used in the allotype suppression studies. BALB/c, the strain generally used as the maternal or antiallotype donor carries Ig-1a and Ig-4a allotypes. C57BL/10, SJL, and several other strains generally used as paternal strains carry Ig-1b and Ig-4b allotypes. Referred to collectively, the immunoglobulins produced by BALB/c (IgG_1, IgG_{2a}, IgG_{2b}, and IgA of allotype "a") are called Iga globulins and the immunoglobulins produced by C57BL/10 or SJL are referred to as Igb globulins. The corresponding shorthand notation for the gene clusters are Ig^a and Ig^b. Low levels of Ig-1b or Ig-4b are readily measurable in the presence of large amounts of Iga globulins by radioimmune assay (Herzenberg and Herzenberg, 1973). For semiquantitative work, we estimate Ig-1b by immunodiffusion in agar gels.

Origins of Immunoglobulins in Young Mice

The young mouse starts to synthesize detectable amounts of its own IgG immunoglobulins sometime around weaning. Prior to this time its circulating IgG comes from maternal IgG which is first passed to the young *in utero* and then passed continually over roughly the first 16 days of life via nursing (Brambell, 1970). In the weanling (about 3 weeks of age), the majority of circulating IgG is still of maternal origin; however, this passively transferred globulin disappears over the next 5 to 8 weeks and is replaced by its natively synthesized counterpart (Herzenberg *et al.*, 1967).

Thus, in heterozygous progeny ($Ig^a.Ig^b$) made by mating BALB/c (Ig^a) females to C57BL/10 (Ig^b) males, most of the IgG in circulation at 3 weeks of age is maternally derived and therefore Iga allotype. This passively transferred immunoglobulin is eliminated at an exponential rate with a half life of approximately 5 to 7 days. Although it is largely gone when the progeny have reached 8 weeks of age, traces may still be found as late as 12 weeks (Herzenberg and Herzenberg, 1966; Herzenberg *et al.*, 1967, Warner and Herzenberg, 1970).

Replacement of the passively acquired maternal IgG by native synthesis begins about 3 weeks of age. Paternal allotypes (for example, Ig-1b in the heterozygote described above) first appear in circulation sometime between 3 and 5 weeks. Levels then continue to rise until about 12 weeks, when stabilization begins to occur at about the expected adult level (see Fig. 1). Synthesis of the immunoglobulin carrying the maternal allotype is more difficult to measure in young animals because of the large amount of maternally derived IgG present; however, it may be presumed to follow the paternal allotype in that levels of both allotypes in 8-week and older progeny are similar and immunization of progeny starting at 3 weeks yield antibody of both allotypes (unpublished observations).

SHORT-TERM ALLOTYPE SUPPRESSION

Allotype suppression interferes with normal pattern of development described above. Exposure of the neonatal mouse to antibody to the paternal

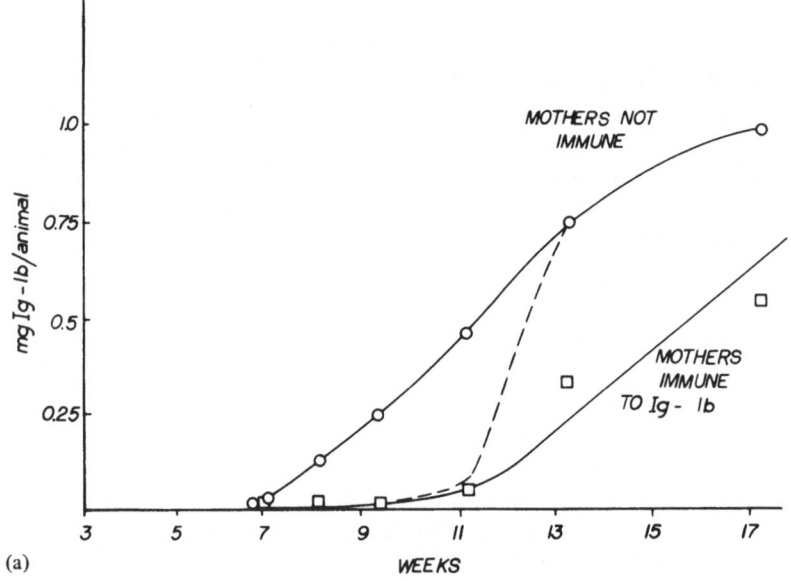

(a)

Figure 1. Increase in allotype levels with age in suppressed and normal progeny. Allotype levels in serum were estimated by radioimmune assay. Calculations for total mg allotype/animal were based on an estimated immunoglobulin space equal to 8.8% body weight.

Figure 1a is reproduced with some modifications from an earlier publication (Herzenberg et al., 1967). Progeny were C57BL/10 × BALB/c hybrids. Dashed curve was calculated on the basis of 25 mg of Ig-1b removed (by maternal antibody), with rate of production set equal to that estimated for controls by equation (1) below. A half-life of 6 days was used. Corrections for the amount of Ig-1b withdrawn in weekly serum sampling were made.

For $t = 0, 1, 2 \ldots .179$, the rate of production of Ig-1b at time t (PRO_t) was found by equation (1) and substituted in equation (2) to determine the amount of Ig-1b expected at time t (Calc Ig_t).

allotype on either IgG_1 or IgG_{2a} globulins specifically delays the onset of synthesis of the IgG_1 or the IgG_{2a} carrying the allotype generally for about 3 weeks. After that, in all strain combinations tested, synthesis of the suppressed allotype or allotypes begins and serum levels climb at a rate similar to that in unsuppressed mice 3 weeks younger.

Most of the data on allotype suppression in mice were collected using BALB/c (Iga) as the mother and the Ig-1b allotype derived from a variety of Igb strains as the suppressed allotype. This particular combination was dictated by the relative ease with which BALB/c mice could be consistently and strongly immunized with Ig-1b. We have now shown, however, that production of Ig-4b, Ig-1a, and Ig-4a is suppressed in similar fashion when neonatal progeny of the appropriate cross are exposed to antibody to the appropriate paternal allotype. The data in Table I summarize these experiments.

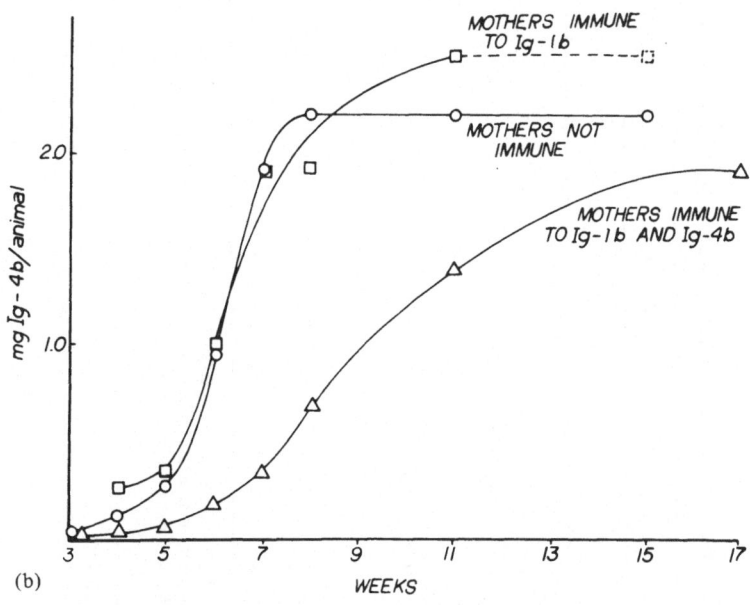

(b)

(1) $\quad PRO_{(t+1)} = (Ig_{(t+1)} - Ig_t) + \left(\frac{\ln 2}{T} + k\right) Ig_t$ and

(2) $\quad Calc\ Ig_{(t+1)} = Calc\ Ig_t + q \cdot PRO_t - \left(\frac{\ln 2}{T} + k\right) Calc\ Ig_t - \theta$

where Ig_t is the observed Ig-1b level in control at time t; T is the half-life in days (taken as 6); k is the fraction of total Ig-1b removed by sampling averaged per day (taken as 0.1/7); q is the fraction by which the rate of production (PRO) is altered; and θ is the amount of Ig-1b withdrawn at $t = 0$, i.e. the amount removed by maternal antibody.

Figure 1b, which shows Ig-4b levels, was drawn from data obtained with a separate group of progeny, in this case (SJL × BALB/c) hybrids.

Table I. Onset of Allotype Synthesis in Suppressed and Normal Mice[1]

Father		Mother			Weeks of age at onset of allotype synthesis			
Strain	Allotype	Strain	Allotype	Immune to	Ig-1a	Ig-4a	Ig-1b	Ig-4b
LP;BAB/14 C57BL/10; CWB/13 101; SJL	Ig^b	BALB/c	Ig^a	Ig-1b			8–10	3–6
Same strains	Ig^b	BALB/c	Ig^a	Nonimmune			3–6	3–6
SJL	Ig^b	BALB/c	Ig^a	Ig-1b + Ig-4b			8–10[2]	8–10
BALB/c	Ig^a	SJL	Ig^b	Ig-1a + Ig-4a	7–9	9–11		
BALB/c	Ig^a	SJL	Ig^b	Nonimmune	3–5	3–5		

[1] A minimum of 20 progeny were used from each mating. Onset of allotype synthesis was scored as the week at which allotype was first seen in immunodiffusion (~0.05 mg/ml). LP, C57BL/10, 101, and SJL were obtained from Jackson Laboratories; BALB/c was obtained from the N.I.H.; BAB/14 is the inbred derivative of 14th backcross generation of a strain congenic with BALB/cN but carrying the Ig^b alleles (originally provided by Dr. Michael Potter); CWB/13 is the inbred derivative of the 13th backcross generation of a strain congenic with C3H.SW (C3H.SW (C3H-H-2^b/SnHz) also carrying the Ig^b alleles.

[2] Some animals (~5%) never show Ig-1 b synthesis.

Since the period of complete suppression is short, it was necessary to show that the absence of circulating allotype was not due mainly to the elimination of newly synthesized allotype resulting from combination with the maternal antibody. The data in Fig. 1a (Herzenberg *et al.*, 1967) show the increase of Ig-1b with age in the sera of a litter of normal animals and a litter of suppressed animals together with a computed curve showing the expected Ig-1b levels if synthesis in the suppressed mice had occurred at the same rate as in normal mice, and maternal antibody merely absorbed the produced immunoglobulin. The "expected" curve shows the level of Ig-1b remaining below the detection threshold for several days longer than normal until the maternal antibody is exhausted. The computed level then rises rapidly to become indistinguishable from levels in normal mice. In contrast, the curve for levels in suppressed mice rises slowly and merges with the levels for normals only when the mice have reached the range for stabilization of adult levels.

Confirmation of this theoretical demonstration of the delay in onset of synthesis of the suppressed allotype comes from the demonstration of small amounts of antiallotype antibody in suppressed mice as late as 8 weeks of age. By this time, if allotype synthesis had been proceeding at a normal rate, enough allotype would have been produced to absorb the original maternal antiallotype antibody several hundred times over (Herzenberg and Herzenberg, 1965; Herzenberg *et al.*, 1967).

Specificity of Suppression

The specificity of antibody to which the young animal is exposed determines the immunoglobulin which is suppressed. This is shown most clearly by the data in Fig. 1b which show levels of Ig-4b with time in three groups of animals: progeny of nonimmune mothers, progeny of mothers immune to Ig-1b, and progeny of mothers immune to Ig-1b and Ig-4b. Suppression for Ig-4b occurs only in the progeny of mothers immune to Ig-4b. Data for suppression of Ig-1b in these animals is not presented; however, progeny of all mothers immunized to Ig-1b showed short-term suppression for that allotype.

Suppression of Antibody Carrying the Suppressed Allotype

Studies on suppression of production of antibody to sheep erythrocytes (SRBC) were conducted with short-term suppressed animals and normal controls. Animals were injected with SRBC at 21 days of age and again at 35 days. At 45 days they were sacrificed and the number of cells in the spleen producing anti SRBC antibody carrying Ig-1a and Ig-1b counted using a localized gel hemolysis assay (Jerne assay) modified to permit estimation of indirect plaques developed with specific antiallotype antibody. Controls produced slightly more

Ig-1a than Ig-1b PFC. The suppressed animals produced few, if any, Ig-1b PFC, although they produced roughly the same number of Ig-1a PFC as the normal controls (see Fig. 2).

It is interesting to note that there was no discernible trend toward increased production of Ig-1a PFC in the suppressed mice, suggesting that at least at this stage, there is no compensating production of the alternate allotype. Direct measurement of Ig-1a levels in suppressed mice past the age when presence of maternal Ig-1a is a significant contribution to the serum Ig-1a also failed to show any evidence of compensation. We also failed to detect a compensatory rise in serum Ig-1a globulins in heterozygotes suppressed for Ig-1b (unpublished observation) although such a rise was detected in suppressed rabbits (Mage and Dray, 1965).

The above essentially summarizes what is currently known about short-term allotype suppression in mice, with the exception of one curious and as yet unexplained observation on the onset of immunoglobulin synthesis both in normal and suppressed mice. Pooling the data for the time of appearance of the first detectable levels of Ig-1b as a function of age in the large group of normal (C57BL/10 X BALB/c)F$_1$ mice studied in these experiments, we found that the range for time of onset varied over a period of several weeks. The range for individual litters, however, was considerably narrower than for the population as a whole. Frequently we found that all the mice in one litter showed detectable Ig-1b before any of the mice in another litter, to all accounts identical, became Ig-1b positive. The similar results with the suppressed population could be dismissed as due to differences in the amount or quality of suppressing antibody delivered by the various mothers; however, since normal controls also clearly showed a closer correlation of time on onset of immunoglobulin synthesis within litters this finding perhaps suggests the existence of a more general basic mechanism regulating initiation of synthesis (Herzenberg *et al.*, 1967).

The simplest explanation for short-term suppression is the elimination or diversion of precursor cells due to reaction with the maternal antiallotype antibody. Once the antibody disappears, or drops below a critical level, synthesis of the suppressed allotype is initiated and then develops from that time according to the normal timetable. How the precursors are removed or diverted, however, is as yet unclear.

CHRONIC ALLOTYPE SUPPRESSION

Immunologic Abnormalities of SJL/J Mice

Our studies on allotype suppression in mice took a different tack with the discovery that progeny produced by mating SJL/J (also Igb) males to BALB/c females immunized to Ig-1b showed not only short-term suppression for Ig-1b,

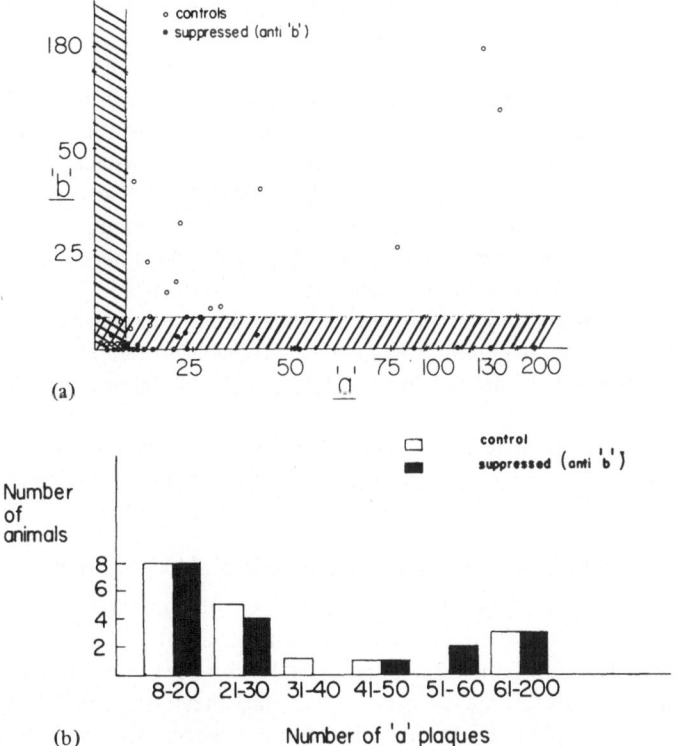

Figure 2. Lack of compensation for suppressed allotype. Figs. 2a and 2b are drawn from the same data. C57Bl/10 ♂ X BALB/c ♀ litters of hybrids from normal mothers or mothers immune to Ig-1b were immunized with 4×10^8 SRBC at 21 and 35 days of age. Animals were sacrificed at 45 days of age and their spleens assayed for direct PFC and indirect PFC developed with anti-Ig-1a and anti-Ig-1b.

In Fig. 2a, the number of "b" allotype plaques in each animal is plotted as a function of the number of "a" allotype plaques in the same animal.

In Fig. 2b, the similar distribution of "a" allotype plaques in suppressed and normal progeny is shown.

but also chronic long-term suppression in which more than half the progeny at 6 months of age had no detectable Ig-1b in circulation (Jacobson and Herzenberg, 1972). This strain combination was selected for study because SJL/J inbred animals show severe abnormalities of the immune system. Not only do SJL/J animals show significant enlarged lymph nodes from birth (Old and Carswell, personal communication), but virtually all mice over the age of one year develop a pleiomorphic reticulum cell sarcoma [classified as Type B by Dr. Thelma Dunn (Dunn and Derringer, 1968)]. Animals greater than 6 months of age also show marked gammopathies, ranging from virtual absence of all immunoglobulin

classes to extraordinary elevations of immunoglobulins of one or more immunoglobulin classes (Wanebo *et al.*, 1966).

While the elevated immunoglobulins in SJL often appear similar to the
restricted electrophoretic mobility "spike" seen in animals with plasmacytomas,
the progressive increase in the protein level with growth of the tumor seen with
plasmacytomas is often not observed in SJL disease. Instead, "spikes" may
appear and rise to quite high levels only to disappear again. New spikes may arise
or the animal may show a general elevation of immunoglobulins or a depletion
of same. While some animals never show "spikes" others may show several, in
sequence or at the same time (unpublished observation).

The mechanisms which regulate this discoordinated immunoglobulin synthesis in SJL mice are at present completely unknown and relatively unstudied. It
has been observed, however, that the IgG_{2a} and IgG_1 immunoglobulin classes
appear to be primarily affected. We have recently shown that SJL mice are
excellent producers of antiallotype antibody, and we have found that some mice
produce restricted heterogeneity antibodies to these antigens (unpublished observation).

Chronic Allotype Suppression in (SJL × BALB/c) Hybrids

Aware, then, that SJL mice show immunologic abnormalities suggestive of
regulatory defects, we mated males of this strain to both normal BALB/c
females and BALB/c females immune to Ig-1b allotypes and followed the onset
of Ig-1b synthesis in the progeny as we had previously with C57BL/10 ×
BALB/c progeny. No significant differences between the two hybrids were
observed during the short-term suppression period, i.e., for the first 8 to 11
weeks. The curves for onset of Ig-1b synthesis in the normal SJL × BALB/c
progeny superimposed on the curve for normal C57BL/10 × BALB/c as did the
early portion of the curves for onset of synthesis in the two types of suppressed
progeny. (Jacobson and Herzenberg, 1972) As time progressed, however, the
SJL × BALB/c progeny from immune mothers began to show marked differences in the pattern of recovery from suppression compared to their suppressed
C57BL/10 × BALB/c counterparts.

To begin with, several suppressed progeny from the SJL × BALB/c cross
never showed detectable Ig-1b levels in circulation, although they were tested
weekly until over 30 weeks of age. Other progeny which appeared to have
recovered from suppression and had initiated Ig-1b synthesis reversed field and
stopped production, so that their levels once again dropped below detectability.
From 10 to 24 weeks of age many of the progeny alternated between synthesis
and nonsynthesis, thus displaying irregular variations in Ig-1b, with shifts from
undetectable levels to normal adult levels and back again being not uncommon.

At about 20 to 24 weeks of age, the Ig-1b levels appeared generally to
stabilize with about half the progeny showing no detectable Ig-1b and the other
half ranging from trace amounts to full adult levels. While some shifting still

occurred after this time, by and large, animals which showed no detectable Ig-1b at 6 months of age tended to remain suppressed (Jacobson and Herzenberg, 1972). These animals, which were dubbed "chronically suppressed," were used in the subsequent experiments which led to the discovery of a thymus-derived cell (T-cell) responsible for this form of allotype suppression.

Examination of the SJL × BALB/c hybrid for abnormalities of the immune system similar to those seen in SJL shows the hybrid to be somewhat abnormal but to a much lesser extent than the parental SJL. The hybrid does not develop tumors, nor does it develop the sharp restricted mobility immunoglobulin "spikes" characteristic of the parental serum. There is, however, a tendency toward generalized elevation of immunoglobulin levels. No differences in serum electrophoretic patterns were observed between suppressed and normal progeny except for the absence of the suppressed allotype (unpublished observation).

SJL Genome and Chronic Suppression

The importance of the SJL genome to the development of chronic allotype suppression is demonstrated by the data in Table II. Of 7 Igb strains tested, only

Table II. Chronic Suppression of Ig-1b Immunoglobulin Synthesis[1]

F₁ hybrid		No. suppressed/total (at 7 months)	
Father (Ig^b)	Mother (Ig^a)	Mother immune to Ig-1b	Nonimmune mother
SJL	BALB/c	100/199	0/152
LP	BALB/c	0/23	0/10
C57BL/10	BALB/c	0/29	0/6
101	BALB/c	1/17	0/5
BAB/14	BALB/c	0/20	0/10
CWB/13	BALB/c	0/19	0/10
B10.S	BALB/c	1/81	0/21
SJL	129	0/23	

[1] Animals were scored for Ig-1b production by immunodiffusion. B10.S is a strain congenic with C57BL/10 carrying H-2^s (i.e., C57BL/10-H-2^s) obtained from Jackson Laboratories. For other strain descriptions, see legend for Table I.

SJL progeny developed chronic suppression. All others recovered from short-term suppression at approximately the same time and subsequently showed no difference in Ig-1b levels between control and suppressed groups. At 6 months of age, only SJL hybrids were suppressed.

It is possible that the BALB/c genome also contributes an element critical to the establishment of chronic suppression. Progeny of 129 (Iga) mothers immunized to Ig-1b mated to SJL males showed short-term suppression but failed to develop any evidence of chronic suppression, suggesting that not all Iga strains can replace BALB/c. Some caution, however, must be used in the interpretation of this result. It could be due to subtle differences between 129 and BALB/c in quality or quantity of anti-Ig-1b passed from mother to offspring. It would perhaps be better to inject young SJL × 129 hybrids born from normal mothers with a known anti-Ig-1b serum, since we have shown that injection of normal SJL × BALB/c hybrids with anti-Ig-1b is just as effective as maternal transfer in generating chronically suppressed progeny (see Table III); however, to date, neither this experiment nor any experiments with other SJL hybrids have been conducted.

Whether BALB/c is unique in its contribution to the hybrid or not, it would appear that it does make a significant contribution toward the development of chronic suppression. SJL inbred animals exposed to conditions which would suppress hybrids show only short-term suppression. Neither injection of antiallotype antibody into SJL inbreds foster nursed on normal BALB/c mothers nor direct transfer of maternal antibody by foster nursing inbreds on BALB/c mothers immunized to Ig-1b induces chronic suppression in the inbred SJL animals. There was no evidence of chronic suppression in three SJL animals which survived transplantation at the late blastocyst stage into an immunized

Table III. Failure to Develop Chronic Suppression in SJL Inbred Mice[1]

Strain	Treatment	Chronic suppressed total
SJL	Egg transplant into BALB/c immune to Ig-1b	0/3
	Foster nurse on BALB/c immune to Ig-1b	0/37
SJL	Injected with anti-Ig-1b	0/4
(SJL × BALB/c)F$_1$	Injected with anti-Ig-1b	11/20

[1] Animals scored for Ig-1b production by immunodiffusion.

BALB/c mother and grew to adulthood, although the animals were tested regularly until over 30 months of age (see Table III).

There also appears to be a restriction on the class of immunoglobulin which may be chronically suppressed, even in the SJL × BALB/c hybrid. In reciprocal crosses (i.e., SJL females immune to Iga allotypes mated to BALB/c males) chronic suppression for Ig-1a is observed, although many fewer progeny exhibit total suppression at 6 months of age (see Table IV). On the other hand, when mothers of either strain were immunized to Ig-4 allotypes (on IgG_1) as well as Ig-1 allotypes (on IgG_{2a}) the progeny showed chronic suppression only for allotypes determined at the Ig-1 locus. The Ig-4a and Ig-4b did show short-term suppression, but all animals recovered and were producing normal levels of Ig-4 by 6 months of age (see Tables I and IV).

As yet we have very few clues as to where these various genetic observations fit in the overall picture of chronic allotype suppression. Nonetheless, they should be borne in mind during consideration of the following studies in which a T-cell responsible for chronic suppression of Ig-1b production is described, so that a comprehensive hypothesis for the origin of this T-cell may be constructed.

Active Factor Responsible for Chronic Suppression

The first evidence that there was an active factor responsible for allotype suppression came from studies in which lethally irradiated (600R) chronically

Table IV. Failure to Develop Chronic Suppressions for Ig-4a or Ig-4b

Strain	Mother immune to	Number of mice showing suppression at 24 weeks or older/total			
		Ig-1b	Ig-4b	Ig-1a	Ig-4a
(SJL × BALB/c)F$_1$	Ig-1b	105/216[1]	0/17[2]	—	—
	Ig-1b and Ig-4b	8/18	0/18	—	—
	Nonimmune	0/165	0/11[2]	—	—
(BALB/c × SJL)F$_1$	Ig-1a and Ig-4a			24/143	0/79
	Nonimmune			0/19	0/19

[1] Animals scored for Ig-1b, Ig-1a, and Ig-4a production by immunodiffusion. Ig-4b was measured by radioimmune assay. Number of suppressed/total tested.
[2] All animals, tested individually reached adult level by 12 weeks. Pools tested to 36 weeks showed average level equal to adult level.

suppressed SJL × BALB/c hybrids 6 months of age or older were reconstituted with spleen from normal syngeneic donors. Although the grafts were accepted and the animals apparently healthy, no Ig-1b appeared in circulation (Jacobson and Herzenberg, 1972). Thus, normal adult cells capable of producing Ig-1b *in situ* were unable to produce the allotype when transferred into an irradiated suppressed host, suggesting the presence of a radiation resistant factor which could prevent Ig-1b production by the transferred tissue.

Spleen or bone marrow transferred from suppressed donors into nonsuppressed irradiated recipients (in this case BALB/c) also failed to produce Ig-1b (Herzenberg *et al.*, 1971).

BALB/c mice were used as recipients in these experiments (as well as in most of those which follow) because of the difficulties in following de novo Ig-1b production by transferred tissue in an animal with Ig-1b in circulation. Although transferring F_1 tissue into irradiated parents is not always successful, we were fortunate in this strain combination that irradiation of recipients with 600R and transfer of a minimum of 10^7 F_1 cells was fully successful in better than 95% of animals. This is demonstrated in suppressed recipients by the continued production of Ig-4b, a nonsuppressed Igb allotype.

The course of suppression in recipients of suppressed spleen or bone marrow showed a curious pattern. In recipients of suppressed cells, a burst of Ig-1b synthesis almost invariably appeared in the first 2 weeks after transfer. By 6 to 8 weeks after transfer, no detectable Ig-1b is produced in recipients of suppressed tissue, although recipients of normal tissue produce consistently high levels of Ig-1b for the duration of the experiment (at least 20 weeks) and recipients of either suppressed or normal tissues produce high levels of Ig-4b throughout the experiment as well.

Mixture-Transfer Assay for Suppression

The key experiment proving that suppressed mice contain an active, dominant cell-associated factor which suppresses Ig-1b production by normal cells otherwise capable of Ig-1b production was that in which spleen from suppressed hybrids was mixed *in vitro* with spleen from syngeneic normal hybrids prior to transfer into the irradiated BALB/c "indicator" hosts. When 10^7 spleen cells of each type mixed prior to transfer were injected, the levels of Ig-1b in serum of the transferred recipients were indistinguishable from the levels in recipients of 10^7 suppressed cells transferred alone, and considerably below levels in recipients of 10^7 normal hybrid cells. At 6 to 7 weeks post transfer, the recipients of suppressed or of suppressed plus normal cells no longer produced any Ig-1b (see Fig. 3).

In a similar experiment, recipients of 4×10^6 suppressed cells mixed with 1.2×10^7 normal cells were suppressed, although not as well as recipients of 1.2

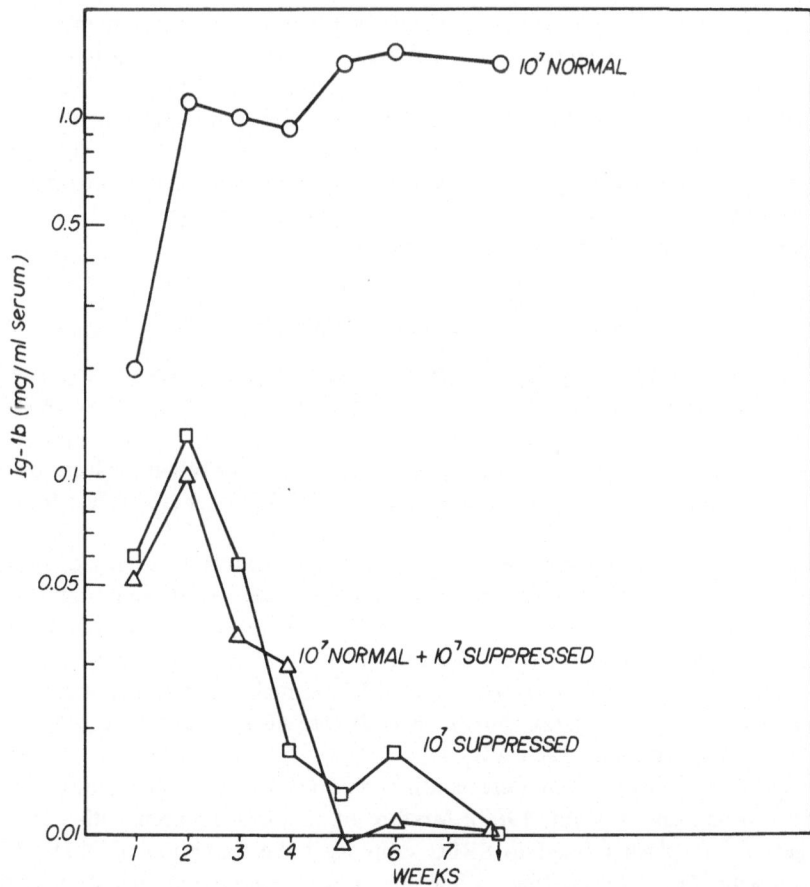

Figure 3. Mixture-transfer assay for suppression of allotype production. Lethally irradiated (600R) BALB/c (Ig^a) were restored with (SJL × BALB/c) hybrid spleen cells approximately 18 hours after irradiation. (○) received 10^7 spleen cells from normal hybrids; (□) received 10^7 spleen cells from chronically suppressed hybrids; and (△) received a mixture containing 10^7 spleen cells from suppressed hybrids and 10^7 spleen cells from normal hybrids. Day 0 = day of transfer. Ig-1b levels were estimated on weekly bleeds by radioimmune assay. Each point is the average of determinations from 5 mice. (Herzenberg *et al.*, 1973).

× 10^7 suppressed cells transferred alone (Jacobson *et al.*, 1972). We have since found that the degree of suppression is more closely related to the number of suppressed cells in the mixture, since results with graded numbers of suppressed cells are roughly similar whether 1.0, 1.2, or even 1.5 × 10^7 normal cells are used in the mixture.

There is considerable variability in the amount of Ig-1b produced in individual recipients of the same suspension of suppressed cells or mixtures of suppressed and normal cells. This is particularly true when marginal numbers of suppressing cells are given (i.e., $3\text{-}5 \times 10^6$ spleen). It is not infrequent to see one or two recipients out of five in such a group become completely suppressed as though these mice had received a full suppressing dose, whereas others in the same group might be only partially suppressed throughout the experiment. Such variability is related perhaps to the escapes from suppression seen in the original suppressed hybrids, both before and after 6 months of age (Jacobson and Herzenberg, 1972, and unpublished observation).

Suppressor T-cells in Lymphoid Tissues

Cells with suppressing activity are found not only in spleen of suppressed hybrids but in thymus, lymph node, and bone marrow. A survey of these tissues in the mixture-transfer assay described above showed that lymph nodes and thymus (parathymic nodes removed) suppress about equally with spleen, on a per cell basis, whereas bone marrow is roughly twofold better (see Tables V and VI).

Experiments with spleen and bone marrow showed that in each of these tissues suppressor activity is associated with T-cells. Cell suspensions from each of the tissues were treated with antiserum to Thy-1b[1] (an antigen found only on thymocytes and T-cells often referred to as theta (Reif and Allen, 1964)) in the presence of complement prior to mixture with normal spleen and transfer into irradiated BALB/c hosts (as above). In each case all suppressing activity was destroyed (see Fig. 4 and Table VII).

The results with spleen were confirmed *in vitro* using Mishell-Dutton cultures (Mishell and Dutton, 1967). Mixture of suppressed spleen with normal syngeneic F_1 spleen primed to SRBC suppressed the formation of Ig-1b PFC while leaving Ig-1a PFC unaffected. Treatment of the suppressed spleen with anti-Thy-1b in the presence of complement prior to mixture and culture destroyed the suppressing activity as it did in the *in vivo* experiments (see Tables VIII and IX).

The demonstration that suppression requires the presence of a T-cell from suppressed animals leaves open the possibility that a bone-marrow-derived cell (B cell) is also required. Such a cell might, for example, produce a suppressing antibody in the presence of T-cells from the suppressed animal. Two lines of evidence, however, make this possibility highly unlikely. First, B-cells generally cooperate with any T-cells if a sufficient number are present. Therefore, transfer of T-cell depleted suppressed spleen should have suppressed, even if somewhat

[1] Nomenclature following recommendation of the Committee on Standardized Nomenclature for the Mouse (Staats, J., 1972).

Table V. Suppressor Cells in Lymphoid Tissues[1]

Normal donor		Suppressed donor		No. of recipients	Ig-1b levels (mg/ml) Weeks after transfer					
Spleen No. of cells		Tissue	No. of cells transferred		1	2	3	4	6	8
10^7		Not done	Not done	3	0.24	>0.38	>0.5	>0.5	>0.5	>0.5
"		Spleen	10^7	4	<0.04	–	–	–	–	–
"		Spleen	10^6	4	0.4	0.13	<0.03	–	<0.02	0.04
"		Thymus	10^7	4	0.02	–	–	–	–	–
"		Thymus	10^6	4	>0.3	>0.3	>0.32	0.12	0.15	0.08
"		Lymph node	10^7	4	0.03	–	–	–	–	–
"		Lymph node	10^6	4	0.4	0.11	0.08	<0.03	<0.02	–

[1] Donors of all cells were (SJL × BALB/c)F$_1$ mice 6–12 months old. Suppressed donors were exposed to maternal anti-Ig-1b perinatally. Ig-1b levels were determined by immunodiffusion. – = <0.01 mg of Ig-1b/ml. Recipients were BALB/c mice irradiated with 600R ~18 hours prior to transfer (Herzenberg et al., 1973a).

Table VI. Suppressor Cells in Bone Marrow[1]

| Number of cells transferred (× 10⁶) | | | | | Mean Ig-1b levels (mg/ml) | | | | |
| Spleen | | Bone marrow | | | Weeks after transfer | | | | |
Normal	Suppressed	Normal	Suppressed	No. of mice	1	2	3	4	6
	12			8	0.2	>0.4	>0.4	>0.5	>0.3
"	3			4	0.1	0.07	<0.02	<0.04	<0.04
"	10			5	0.1	0.03	<0.02	–	–
"		10		4	0.3	0.4	>0.5	>0.5	>0.5
"			1	4	0.07	0.4	0.4	0.3	0.1
"			5	4	0.12	0.07	0.02	–	–
"			10	4	0.06	0.04	0.02	–	–

[1] Donors of all cells were (SJL × BALB/c)F$_1$, mice 6–12 months old. Suppressed donors were exposed to maternal anti-Ig-1b perinatally. Ig-1b levels were determined by immunodiffusion. − = <0.01 mg of Ig-1b/ml. Recipients are BALB/c mice irradiated with 600 R 18 hours prior to transfer (Herzenberg et al., 1973).

Table VII. Anti-Thy-1b (theta) Sensitivity of Suppressor Cells in Bone Marrow[1]

Experiment No.	Spleen Normal	Bone marrow Normal	Bone marrow Suppressed	Treatment	No. of mice	Mean Ig-1b level (mg/ml) Weeks after transfer						
						1	2	3	4	5	6	8
I	12			–	4	0.2	>0.5	>0.5	>0.5	>0.5	>0.4	>0.5
	"	10		–	4	0.4	>0.5	>0.5	>0.5	>0.5	>0.5	>0.5
	"		10	Anti-Thy-1b + C'	4	0.1	>0.5	>0.5	>0.4	>0.4	>0.4	>0.4
	"		10	NMS + C'	4	0.07	0.1	<0.04	<0.02	–[2]	<0.02	<0.04
	"		10	–	4	0.07	0.04	–	–	–	–	–
II	12			–	4	0.1	>0.5	>0.4	>0.5		>0.5	>0.5
	"		9	Anti-Thy-1b + C'	6	0.1	>0.5	>0.5	>0.5		>0.5	>0.5
	"		9	Congenic Anti-Thy-1b + C'	6	0.3	>0.5	>0.5	>0.5		>0.5	>0.5
	"		9	NMS + C'	4	0.1	0.1	0.2	0.2		0.05	0.05

[1] Donors of all cells were (SJL × BALB/c)F$_1$ mice 6 – 2 months old. Suppressed donors were exposed to maternal anti-Ig-1b perinatally. Where indicated under "Treatment," cell suspensions from suppressed donors were incubated with guinea pig serum and anti-Thy-1b or AKR normal serum, at 37°C for 45 min, sedimented, washed, counted, mixed with syngeneic normal cells and injected i.v. Ig-1b levels were estimated by immunodiffusion. Recipients were BALB/c mice irradiated with 600 R ~ 18 hours prior to transfer. In experiment 1, AKR anti-Thy-1b or AKR normal serum was used. In experiment II, congenic anti-Thy-1b (from Dr. E. A. Boyse) was used in addition (Herzenberg et al., 1973).
[2] – = <0.01 mg of Ig-1b/ml.

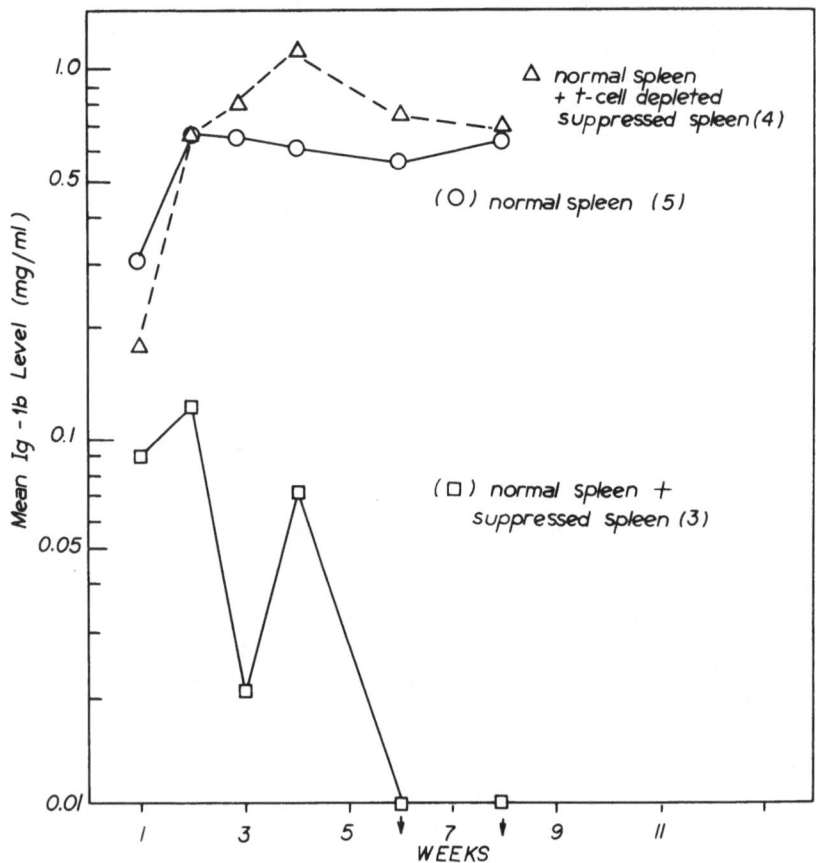

Figure 4. Depletion of suppressor T-cells from spleen by treatment with anti-Thy-1b (anti-θ). Experimental details were the same as described in the legend for Fig. 3. (○) received 10[7] spleen cells from normal (SJL × BALB/c) hybrids; (□) and (△) received a mixture of 10[7] spleen cells from normal hybrids plus 10[7] spleen cells from suppressed hybrids. Cells from suppressed hybrids were treated with anti-Thy-1b plus complement (△) or with AKR normal serum plus complement (□) as described in legend for Table VII (Herzenberg *et al.*, 1973a).

less effectively, when transferred with whole normal spleen. Second, although thymus suppresses about equally to spleen, very few B-cells are found in thymus.

Since bone marrow contains very few T-cells, the demonstration that bone marrow has a high suppressor activity makes the T-cell depletion experiments with bone marrow particularly crucial. The data in Table VII show the results of treatment of bone marrow with two antisera to Thy-1b, one prepared in AKR mice against Thy-1b carried on C3H cells and the other[2] prepared in one

[2] Kindly provided by Dr. E. A. Boyse.

Table VIII. Active Suppression of the Ig-1b Secondary Response to SRBC in Culture[1]

Number of spleen cells cultured ($\times 10^6$)			Allotype developed plaques 10^6 recovered cells			a/b normalized
SRBC primed	Unprimed					
Normal	Normal	Suppressed	a	b	a/b	
20	-	-	908	658	1.4	1
15	5	-	716	343	2.1	1.6
15	-	5	905	83	11	7.7
10	10	-	286	139	2.0	1.5
10	-	10	279	9	33	25

[1] Donors of all cells were (SJL $\times$ BALB/c)F$_1$ mice 6–12 months old. Suppressed donors were exposed to maternal anti-Ig-1b perinatally. The a/b ratios were normalized by setting the ratio for primed cells alone equal to 1 (Herzenberg et al., 1973a).

Table IX. Requirement for T-Cells For Active Suppression in Culture[1]

Numbers of spleen cells cultured ($\times 10^6$)			Treatment of suppressed cells	Normalized a/b allotype ratio of PFC			
SRBC primed	Unprimed			Experiment number			
Normal	Normal	Suppressed		7	8	9	10
20	-	-	None	1 (2.9)	1 (1.4)	1 (2.3)	1 (1.7)
10	-	10	None	6.3	22	5	15
10	-	10	C'	4.7	18	5.9	5.4
10	-	-	C'+ anti-thy-1b	0.67	1.2	1.8	0.77
10	10	-	None	0.67	1.5	1	1.4

[1] Donors of all cells were (SJL $\times$ BALB/c)F$_1$ mice 6–12 months old. Suppressed donors were exposed to maternal anti-Ig-1b perinatally. Where indicated under "Treatment," cell suspensions from suppressed donors were incubated with guinea pig serum and AKR anti-Thy-1b or guinea pig serum alone, 37°C for 45 min, sedimented, washed, counted, mixed with primed normal cells and cultured. Results with AKR anti-Thy-1b were confirmed with congenic anti-Thy-1b in another experiment. The a/b ratios were normalized for each experiment by setting the a/b ratio for primed cells alone equal to 1 (see Table VIII) Total b PFC per 10^6 recovered cells for each experiment: No. 7 = 408, No. 8 = 658, No. 9 = 278, No. 10 = 77 (Herzenberg et al., 1973a).

Table X. Retransfer of Suppressor Cells from Irradiated BALB/c Recipients of a Mixture of Suppressed and Normal Spleen (Mixture-Transfer Recipients)[1]

| Number of cells transferred (× 10⁶) | | | No. of recipients | Mean Ig-1b levels (mg/ml) in serum | | | | | |
| Normal spleen | Suppressed | | | Weeks after transfer | | | | | |
	Spleen	Bone marrow		3	4	5	6	8	12
12			2	>0.5	>0.5	>0.5	>0.5	>0.5	>0.5
	10		3	<0.07	0.01	–	–	–	–
	3		3	0.14	0.11	0.05	–	–	–
		10	3	0.08	0.05	0.04	0.02	–	0.07
		3	3	0.14	0.27	0.11	>0.35	>0.23	>0.07
		1	3	>0.5	>0.4	>0.4	0.14	0.08	0.07

[1] Suppressed donors were BALB/c recipients 11 weeks prior to this transfer of a mixture of suppressed and normal cells as in Fig. 3. All were negative for Ig-1b. Normal donors were (SJL × BALB/c) hybrids. Recipients in this experiment were, as usual, BALB/c irradiated with 600R ~ 18 hours prior to transfer. Ig-1b levels were determined by immunodiffusion. – = <0.01 mg Ig-1b/ml.

member of a pair of Thy-1 congenic strains against the Thy-1b of the other strain. Suppressing activity is destroyed by both sera.

A rough calculation suggests that there is considerably more suppressing activity per T-cell in bone marrow than per T-cell in spleen. Setting a conservatively high estimate of T-cells in bone marrow at 10% and a conservatively low estimate of T-cells in spleen at 30%, the observation that bone marrow suppresses as well as spleen on a total cell basis suggests that the T-cell population in bone marrow is, at a minimum, 3 times more effective in suppressing.

The significance of this concentration of suppressor activity in bone marrow is not clear; however, we have shown recently that bone marrow of BALB/c recipients of mixtures of suppressed and normal spleen (i.e., recipients in mixture-transfer experiments) contains suppressor cells which must have settled there after transfer. To demonstrate this we extended an earlier observation that spleen cells taken from recipients after they were completely suppressed (11 weeks) are able to suppress when repassaged in a mixture-transfer experiment. As the data in Table X show, both bone marrow and spleen from transferred BALB/c recipients suppress about as well as their counterparts taken directly from chronic suppressed hybrids.

Chronic Suppression by Transfer of
Suppressor Cells to Young Syngeneic Hybrids

In the transfer experiments discussed thus far, T-cells from various lymphoid tissues of chronic suppressed SJL × BALB/c hybrids have been shown to actively suppress Ig-1b production by normal syngeneic spleen when the two tissues are transferred together into an irradiated nonsyngeneic host. We have also shown, however, that lymphoid tissues from chronic suppressed donors suppress Ig-1b production when transferred into young, intact syngeneic hybrids.

Table XI. Chronic Suppression by Passage of Suppressor T-Cells into Young Syngeneic Hosts[1]

Recipient	Age at transfer	Suppressor tissue	No. of cells	Chronic suppressed/ total
(SJL × BALB/c)F₁	2–3 weeks	Spleen	1.5×10^7	53/58
,,	,,	Thymus	,,	5/6
,,	,,	Bone marrow	,,	6/9

[1] Animals were scored for chronic suppression at 24 weeks of age.

The data in Table XI show that nearly all young normal SJL X BALB/c hybrids receiving 1.5×10^7 bone marrow, spleen, or thymus from chronically suppressed donors, either i.v. or i.p., are suppressed for Ig-1b production by the time they reach 20 weeks of age. While many more of these secondarily suppressed hybrids fail to initiate Ig-1b production, the rest mimic the primary suppressed donors in that they produce some Ig-1b until about 5 to 6 months of age and only become completely suppressed at that time. Suppressor cells are demonstrable in secondary suppressed hybrids at 6 months of age either by transfer to other syngeneic hybrids or in a mixture-transfer experiment.

Despite the similarities between primary animals suppressed because of exposure to maternal antiserum and secondary suppressed mice suppressed due to transfer of active suppressing T-cells, there exists one basic difference in the pattern of suppression: of the mice initiating Ig-1b production, primary suppressed mice always show the delay in onset of Ig-1b synthesis characteristic of short-term suppression, whereas secondary suppressed mice never do. This is illustrated by the data in Table XII, where weekly test results for representative animals are presented. Some secondary mice never initiate Ig-1b synthesis. All who do, however, do so by 5 weeks of age, whereas primary mice delay until 8 to 10 weeks (see Table I). Termination of synthesis occurs in both types of mice at about 5 to 6 months. Thus, suppressor T-cells may either suppress immediately or remain dormant or only partially active for up to 5 months. Once present, however, they do not appear to need the period of short-term suppression in order to be active, nor do they seem to be able to create that period except by entirely suppressing the recipient.

Role of the Thymus in
Generation and Maintenance of Suppression

In a recent series of experiments, we focused our attention on the *in vivo* characterization of the suppressor T-cell and its relationship to the thymus. While not all of the experiments in this series have been completed as yet, the information which we now have bears presentation here as it is relevant to the consideration of mechanism of chronic suppression.

Although the data are scanty due to poor survival of neonatally thymectomized animals, it would appear that an intact thymus is necessary for the development of chronic suppression. Four neonatally thymectomized animals (NTx) from immune mothers were tested. All recovered from short-term suppression and then maintained continually high levels of Ig-1b until termination of the experiment when they reached 15 months of age. All 6 sham thymectomized mice drawn from the same litters, however, showed evidence of suppression of Ig-1b production.

In contrast, 21/25 ATx progeny thymectomized at 6 to 8 weeks of age born

Table XII. Lack of Short-Term Suppression in Young Hybrid Recipients of Suppressor T-Cells[1]

Recipient	Animal No.	Age of recipient at transfer	Injected with	Ig-1b level in serum — Weeks of age							
				5	6	7	9	11	13	16	20
(SJL × BALB/c)F$_1$	66	2–3 weeks	1.5×10^7	0.05	0.14	0.14	0.14	0.14	0.05	–	–
,,	67	,,	spleen cells	0.14	0.05	0.05	0.05	0.01	–	–	–
,,	70	,,	from chronic	0.05	0.01	–	0.05	0.01	–	–	–
,,	95	,,	suppressed	0.05	0.05	–	–	–	–	–	–
,,	74	,,	F$_1$ donor	>0.5	0.14	0.14	0.14	0.14	>0.5	0.05	0.14
,,	75	,,	,,	>0.5	0.14	0.14	0.05	0.05	0.14	0.01	–
,,	43	,,	,,	0.01	–	–	–	–	–	–	–
,,	90	,,	,,	–	–	–	–	–	–	–	–
,,	–	Not transferred	–	0.14	>0.5	>0.5	>0.5	>0.5	>0.5	>0.5	>0.5

[1] Animals were chosen from colony to show various patterns of secondary suppression. Ig-1b levels were determined by immunodiffusion. – = <0.01 Ig-1b/ml.

of immune mothers developed chronic suppression, suggesting that the thymus is necessary only for development of chronic suppression and not for the expression of suppressor cell activity (see Table XIII). This conclusion is supported by the demonstration that spleen from suppressed donors is active in a mixture-transfer experiment when the BALB/c recipients have been thymectomized one month prior to irradiation and transfer (see Table XIV).

Table XIII. Effect of Thymectomy on Development of Chronic Suppression[1]

	Age at Tx	Chronic suppressed/total
NTx	1–2 days	0/4
Sham N Tx	”	6/6
A Tx	6–8 weeks	21/25
Sham A Tx	”	11/12

[1] Litters of (SJL × BALB/c) hybrids exposed perinatally to maternal anti-Ig-1b were divided equally between sham and thymectomized animals. Most animals classified as chronic suppressed were negative for Ig-1b after 6 months of age. Some showed sporadic low levels of the allotype.

The four neonatally thymectomized animals showed continued high (normal) levels of Ig-1b starting at 10–12 weeks of age, i.e., after short-term suppression was over.

Table XIV. Transfer of Mixture of Suppressed and Normal Spleen into ATx Irradiated BALB/c[1]

Recipient (BALB/c)	Number of cells transferred (× 10⁶)		Number of recipients suppressed/total
	Normal spleen	Suppressed spleen	
ATx	13	10	3/3
Sham	”	”	4/4
Normal	”	”	3/3
ATx	13	-	0/3
Sham	”	-	0/3
Normal	”	-	0/3

[1] Recipients were BALB/c mice thymectomized or sham thymectomized at 12 weeks of age, irradiated (600R) 4 weeks later, and injected with cell suspension ~ 18 hours after irradiation. Suppressed mice showed typical pattern in mixture-transfer experiment (see Fig. 3).

MECHANISM OF CHRONIC ALLOTYPE SUPPRESSION

Most of the studies completed so far on chronic allotype suppression have involved the identification of T-cells as responsible for chronic allotype suppression and the investigation of conditions under which suppression occurs. In addition, we have made some progress toward understanding the mechanism by which T-cells suppress. While the data are still incomplete, when taken in conjunction with what is known about the normal pathway of differentiation of immunoglobulin producing cells and the known properties of other types of T-cells, several interesting possible hypotheses arise. Before proceeding to a discussion of these, however, we will briefly review the events in the B-cell line leading to antibody synthesis and the role of T-cells in the immune system in order to bring together a number of relevant considerations.

B-Cell Differentiation

The normal process of differentiation to synthesis of γG or γA immunoglobulin (or antibody) involves the commitment of an originally totipotent (with respect to species of immunoglobulins) B-stem cell to the production of a large amount of a unique immunoglobulin molecule. During this process, one of the two autosomal chromosomes carrying H-chain determinants is selected, the variable region is determined, and one of the four linked genes for H-chain constant regions (in the mouse Ig-1 to Ig-4, specifying γG_{2a}, γA, γG_{2b}, and γG_1, respectively) paired to it in a manner which allows for the transcription of the entire unit as a single messenger. In similar fashion a unique light-chain messenger is transcribed. Light and heavy chains are then produced, assembled, and exported, while the cell differentiates further to a mature plasma cell. While there is evidence (Pernis *et al.*, 1971; Wang *et al.*, 1970) which indicates that during this process some or all cells may go through a stage of γM production before selection of the final γG or γA class without change in the variable region, this does not substantially alter the above description.

Almost nothing is known of the mechanisms involved in this process. If the insertion of a γM step proves correct, then chromosome exclusion and variable region choice occur earlier than selection of H-chain class. In any event, at the end of the process a single cell produces a unique immunoglobulin whose H-chain is determined by a gene (or genes) on only one of the two parental chromosomes (Pernis *et al.*, 1965). No other such system for exclusion of autosomal genes is known in mammalian cells.

In an allotype heterozygote, such chromosomal (or allelic) exclusion leads to the presence of two populations of immunoglobulin-producing cells for any given class, one making immunoglobulins of paternal allotype and the other of maternal allotype. Usually an animal has a characteristic ratio of cells producing each of the parental allotypes, and circulating immunoglobulins reflect this cellular ratio (Cebra, 1968). While there is little understanding at present of how this ratio is maintained, the regularity with which certain allotype (and classes) predominate over others suggests that there is more than just random selection operating.

It is usually assumed that all immunoglobulins in circulation in normal animals are antibodies produced in response to antigenic stimulation. This assumption is buttressed by the demonstration that animals raised in a germ-free environment show very low IgG levels (Gustafsson and Laurell, 1959). Although the low levels could be explained by factors other than lack of antigenic exposure, the studies with germ-free animals suggest that the presence of an immunoglobulin molecule in circulation is evidence of antigenic stimulation, i.e., that a progenitor B-cell committed to production of that immunoglobulin was stimulated by antigen to give rise to cells producing the immunoglobulin.

T-Cell Functions

Combination of B-cells with antigen is a necessary but generally not sufficient condition for antibody production to ensue.[1] The antigen driven differentiation of B-cells from precursors to IgG antibody producing cells most often requires interaction with a (thymus-derived) "cooperating" T-cell capable of recognizing either the antigen or a carrier to which the antigen has been attached. Some antigens are known which stimulate antibody production in the apparent absence of T-cells. For example, neonatally thymectomized or irradiated adult thymectomized mice reconstituted with either fetal liver or bone marrow, respond to polymerized flagellin, as do genetically athymic (nu/nu) mice. Since a small number of Thy-1 (theta) positive cells, presumably T-cells, are always found in these animals and polymerized flagellin is a very good antigen, the possibility formally remains that thymic independent antigens are those capable of extraordinarily efficient use of cooperators (Rajewsky et al., 1969; Miller and Mitchell, 1969; Davies, 1969; Claman and Chaperon, 1969; Taylor, 1969, Mäkelä et al., 1971; Warner, 1972; Mitchison, 1967; Paul et al., 1967).

Interestingly, T-cell depleted animals such as those described in the preceding paragraph produce substantial levels of IgG even though the IgG antibody response shows a virtually absolute dependence on T-cell cooperation. T-cell depleted animals have been shown to respond to antigens with IgM antibody but not with IgG antibody production. This again raises the question of whether all

[1] A complete review with extensive referencing on T- and B-cell interactions is beyond the scope of this work. The short list of references presented at the end of each paragraph is intended to be minimal rather than comprehensive.

IgG is, in fact, produced in response to antigenic stimulation (Wortis, 1971; Tyan and Herzenberg, 1968; Warner, 1972; Grumet, 1972; Mitchell *et al.*, 1972*a*).

The cooperating T-cell has been extensively studied over the last several years, but as yet the mechanism of cooperation has not been firmly established. For our purposes here it is sufficient to state that (at least for most antigens) B-cells capable of binding the antigen must interact with T-cells capable of recognizing the antigen, although the two cell types probably do not recognize the same antigenic determinants. This interaction could be directly between B- and T-cells or between B-cells and a factor produced by T-cells stimulated by antigen (Feldmann, 1972; Iverson, 1972).

T-cells serve a second major function in the immune system. They are the effectors of cellular immunity. T-cell depleted animals are unable to reject homografts or to show other manifestations of cellular immunity, such as delayed hypersensitivity. These functions may be restored in depleted animals by reconstitution with thymus, spleen, or lymph nodes from normal animals. Reconstitution with bone marrow, which contains many fewer T-cells, is effective but only marginally so (Warner *et al.*, 1962; Raff, 1971).

Immunologic memory appears to be carried in both T- and B-cell lines. Although in many cases a primed B-cell population can produce a secondary response in cooperation with a sufficient number of unprimed T-cells, priming renders the T-cell population far more effective for cooperation. Similarly, although an allograft will be rejected by an animal never previously exposed to the allograft antigens, the rejection of a second graft is considerably more rapid and vigorous. Spleen and lymph node appear to be the principal location of both B- and T-cell populations carrying immunologic memory. The thymus and bone marrow seem to serve more as reservoirs of stem and progenitor cells, since transfer of these tissues from primed animals mainly yields a primary type response (Jacobson *et al.*, 1970, Mitchell *et al.*, 1971, Mitchell *et al.*, 1972*a*; Cunningham and Sercarz, 1971; Davies, 1969; Raff, 1970).

Suppression of Immunoglobulins in Other Systems

Various types of suppression of antibody or immunoglobulin synthesis have been reported by other laboratories in addition to the short- and long-term allotype suppression described earlier in this chapter.

Injection of neonates with heterologous anti-immunoglobulin antibody specific for a particular immunoglobulin class suppresses the production of antibodies and immunoglobulin of that and other classes perhaps by a mechanism similar to short-term suppression (Manning and Jutila, 1972; Lawton *et al.*, 1972). The suppression lasts for shorter or longer periods and covers other classes, depending on the specificity of the antiserum and the injection protocol. Similarly, treatment of spleen cell cultures with heterologous anticlass antibody suppresses the *in vitro* anti-SRBC response in that class (Pierce *et al.,* 1972). A "feedback" inhibition of the IgM response to a particular antigen as the result of presence of IgG antibody to the same antigen has also been shown, but whether this relates to suppression of immunoglobulin synthesis by anti-immunoglobulin reagents is unclear (Henry and Jerne, 1967).

Examples of active cellular suppression of antibody response, which is perhaps analogous to T-cell mediated chronic allotype suppression, have recently been reported. Two of these, which have been well documented, are the responses to polyvinylpyrollidone and to pneumococcal polysaccharide, both "thymic independent" antigens (Baker *et al.,* 1970; Kerbel and Eidinger, 1972). The suppression in these cases has been interpreted to be T-cell mediated suppression of IgM response. No IgG response occurs. Evidence for "active tolerance" to T-dependent antigens appears to be more difficult to obtain; however, data suggesting this may occur for IgE antibody in rats (Okamura and Tada, 1971), and for a variety of other systems in mouse (Gershon, 1973), have been reported.

The demonstration of apparent analogies to chronic allotype suppression suggests that perhaps the T-cell mediated suppression demonstrable in SJL X BALB/c hybrids may have a broader biological significance than its restriction to one class of immunoglobulin and one hybrid cross would indicate. It is intriguing to speculate that suppressor cells play a role in the regulation of antibody synthesis and overall immunoglobulin levels, but evaluation of this possibility will have to wait until there is more evidence with which to establish a firmer concept of the mechanism(s) of suppression.

In chronic allotype suppression, we have established that exposure to antiallotype antibody is necessary for the development of chronic suppression. Once the suppressor T-cell population is established, however, its maintenance and activity do not require the continued presence of antiallotype antibody.

The suppressor T-cells could be required as cooperators for B-cells primed to produce an unknown antibody which then is the suppressing agent. This is unlikely, however, since (1) the thymus, which contains few B-cells, is as good a source of suppressor activity as spleen; (2) T-cell depleted suppressor spleen does not suppress, although it is in the presence of an abundance of T-cells from a concomitantly transferred normal spleen population; and (3) no evidence for a circulating suppressing factor has been found.

A more likely interpretation of the data is that the suppressor T-cell exerts its influence by interaction with a precursor cell originally destined to produce the suppressed allotype. The suppressor cell may either kill the precursor, hold it static by preventing its differentiation to immunoglobulin production, or divert it to another pathway of differentiation. This interaction could be a direct T-cell to B-cell interaction (e.g., at a membrane level), or it could be mediated either by a factor elaborated by the suppressor or other cells activated by the suppressor. In either case, the requirement for suppressor T-cells does suggest that if this is the case, then the T-cell must initiate the interaction.

Since the suppression is specific for Ig-1b production in an Ig^a/Ig^b heterozygote, it is likely that the suppressor T-cells act on B-cells which have differentiated to a point at which they are committed to Ig-1b production and are recognizable as such. This is most likely after allelic exclusion has taken place and the cell is committed to production of a unique antibody molecule.

Antibody forming cell precursors are known to synthesize small amounts of the antibody molecule to which the cell is committed and to display this antibody on the cell surface, where it can be detected either by antigen binding or heterologous antiallotype and anti-immunoglobulin reagents (Wigzell *et al.*, 1971; Rabellino *et al.*, 1971; Raff *et al.*, 1970; Julius *et al.*, 1972). Short-term suppression probably results from combination of the exposed antibody with antiallotype or anticlass specific antibody. The marker which the T-cell suppressors recognize must be somewhat more complex than the Ig-1b allotype as it occurs in circulation, since large amounts of circulating Ig-1b do not block the onset of suppression. We have proposed that Ig-1b bound to the cell surface displays or creates a new antigen, which is the recognition clue for the suppressor T-cell, but this marker could be antigenically distinct from the free Ig-1b molecule and simply occur uniquely on Ig-1b committed B-cells.

Suppressor T-Cells as Killers?

Perhaps the most significant question still to be answered about suppressor T-cells is the identification of their normal role in the animal. A conservative hypothesis pictures these cells as part of the population of T-cells responsible for cellular immunity (immune surveillance). It is possible that exposure to antiallotype antibody removes Ig-1b precursors from the young animal for a sufficient period past the "tolerance" limit so that new Ig-1b precursors, when they appear, are no longer recognized as self. T-cells seeing these "nonself" cells become primed to them as if to an allograft. Once this occurs, new Ig-1b precursors will be eliminated as they arise by the primed T-cells acting in their normal surveillance role.

This hypothesis has much to recommend it in that it assigns a role to suppressor T-cells consistent with a known T-cell function; however, a number of accommodations must be made in order to make this hypothesis consistent with all the data. A seesaw balance between rejecting T-cells and Ig-1b precursors which tips towards rejection when the animals reach 6 months of age must be postulated. Otherwise, if there is a sensitized T-cell population able to reject Ig-1b precursors as a foreign graft, why does Ig-1b synthesis become established in most animals prior to 6 months of age, and complete rejection only occur in animals over 6 months of age? Similarly, why is a partially suppressed Ig-1b level frequently maintained, not only in young animals, but often for the life of those animals over six months of age who do not become completely suppressed. While a balanced rejection state in which antibody to cellular antigens ("blocking antibody") prevents rejection by T-cells has recently been suggested in other systems (Hellström, 1972), evidence for its existence as a general phenomenon applicability here is still lacking.

Another inconsistency is the demonstration of high suppressor activity in bone marrow which is in general a poor source of cells for cellular immune reactions. This finding can be reconciled with the hypothesis by postulating that suppressor T-cells have specifically migrated into the bone marrow in large numbers because target cells occur there; however, such arguments do raise some serious, albeit not fatal objections, to the hypothesis. Additional questions are why chronic suppression only occurs in SJL × BALB/c hybrids and why only for γG_{2a} globulins.

Suppressor T-Cells as Regulators?

A more novel approach to the mechanism of chronic allotype suppression is to focus on the inherent regulatory role of T-cells in the differentiation of B-cells from precursors to IgG antibody producing cells. Since this differentiation generally requires the cooperation of a T-cell, antibody production may be limited not only by the number of B-cell precursors able to differentiate to produce antibody to a given antigen, but as well by the number of T-cells available to cooperate with the B-cell precursors in order to facilitate their differentiation to antibody forming cells. Put another way, the requirement for cooperation with T-cells before antibody production can proceed creates a pressure point at which the extent of the antibody response may be controlled by the availability of cooperating T-cells.

While this type of T-cell control over B-cell function is essentially passive, i.e., a decrease of cooperators results in a decrease of the response, it is possible that another class of T-cells exists which actively regulates the flow of B-cells from precursors to antibody forming cells, perhaps by preventing or aborting cooperation. The data we have presented on suppression of Ig-1b synthesis are as well explained by postulating that the T-cell responsible for the active suppression of Ig-1b is one of a group of many specific suppressor (regulator) T-cells, collectively responsible for the active control of the levels of antibody of the various classes in serum.

A simple model for the mechanism of this kind of regulation could be competition for B-cells between cooperators and suppressors, where blocking of the interaction between cooperators and B-cells by suppressors results in prevention of further differentiation of the B-cell. Under ordinary circumstances, the presence of suppressors and cooperators adheres to a finely tuned balance which maintains the relatively uniform immunoglobulin levels found in mice of the same age and strain. The presence of antiallotype serum in the young animals, however, could shift this balance in favor of overregulation of Ig-1b synthesis. In SJL X BALB/c animals which, like the SJL parent, show an abnormal regulation of IgG immunoglobulin synthesis, this early shift could result in the establishment of an overdeveloped population of regulator (suppressor) T-cells which specifically suppress Ig-1b precursors from differentiating to producers.

While the animal is young and its immune response is at its peak, cooperators would be expected to have a numerical advantage and, therefore, be able to override suppressors. On the other hand, during periods of relative immunologic inactivity suppressors would once again be dominant.

As the animal ages and cooperator function declines, the degree of overregulation originally established would determine whether the animal will become completely or partially suppressed.

A competition model such as this depends on the validity of assuming that all B-cell differentiation to IgG production is T-cell dependent, a point which is hardly well established. The inability to obtain chronic suppression for γG_1 could be explained, however, if the γG_1 production were not entirely T-cell dependent, whereas the γG_{2a} production was.

This model is admittedly fanciful. Nevertheless, it does deal more easily with some of the objections to viewing chronic allotype suppression as an induced autoimmunity. No telling argument currently exists for determining which of the two hypotheses is correct, and we therefore leave the decision up to the personal preference of the reader until decisive evidence bearing on the question is available.

ACKNOWLEDGMENTS

Since allotype suppression in the mouse has been a major area of interest in our laboratory for several years, virtually all of our students, fellows, and technical staff have contributed in some measure to the progress made on the problem. In addition to those who have published papers on allotype suppression from this laboratory or in collaboration with us, (Ethel Jacobson, Roy Riblet, Eva Chan, Myrnice Ravitch, Edna Rivera, and Robert Goodlin), significant experimental work was done here by Alastair Cunningham, Charles Metzler, Katherine Bechtol, and by Robert Mishell in his own laboratory. Derek Hewgill prepared many of the absorbed antisera and purified proteins used as reagents for the study.

We would particularly like to call attention to the contribution of F. Timothy Gadus, who not only bled, tested, and kept track of the thousands of mice studied in this project, but also, over the last year, helped to plan and execute several of the key transfer experiments. Mr. Gadus' mastery of the complex logistics required to provide an adequate supply of chronic suppressed mice is in itself worthy of note.

We would also like to thank Phillipa Meyering, our very able secretary, for her unstinting help in the preparation of this manuscript and in general for her help over the years in smoothing the administrative burdens which otherwise would have detracted from our ability to work in the laboratory.

REFERENCES

Appella, E., Mage, R. G., Dubiski, S., and Reisfeld, R., 1968. *Proc. Nat. Acad. Sci.* **60**:975.

Baker, P. J., Stashak, R. W., Amsbaugh, D. F., Prescott, B., and Barth, R. F., 1970. *J. Immunol.* **105**:1581.

Brambell, F. W. R., 1970. *The Transmission of Passive Immunity from Mother to Young.* American-Elsevier, New York.

Cebra, J. J., 1968. *Symp. Intern. Soc. Cell Biol.* **7**:69.

Claman, H. N., and Chaperon, E. A., 1969. *Transpl. Rev.* **1**:92.

Cunningham, A. J. and Sercarz, E. E., 1971. *Eur. J. Immunol.* **1**:413.

David, G. S., and Todd, C. W., 1969. *Proc. Nat. Acad. Sci.* **62**:860.

Davies, A. J. S., 1969. *Transpl. Rev.* **1**:43.

Dray, S., 1962. *Nature* **195**:181.

Dubiski, S., 1967. *Nature* (London) **214**:1365.

Dunn, T. B., and Derringer, M. K., 1968. *J. Nat. Cancer Inst.* **40**:771.

Feldmann, M., 1972. *J. Exp. Med.* **136**:737.

Gershon, R. K., 1973. *Contemporary Topics in Immunobiology,* Vol. 3. Plenum Press, New York.

Grumet, F. C., 1972. *J. Exp. Med.* **135**:110.

Gustafsson, B. E., and Laurell, C. B., 1959. *J. Exp. Med.* **110**:675.

Harrison, M. R., Mage, R. G., and Davie, J. M., 1973a. *J. Exp. Med.* **137**:254.

Harrison, M. R., Jones, P. P. and Mage, R. G., 1973b. *J. of Immunol.* **111**:1595.

Hellström, K. E., and Hellström, I., 1972. In *Ontogeny of Acquired Immunity: A Ciba Foundation Symposium,* Assoc. Sci. Publ., New York, p. 133.

Henry, C., and Jerne, N. K., 1967. In J. Killander (ed.), *Gamma Globulins Nobel Symp.,* Vol. 3, Almquist and Wiksell, Stockholm, p. 421.

Herzenberg, L. A., 1972. In *Ciba Foundation Symposium: Ontogeny of Acquired Immunity.* Associated Scientific Publishers, New York. pp. 106–112.

Herzenberg, L. A., and Herzenberg, L. A., 1973. In D. M. Weir (ed.), *Handbook of Experimental Immunology,* 2nd ed., Blackwell Scientific Publications. Oxford, pp. 13.1–13.18.

Herzenberg, L. A., and Herzenberg, L. A., 1966. In *Proceedings of Symposium on the Mutational Process,* Czechoslovakian Acad. Sciences, Praha, pp. 227–232.

Herzenberg, L. A., Chan, E. L., Ravitch, M. M., Riblet, R. J., and Herzenberg, L. A., 1973. *J. Exp. Med.* **137**:1131.

Herzenberg, L. A., Jacobson, E. B., Herzenberg, L. A., and Riblet, R. J., 1971. *Ann. N.Y. Acad. Sci.* **190**:212.

Herzenberg, L. A., McDevitt, H. O., and Herzenberg, L. A., 1968. *Ann. Rev. Genet.* **2**:209.

Herzenberg, L. A., Herzenberg, L. A., Goodlin, R. C., and Rivera, E. C., 1967. *J. Exp. Med.* **126**:701.

Iverson, G. M., 1972. In Silvestri (ed.), *Lepetit Symposium,* North Holland Publishing Co., Amsterdam.

Jacobson, E. B., and Herzenberg, L. A., 1972. *J. Exp. Med.* **135**:1151.

Jacobson, E. B., Herzenberg, L. A., Riblet, R. J., and Herzenberg, L. A., 1972. *J. Exp. Med.* **135**:1163.

Jacobson, E. B., L'age-Stehr, J., and Herzenberg, L. A., 1970. *J. Exp. Med.* **131**:1109.

Julius, M. H., Masuda, T., and Herzenberg, L. A., 1972. *Proc. Nat. Acad. Sci.* **69**:1934.
Kerbel, R. S., and Eidinger, D., 1972. *Eur. J. Immunol.* **2**:114.
Kim, B. S., and Dray, S., 1973. *Eur. J. Immunol.*
Lawton, A. R., Asofsky, R., Hylton, M. B., and Cooper, M. D., 1972. *J. Exp. Med.* **135**:277.
Lummus, Z., Cebra, J., and Mage, R. G., 1967. *J. Immunol.* **99**:737.
Mage, R. G., 1967. *Cold Spring Harbor Symp. Quant. Biol.* **32**:203.
Mage, R. G., and Dray, S., 1965. *J. Immunol.* **95**:525.
Mäkelä, O., Cross, A., and Kosunen, T. U., 1971. *Cell Interactions and Receptor Antibodies in Immune Responses.* Academic Press, London.
Manning, D. D., and Jutila, J. W., 1972. *J. Exp. Med.* **135**:1316.
Miller, J. F. A. P., and Mitchell, G. F., 1969. *Transpl. Rev.* **1**:3.
Mishell, R., and Dutton, R., 1967. *J. Exp. Med.* **126**:423.
Mitchell, G. F., Chan, E. L., Noble, M. S., Weissman, I. L., Mishell, R. I., and Herzenberg, L. A., 1972*a. J. Exp. Med.* **135**:165.
Mitchell, G. F., Grumet, F. C., and McDevitt, H. O., 1972*b. J. Exp. Med.* **135**:126.
Mitchell, G. F., Mishell, R. I., and Herzenberg, L. A., 1971. In B. Amos (ed.), *Progress in Immunology,* Vol. 1. Academic Press, New York, p. 323.
Mitchison, N. A., 1967. *Cold Spring Harbor Symp. Quant. Biol.* **32**:432.
Okamura, K., and Tada, T., 1971. *J. Immunol.* **107**:1682.
Old, L. J., and Carswell, E., personal communication.
Paul, W. E., Siskind, G. V., Benacerraf, B., and Ovary, Z., 1967. *J. Immunol.* **99**:760.
Pernis, B. G., Chiappino, A. S. K. and Gell, P. G. H., 1965. *J. Exp. Med.* **122**:853.
Pernis, B., Forni, L., and Amante, L., 1971. *Ann. N.Y. Acad. Sci.* **190**:420.
Pierce, C. W., Solliday, S. M., and Asofsky, R., 1972. *J. Exp. Med.* **135**:698.
Rabellino, E. Colon, S., Grey, H. M., and Unanue, E. R., 1971. *J. Exp. Med.* **133**:156.
Raff, M. C., 1971. *Transpl. Rev.* **6**:52.
Raff, M. C., 1970. *Nature* (London) **226**:1257.
Raff, M. C., Sternberg, M., and Taylor, R. B., 1970. *Nature* **225**:553.
Rajewsky, K., Chirrmacher, V., Nase, S., and Jerne, N. K., 1969. *J. Exp. Med.* **129**:1131.
Reif, A. E. and Allen, J. M., 1964. *J. Exp. Med.* **120**:413.
Staats, J., 1972. *Cancer Res.* **32**:1609.
Taylor, R. B., 1969. *Transpl. Rev.* **1**:114.
Tyan, M. L., and Herzenberg, L. A., 1968. *J. Immunol.* **101**:446.
Wanebo, H. J., Gallmeier, W. M., Boyse, E. A., and Old, L. J., 1966. *Science* **154**:901.
Wang, A. C., Wilson, S. K., Hopper, J. E., Fudenberg, H. H., and Nisonoff, A., 1970. *Proc. Nat. Acad. Sci.* **66**:337.
Warner, N. L., 1972. *Contemporary Topics in Immunology* Vol. 1, p. 87. Plenum Press, New York.
Warner, N. L., and Herzenberg, L. A., 1970. *J. Exp. Med.* **132**:440.
Warner, N. L., Szenberg, A., and Burnet, F. M., 1962. *Aust. J. Exp. Biol.* **40**:373.
Wigzell, H., Andersson, B., Mäkelä, O., and Walters, C. S., 1971. In O. Mäkelä, A. Cross, and T. V. Kosunen (eds.), *Cell Interactions and Receptor Antibodies in Immune Responses,* Academic Press, New York.
Wortis, H. H., 1971. *Clin. Exp. Immunol.* **6**:305.

Chapter 3

On the Relationship Between Cellular and Humoral Antibodies

Hans Wigzell

Department of Tumor Biology
Karolinska Institutet
Stockholm, Sweden

INTRODUCTION

Lymphocytes and their descendants constitute the pool of specific immuno-competent cells, carrying the information to react in a selective manner against foreign material, antigen. At least two major groups of lymphocytes can be recognized, namely, s.c. B and T lymphocytes (*Trans. Rev.*, 1969; Cooper *et al.*, 1966). B cells derive their name from their site of immunological maturation in birds, namely the bursa of Fabricius (Cooper *et al.*, 1966), but the corresponding site in mammals is still under dispute. B lymphocytes are known to provide the precursor cells for production of conventional humoral antibodies if properly stimulated, but other functions of these cells have recently been suggested as well (Harding *et al.*, 1971; Perlmann *et al.*, 1972). T cells, on the other hand, have never been found to release antibodies at a high rate, and some workers have failed to identify any immunoglobulin-like material on or in such cells (Raff *et al.*, 1970; Pernis *et al.*, 1970; Coombs *et al.*, 1971; Kincade *et al.*, 1971). They are called T cells as they would seem to be derived from and to mature immunologically within the thymus, (Blomgren and Andersson, 1971). Their major functional capacity is to be the initiator and mediator of cell-mediated immune reactions involving delayed hypersensitivity reactions and transplantation rejection systems, but they can also function as "helper" cells for B cells in the function of the latter cells as humoral antibody producers (*Trans. Rev.* 1969; Mitchison, 1971). In this chapter, most of the works reported will deal with cellular *vs.* humoral antibodies in B cell systems, although a minor part will also deal with T lymphocytes.

CELLULAR AND HUMORAL
ANTIBODIES PRODUCED BY B CELLS

Identification of the Antigen-Binding,
Cellular Receptor as an Immunoglobulin

In virtually all theories of immunological recognition of cells the antigen-binding receptor(s) is supposed to be on the outside of the cells, thus enabling swift access even to antigenic macromolecules or particles. That lymphocytes can bind antigen to their outer surface in a selective manner has been known for a long time (Mäkelä and Nossal, 1961), and using isotope labeled antigens it has been possible to study such binding in detail (Davie and Paul, 1971a,b; Roelants, 1972).

B cells can be distinguished from T cells both by morphological and functional criteria: One feature differentiating B from T lymphocytes would seem to be the higher surface concentration of immunoglobulin on the former cells (Raff et al., 1970; Pernis et al., 1970; Raff and Wortis, 1970; Rabellino and Grey, 1971; Unanue et al., 1971; Fröland et al., 1971; Wilson and Nossal, 1971; Cooper et al., 1971). In fact, although certain opposite findings have been reported (Hämmerling and Rajewsky, 1971; Marchalonis et al., 1972a), it is the view of this author that this is a highly useful marker to differentiate, in a simple way, on morphological grounds a B cell from a T cell. The distribution pattern of immunoglobulin in the cellular population of lymphocytes strongly suggests that the predominant immunoglobulin molecules present on a lymphocyte of B cell type are indeed products of the cell itself (Pernis et al., 1970; Coombs et al., 1971; Kincade et al., 1971; Davie et al., 1971; Fröland and Natvig, 1972b). Thus, in the normal case a single cell will only express one heavy and one light chain type on its surface immunoglobulin, and will also express only one out of two possible alleles (Davie et al., 1971; Fröland and Natvig, 1972b). If the antigen-binding structures on the lymphoid cells had antigenic similarities to humoral immunoglobulin molecules, one would anticipate that anti-immunoglobulin sera of suitable specificity should block the attachment of antigen. This has been shown to be true in several systems, suggesting a close relationship if not identity between the surface immunoglobulin and the antigen-binding structures on the cell (Davie and Paul, 1971a,b; Singhal and Wigzell, 1971; Walters and Wigzell, 1970). More direct identification of the antigen-binding receptor as an immunoglobulin comes from experiments where immune cells were preincubated with anti-immunoglobulin class specific sera before filtering such cells through antigen-coated columns (Walters and Wigzell, 1970). Such columns are known to normally retain B lymphocytes according to their potential immune capacity (Walters and Wigzell, 1970; Wigzell, 1970). Here it could be shown that incubation with an antigamma-1 specific serum would allow the potential gamma-1 antibody producing cells against the column antigen to go through the antigen-coated column, whereas in the same population potential gamma-2a antibody-producing cells were retained in the expected fashion. Exactly opposite results were obtained when using an antigamma-2a serum. Experiments were subsequently carried out using antilight chain and antipolyvalent immunoglobulin sera. The results were quite conclusive, demonstrating that at least in the immune cell population the antigen-binding receptor on the B memory cell had the same antigen-binding specificity and the same heavy and light chain in the immunoglobulin molecule as would be present in the potential product, the humoral antibody of that cell (Walters and Wigzell, 1970; Wigzell, 1970). It would thus seem clear that the antigen-binding receptor present on a B lymphocyte is an immunoglobulin-like molecule.

Orientation and Chemistry
of Membrane-Bound Immunoglobulin

Antibodies made specific for various parts of humoral immunoglobulin molecules are useful in the analysis of the orientation of membrane-bound immunoglobulin. Antibodies directed against the Fab or Fc regions of immunoglobulin have been shown capable of binding to the lymphocyte-bound immunoglobulin as indicated by induction of cellular division (Sell, 1970) or direct visualization (Pernis et al., 1970; Coombs et al., 1971; Kincade et al., 1971). Often such reactions were weaker or more difficult to obtain when using anti-Fc sera. It is now possible, however, to be more precise in such studies using antisera made specific for the various homology regions of the heavy chain of the immunoglobulin molecule. The heavy chain can be divided into three constant homology regions, CH1-3, where CH3 is the C-terminal piece of the Fc (Asofsky et al., 1969). Using antibodies against antigens on CH2 it was possible to obtain the same staining as with antibodies against intact Fc-pieces of that immunoglobulin class, reaching the same number of membrane-positive cells in fluorescent antibody tests (Fröland and Natvig, 1972a,b). However, when using antisera specific for antigens present on CH3 no cellular staining was observed (Fröland and Natvig, 1972a,b). It is known that in the creation of the CH3 specific antigens both the first 12 C-terminal amino acids and a region involving the amino acids in position 355-358 [Eu numbering (Edelmann et al., 1969)] do participate (Natvig and Turner, 1971). It would thus seem clear that the cell-bound immunoglobulins display a strictly ordered orientation with the Fab-part outward from the cell and with the Fc C-terminal end closest to the membrane, possibly with an unidentified part within or shielded by membrane components. This would be the expected way of displaying a receptor with antigen-binding capacity to obtain maximum binding efficiency. Antibodies as means for the analysis of other macromolecules are rather blunt tools suffering from problems of macromolecular steric hindrance and, although the above data are conclusive as to the orientation of the membrane-attached immunoglobulin molecules, they do not inform us as to the chemistry of the site of immuno-globulin attachment to the cell membrane. One approach to study this has been made using lactoperoxidase methods, whereby cell surface molecules can be radioactively labeled by iodine (Phillips and Mollisen, 1971; Marchalonis et al., 1971; Baur et al., 1972). Serum immunoglobulin molecules can be tagged with iodine and the relative amount of label attached to the subsequently isolated heavy vs. the light chain can be analyzed. In a similar way, membrane-bound immunoglobulin on lymphoma or B cells can be tagged in situ, whereafter the immunoglobulins are solubilized and split into free chains, and the ratio of the label attached to the two chains compared. Studying IgM in serum vs. membrane IgM [the major cell surface immunoglobulin on small B cells (Baur et al., 1971)] it was found that they displayed identical ratios of iodine on heavy vs. light chains (Vitetta et al., 1971; Marchalonis et al., 1972b). This was interpreted to mean that the cellular IgM was attached to the cell membrane by a very small piece, since otherwise the iodine labeling on the heavy chain of the cellular IgM should have been lower than that of humoral IgM. However, it is not clear how deep in the cell membrane activated iodine molecules might penetrate during the lactoperoxidase labeling and thereby label suitable residues on proteins.

The actual site through which immunoglobulin produced by a cell is kept to the outer surface of that cell is poorly defined. Several cell types have been shown capable of binding particularly 7S immunoglobulin from the surrounding fluid via a membrane-bound, Fc-binding receptor (Uhr and Phillips, 1966; LoBuglio et al., 1967; Huber and Fudenberg, 1968; Basten et al., 1972). However, most of the binding forces involved when binding free 7S IgG mole-cules to B lymphocytes would seem to be very low, and attached IgG molecules can seemingly be easily washed away (Basten et al., 1972). If multivalent aggregates are made between antibodies and antigen, the binding would seem to be significantly enhanced (Basten et al., 1972; Phillips-Quagliata et al., 1971). The binding sites on mast cells for IgE (Ishizaka and Ishizaka, 1968; Becker and Austen, 1966) might constitute another Fc-receptor, where the binding forces would be of a higher order of magnitude (Becker and Austen, 1966). Judging from enzymatic attempts to destroy such Fc-receptors on cell surfaces, they might very well be of a phospholipid nature (Howard and Benacerraf, 1966; Cline and Warner, 1971). The meagre data that exists on the surface binding of Ig-molecules on the actual cell of production would suggest that surface Ig-mole-cules are bound to lipids (Vitetta and Uhr, 1972a). Although isolation of specific, antigen-binding immunoglobulins from the membranes of immunocom-petent cells is still lacking, attempts to isolate surface immunoglobulin from either normal B lymphocytes or from B lymphomas have been quite successful (Baur et al., 1972; Baur et al., 1971; Vitetta et al., 1971; Marchalonis et al., 1972b; Vitetta and Uhr, 1972a; Klein et al., 1970; Klein and Eskeland, 1971).

Here, IgM has been found to be the dominating immunoglobulin class extractable from the membranes of normal B lymphocytes in the systems analyzed so far (Baur *et al.*, 1971; Vitetta *et al.*, 1971; Marchalonis *et al.*, 1972*b*; Vitetta and Uhr, 1972*a*). Also, IgM is the most frequent surface immunoglobulin class on the membrane of B cell lymphomas (Klein *et al.*, 1970; Klein and Eskeland, 1971). This IgM shows certain nonconventional features, especially with regard to molecular size. In no case so far has 19S IgM been isolated from the membranes of either B lymphocytes or from IgM-membrane positive lymphomas, but the molecular size has always been of a 7-8S IgM (Vitetta *et al.*, 1971; Marchalonis *et al.*, 1972*b*; Klein and Eskeland, 1971). It has previously been shown that myelomas producing 19S IgM do not assemble 7S IgM to 19S IgM until the very last stage of secretion, that is at the level of the outer cell surface (Askonas and Parkhouse, 1969; Parkhouse, 1971; Andersson and Melchers, 1973), and such assembling steps would seemingly be lacking on B lymphocytes. That isolated IgM from normal B cells or lymphomas are actually being produced by the cells themselves has been shown or indicated by several experiments. Although the IgM would seem to be the dominating membrane immunoglobulin class on B lymphocytes, and thus also should be the dominating antigen-binding receptor class on normal B lymphocytes, there is no doubt that e.g. IgG can also function as an antigen-binding receptor on the outer membrane (Davie and Paul, 1971*a,b*; Walters and Wigzell, 1970). It would seem that "virgin" B lymphocytes not yet stimulated by antigen would preferentially use IgM as receptor molecules, whereas immune cells might preferentially use other immunoglobulin classes.

Studies on immunoglobulin molecules on B lymphocytes indicate a rapid turnover of membrane material at $37°C$, with a half-life of maybe only a few hours (Vitetta and Uhr, 1972*a*; Lerner *et al.*, 1972). If experiments are carried out using radioactive amino acids for internal labeling coupled with lactoperoxidase mediated iodination of the outer surface proteins, studies can be made on the distribution forms of immunoglobulin secreted according to classical ways, like conventional humoral antibodies in comparison to the behavior of the membrane attached immunoglobulins (Andersson and Melchers, 1973). Here it can be shown that although the membrane immunoglobulins display a rapid turnover, they are substantially more "long lived" on the cell of production than are immunoglobulins destined for secretion and produced by the same cells (Andersson and Melchers, 1973). Several examples are known where cells can display membrane-bound immunoglobulins and at the same time secrete molecules of the same immunoglobulin class at high rate (Singhal and Wigzell, 1971; Baur *et al.*, 1972; Lerner *et al.*, 1972; Reif, 1970). This would exclude simple theories trying to distinguish between antigen-binding cells and antibody-releasing cells as being due to a difference in production rate of antibody coupled with an absence of immunoglobulin-binding structures on the outer membranes of the latter cell type.

Chemical analysis of membrane-attached immunoglobulins from B lymphocytes or lymphomas have failed to disclose any difference in the composition of the isolated heavy and light chains of membrane IgM in comparison to serum IgM from the same species (Baur *et al.*, 1972; Klein and Eskeland, 1971). Release of membrane IgM can be accomplished by a variety of methods, such as freezing and thawing without allowing the temperature to rise above 4°C (Klein and Eskeland, 1971), suggesting that integrity of the membrane is essential for the maintenance of the cell-bound characteristic of this Ig molecule. If cells are incubated at 37°C, it can be shown that B lymphocytes do shed some of their membrane IgM in the form of a complex with lipids, thus making it a large "molecule," now with a density of a lipoprotein (Vitetta and Uhr, 1972*a*,*b*). Treatment with detergent reduces the size to a 7-8S IgM with the expected density of such a molecule (Vitetta and Uhr, 1972*a*,*b*). In summary, then, the surface immunoglobulin on B lymphocytes is attached via its Fc C terminal end, and with its Fab-ends outward. A minor piece of the Fc might be shielded in the membrane, possibly via the attachment to lipid groups. Shedding of surface IgM can be shown to take place in the form of a complex with lipids. It has been suggested (Vitetta and Uhr, 1972*a*) that such molecules might function as the natural antibodies postulated in certain immunological theories (Jerne, 1955). No evidence exists for or against this hypothesis.

Distribution and Density of
Membrane-Bound Ig or Antigen-Binding Receptors

The appearance of immunoglobulin positive cells during ontogeny would seem to parallel the development of capacity to produce humoral antibodies, although direct proof for this is difficult to obtain (Thorbecke *et al.*, 1968; Kincade and Cooper, 1971; Toivanen *et al.*, 1973). In the mouse it is relatively easy to study the appearance of humoral antibody forming capacity against thymus independent antigens of various cell populations by the use of *in vivo* transfer systems into lethally X-irradiated recipients. Here it can be shown that there exist in the bone marrow few mature, immunocompetent B cells, but a relatively high proportion of cells ready to differentiate into such cells (*Trans. Rev.*, 1969). In the spleen, on the other hand, there seem to be relatively the opposite ratios. If a comparison is made between the capacity to produce humoral antibodies of normal bone marrow and spleen cells with time after administration to irradiated recipients, it can be seen that the antibody response against the thymus independent antigens is coming up faster and reaches a higher plateau level when using spleen cells (Andersson, in prep.). This merely supports the previous notion that spleen cells in comparison to bone marrow cells are richer in the percentage of mature B cells. If, however, before transfer the cells are passed through an anti-immunoglobulin coated column known to remove mature B cells (Wigzell, 1970), the antibody response will come later, but there would now seem to be a somewhat better antibody response provided for by the bone marrow cells in comparison to the spleen cells (Wigzell, in prep.). This would suggest that immature B cells do not have enough immunoglobulin on their surface to become retained by the columns; in fact it is dubious if they have any immunoglobulin on their surfaces at all (Ada, 1970). If we accept that immunocompetence of B cells goes hand in hand with appearance of surface immunoglobulins functioning as antigen-binding receptors, it is important to know the distribution pattern with regard to surface immunoglobulin among B lymphocytes at different stages of differentiation after contact with antigen. By following the capacity to bind antigen to cells *vs.* the capacity of the same cells to produce humoral antibodies as measured by hemolytic plaque formation, it becomes apparent that with time after induction of the immune process it becomes more difficult to demonstrate antigen-binding capacity on antibody-releasing cells (McConnell, 1971). Also, in certain systems, where specific retention of antigen-binding cells was estimated using antigen-coated fibers, no specific retention at all was recorded for high rate antibody-producing cells (Edelmann *et al.*, 1971). Furthermore, it has been reported that plasma cells have no surface immunoglobulins as detected by immunofluorescent antibody tests (Pernis *et al.*, 1970; Pernis *et al.*, 1971). However, the above results can all be explained on the basis of sensitivity of the various tests employed. If secretion of antibody from the cell is not stopped during the measurements, it is quite possible that secreted Ig will bind the specific ligand for the membrane-attached Ig, thus producing a false negative cell. Antigen-coated bead columns can be shown quite capable of specifically retaining antibody-producing cells even quite late after immunization, especially if separation is carried out at 4°C (Wigzell, 1970; Wigzell and Andersson, 1969; Truffa-Bachi and Wofsy, 1970). Furthermore, it is possible to selectively suppress the growth of mouse myeloma cells by immunization with the respective myeloma protein, thus evoking anti-idiotype specific antisera against such proteins (Lynch *et al.*, 1972). Also, anti-immunoglobulin antibodies have been shown capable of lysing, together with complement, certain plasma cell tumors in the mouse (Rabellino *et al.*, 1971). By the use of the lactoperoxidase method, direct labeling and isolation of surface immunoglobulin from myeloma cells has been reported (Baur *et al.*, 1972). Thus, even plasma cells can express surface immunoglobulin like the small B lymphocytes. It would thus seem likely that most if not all of the cells belonging to the B cell series maintain the capacity to display surface-bound immunoglobulin after reaching immunological maturation and even when differentiating further. This would mean that the B cell series, even at a high rate of antibody production at the single cell level, mostly keep the membrane-bound, antigen-binding receptors through which further regulation by antigen of cell function might proceed.

Estimates of the number of Ig molecules or antigen-binding receptors on single cells seem to match quite well (Klein *et al.*, 1970; Lerner *et al.*, 1972; Rabellino *et al.*, 1971; Davie and Paul, 1972*a*). Attempts to measure the actual number of surface immunoglobulin molecules on a small B lymphocyte have yielded figures ranging from 5×10^4 to 2×10^5 molecules (Klein *et al.*, 1970; Lerner *et al.*, 1972; Rabellino *et al.*, 1971). Using radioactively labeled antigen at saturating concentrations for high avidity cells, a similar number of antigen-binding receptors could be demonstrated on small lymphocytes (Ada, 1970; Davie and Paul, 1972*a*). In this last system only cells with high surface immunoglobulin concentration could be shown to demonstrate detectable antigen binding, thus demonstrating the B cell specificity of the reaction measured (Davie and Paul, 1971*a,b*). It would thus seem that the majority, if not all, of the surface immunoglobulin molecules on the outer membrane of a B lymphocyte are of one immunoglobulin class and with the same antigen-binding specificity.

Is there any increase in the density or number of antigen-binding sites per cell after immunization? Approaching this question using radioactively labeled antigen or anti-immunoglobulin antibodies, there does not seem to be any detectable increase in the number or density of antigen-binding receptors on B lymphocytes after immunization (Ada, 1970; Davie and Paul, 1972*a*). In fact, slightly decreased figures as far as density goes have been reported for the large B lymphoblasts appearing shortly after administration of antigen (Ada, 1970). No support exists for the view that a "virgin" small B lymphocyte would have a different concentration of surface immunoglobulin in comparison to a "memory" B cell.

There are limitations to experiments trying to define the number of immunoglobulin molecules on a single cell. Primarily they reside in the problem of redistribution and possible loss of surface immunoglobulin (Taylor *et al.*, 1971; Unanue *et al.*, 1972). Lymphocytes studied at $37°C$ using antigen or anti-immunoglobulin antibodies in the medium can be shown to display a change in the distribution pattern of surface molecules reactive with antigen or anti-Ig sera, going from a diffuse membrane distribution to a patchy distribution, to be followed by the accumulation of the relevant surface molecules at one pole of the cell (Taylor *et al.*, 1971). Subsequent to this, the immunoglobulins are lost from the surface of the cell, removed by endocytosis or shedding (Taylor *et al.*, 1971; Unanue *et al.*, 1972). This would yield a cell temporarily stripped from that particular surface component but leaving other structures intact on the surface (Taylor *et al.*, 1971; Preudhomme *et al.*, 1972). The functional importance of this capping phenomenon is unknown. Thus, absolute numbers of surface molecules on a cell should be regarded with caution in view of the above described phenomenon.

The Relationship Between Immunoglobulin Heavy Chain
Class in Receptor and Humoral Antibody Produced by the Same Cell

During ontogeny there is first an appearance of IgM containing cells to be followed by the appearance of IgG cells (Kincade and Cooper, 1971). Administration of anti-IgM serum early during ontogeny administered at a time when only IgM cells have developed will reduce both IgM and IgG antibody production later in the life of that individual if, simultaneously, steps are taken to stop further production of new B cells from stem cells (Kincade et al., 1970). If on the other hand anti-IgM serum is given at a later stage, when IgG cells have appeared as well as IgM cells, there will only be a selective depression of IgM antibody forming capacity (Kincade et al., 1970). This would suggest that the IgG precursor antibody forming cells have to pass through a stage of expressing IgM on the surface before expressing IgG. Similarly, it is well known that during primary immunization IgM antibody formation precedes IgG formation, suggesting that IgM producing cells might switch into IgG synthesizing cells. Direct demonstration of such cells caught in the actual switching process have been claimed using either tests for specific antibody forming capacity (Nossal et al., 1971; Greaves, 1971) or indirect fluorescent antibody tests (Pernis et al., 1971). In the latter case studies were carried out on rabbit lymphoid cells, thus allowing the use of antiallotype sera specific for markers on either the constant or variable part of the heavy chain as well as on the constant part of the light chain (Kelus and Gell, 1967). Here it was found that after immunization during the period of switch from IgM to IgG antibody synthesis, single immunoglobulin-positive cells were found expressing IgM on the surface but with IgG inside in the cytoplasm (Pernis et al., 1971). Allotype studies suggested that the same light chains were present in both Ig classes in the same cell, and the same allotype marker for the variable part of the heavy chains was found indicating that in these cells IgM and IgG molecules were simultaneously produced with the same light and heavy peptide chains except for the constant regions of the respective heavy chains (Kelus and Gell, 1967). In the mouse, experiments have been done demonstrating that if anti-IgM antibodies or anti-IgG are administered during or before a primary immune response (Lawton et al., Manning and Jutila, 1972) anti-IgM antibodies will suppress both IgM and IgG production, whereas anti-IgG antibodies will only depress IgG antibody synthesis. However, if the same experiment is carried out in a secondary immune response system the emerging picture is different; here anti-IgM will only depress IgM formation and not IgG synthesis whereas, before, anti-IgG antiserum would only suppress IgG production (Pierce et al., 1972). This would suggest that the surface Ig classes differ when comparing normal and immune cells. Direct demonstration that the antigen-binding receptor in immune B cells has the very same heavy chain as will be present in the humoral antibody produced by the same cells was provided for by the previously reported work (Walters and Wigzell, 1970), using anti-class specific immunoglobulin sera to block the antigen-binding receptor of memory B cells. After incubation with anti-gamma-1 and -gamma-2a, respectively, specific sera immune cells were filtered through antigen-coated columns whereafter the potential gamma-1 and gamma-2a antibody forming capacity against the column antigen was tested using control or column-passed cells. Here, anti-gamma-1 incubation would selectively let through gamma-1 memory cells whereas gamma-2a memory cells for the column antigen were retained in the normal fashion. As exactly opposite results were obtained when using the anti-gamma-2a serum the conclusion must be that the same heavy chain is present in the membrane-bound, antigen-binding structures as in the humoral antibodies coming from the same B memory cell. The above data, in conjunction with the finding that in the average lymphoid cell population in the mouse IgM is the predominant immunoglobulin class directly demonstrable (Baukhurst and Warner, 1971) or extractable (Vitetta et al., 1971) from small lymphocytes, would suggest that IgM does also constitute the dominating receptor class present on most virgin B lymphocytes. After immunization, cells with other heavy chain receptors in their surface receptors will appear with corresponding changes being reflective in their potential humoral antibody-forming capacity. It should be realized, though, that in guinea pigs there is evidence that B lymphocytes from normal individuals and thus of presumed "virgin" type for certain antigen might use IgG as their dominant surface receptor for antigen (Davie and Paul, 1971a,b).

In summary, it would thus seem likely that a cell can shift from expressing IgM to IgG or other immunoglobulin classes as its membrane receptor for antigen. Such a shift can take place under the influence of a physiological mechanism, initiated or not (Kincade and Cooper, 1971) by specific antigen. Mostly, the antigen-binding receptor and the subsequently produced humoral antibody coming from the same cells will have the same chemistry with regard to heavy and light chain classes. However, at certain stages during an early, primary immune response this rule would not seem to hold since cells here can be found which have on their surface immunoglobulins of an "earlier" class, IgM, while in the cytoplasm IgG antibodies will be found, that is, antibodies of a "later" kind. Indirect evidence from myeloma studies (Penn et al., 1970) and studies on "switching" cells (Nossal et al., 1971; Greaves, 1971) would suggest that IgM and IgG molecules produced by the same cell have the same antigen-binding specificity.

The Antigen-Binding Specificity of Surface Antibodies in Comparison to Humoral Antibodies Produced by the Same Cell

One characteristic which lends itself well to study with regard to antigen-binding characteristics of cell-bound vs. humoral antibodies is the binding efficiency or avidity. It is well known that the humoral antibody response against most immunogens is highly heterogenous with antibodies of widely different binding efficiency (Eisen and Siskind, 1964). Normally there is production early in the immune response of antibodies with a low avidity to be followed later in the immune response of antibodies with a higher average binding efficiency. It is possible to study the avidity of the cell-bound receptor for antigen by several approaches (Davie and Paul, 1971a; Wigzell, 1970; Davie and Paul, 1972a; Andersson, 1972b; Rutishauser et al., 1972). One approach is to use radioactively labeled antigen with increasing concentrations of the antigen when incubating with cells, followed by subsequent washing and test for uptake using autoradiography (Davie and Paul, 1971a; Ada, 1970; Davie and Paul, 1972a). This approach has clearly demonstrated that the term antigen-binding cell in numerical terms is meaningless if the actual concentration of antigen during the experiment is not reported. With increasing concentrations of antigen there is a corresponding increase in the number of cells being classified as positive with no saturation point being reached (Davie and Paul, 1971a; Ada, 1970; Davie and Paul, 1972a). This concentration dependency would seem to reflect the avidity of the antigen-binding receptors on these cells, and if immune cells are used they can be shown to contain an increased proportion (in comparison to normal cells) of cells being stained by antigen at low concentration (Davie and Paul, 1972a). The concentration of antigen in the in vitro uptake studies, above which no increase in the number of cells will take place during in vivo immunization, would seem to set the concentration limit above which antigen-binding cells, although taking up antigen in vitro to a detectable degree, had not been switched on in vivo by antigen into cellular proliferation (Davie and Paul, 1971a; Davie and Paul, 1972a). A direct comparison between the avidity of antigen-binding receptor on cells (using uptake of radioactive antigen coupled with attempts to block this uptake with free hapten) in an immune population has demonstrated that high avidity cells exist already in normal cell populations although at a very low frequency (Davie and Paul, 1971a; Davie and Paul, 1972a). Upon immunization both low and high avidity cells increase in numbers but gradually, as antigen concentration is decreasing, there would seem to be a preferential proliferation of the high avidity, antigen-binding cells (Davie and Paul, 1972a). A positive correlation exists between the increase in avidity of the average, antigen binding cell and the corresponding increase in binding efficiency of the humoral antibodies produced by single cells in the same individual (Davie and Paul, 1972a,b). A similar increase in the avidity of antigen-binding cells with time after immunization can be observed using antigen-coated beads (Wigzell, 1970; Andersson, 1972b) or fibers (Rutishauser et al., 1972). By the use of antigen-coated columns a selective depletion of memory B cells capable of producing high-avidity antibodies against the column antigen can be demonstrated, directly suggesting that the avidity of the antigen-binding surface receptor is similar, if not identical to that of the eventual product, the humoral antibody coming from the same cell (Andersson, 1972b). As has already been described, the observed increased binding efficiency of immune cells cannot be ascribed to an increase in the number of antigen-binding receptors with immunization (Ada, 1970; Davie and Paul, 1972*b*), but is most easily explainable on the basis of selection of cells with high avidity receptors.

Another comparison between cellular *vs.* humoral antibodies can be made, namely as to their capacity to react with small chemical groups present on a large molecule. If an individual is immunized with a hapten-protein conjugate the antibody response against such an immunogen will be complex consisting of three major groups of antibodies, specific for the hapten, for the protein, and for the actual hapten-protein conjugate (Paul *et al.,* 1966). If cells immune against a hapten-protein conjugate are filtered through a column coated with that hapten alone or hapten coupled to another molecule (Wigzell, 1970; Wigzell and Mäkelä, 1970; Davie and Paul, 1970), specific retention of antihapten memory B cells will take place. Fractionation through a column coated with the protein only will only retain antiprotein B cells. If the cells are filtered through a column coated with the actual hapten-protein conjugate that was used for immunogen, all antibody forming capacity against that conjugate is removed from the passing cells (Wigzell and Mäkelä, 1970; Davie and Paul, 1970). However, if such a filtration is done in the presence of free hapten, potential antihapten antibody producing cells will go through, whereas cells potentially able of producing antibodies against the protein (Wigzell and Mäkelä, 1970; Rubin and Wigzell, 1973) or against the new determinants arising as a consequence of the hapten-protein coupling reaction (Rubin and Wigzell, 1973) are retained in the normal fashion. Thus, the antigen-binding receptor on a B lymphocyte does have an antigen-binding site of a similar size or specificity as has the humoral antibody coming from the same cell.

A Speculative Comparison of the Competitive
Capacity for Antigen of Cellbound *vs.* Humoral Antibodies

Administration of a small amount of antigen to an already immunized individual will normally result in a secondary humoral antibody response signifying that the cellular immune system is successfully competing with the circulating antibodies for the administered immunogen. This competition for antigen is a most complex process where cells of different types like macrophages, T, and B lymphocytes are involved and where humoral factors such as antibodies and complement very likely play important roles. I will here only try to speculate on, in an artificially isolated manner, the competitive capacities for antigen of humoral *vs.* cellular antibodies. First, let us consider the matter of local concentration of antigen-binding molecules, which would allow the creation of several bonds between a multivalent antigen and antibodies. Such a creation of several binding sites between two molecules can be shown to increase the binding forces in an exponential way (Hornick and Karush, 1969), making multivalence a most powerful tool in the creation of strong bonds between macromolecules. Humoral antibodies are randomly oriented in space in contrast to the cellular antibodies which are regularly arranged with their Fab-end outward. Assuming a number of 10^5 antibody molecules per small lymphocyte (Rabellino *et al.*, 1971) and an even distribution pattern of such molecules on the cell surface, this would correspond to a molecular number of around 1-4 × 10^4 molecules per cu. micron. Now it is known that the cell-bound antibodies are mobile while still remaining bound to the membrane (Taylor *et al.*, 1971; Unanue *et al.*, 1972) and multivalent antigens can be shown to cause local spots of highly aggregated surface antibodies probably increasing the above concentration figure to maybe 5–10 times that number. This very local high concentration of regularly arranged antibodies on the cell surface will constitute a formidable spot of antigen-binding molecules competing favorably with the circulating antibodies, especially if confronted with multivalent antigens (Davie and Paul, 1972*b*). The average antigen-binding efficiency of the isolated cellular antibody molecule in comparison to the humoral might also be considered to be at least equal, as proliferation of cells going to produce antibodies of higher and higher avidity will occur before the production of such humoral antibodies. Cells of B memory type can be shown to recirculate in the blood, thus making the time factor to reach contact between antigen and antibody not too unfavorable for the cellular *vs.* the humoral antibody.

In summary, although it is realized that induction of antibody formation is a complicated process, a speculative comparison between humoral and cellular antibodies in their competitive capacity for antigen has been made. The concentration, arrangement, and membrane mobility of cellular antibodies will make them superior to humoral antibodies when competing for antigen.

The Role of Cellular Antibodies in the Induction of Humoral Antibody Formation

As the immunocompetent B cells always seem to have antigen-binding receptors expressing the potential immune reactivity of the cell, it would seem logical that they play a mandatory role in the induction of the immune response. They are present on the outer surface of cells, making them able to combine quickly, even with particulate antigen. The actual role of the cellular antibody during a switch onto humoral antibody formation, however, is unknown. The fact that they are primarily located on the outer cell membrane is not informative as to whether the actual triggering is initiated at this location. Antigen–antibody complexes can be shown to be created on the surface of the cells to later become ingested by endocytosis into the interior of the cell (Unanue *et al.*, 1972). It is possible that the actual induction takes place in the cytoplasm, and a special subfraction of cellular antibodies has been described and assumed to have some role in this inductive process (Merler and Silberschmidt, 1972). As studies with humoral antibodies have failed to indicate any transmittance of allosteric changes from the Fab-region down into the Fc-region as a consequence of antigen-binding, theories on allosteric transformation as an inducer to high rate antibody formations have failed to receive experimental support (Ashman *et al.*, 1971; Ashman and Metzger, 1971). Rather, aggregation and cross-linkage of surface Ig have been implied as activating or inactivating immunocompetent B cells (Fanger *et al.*, 1970). Aggregated humoral immunoglobulin will activate the complement system (Ishizaka *et al.*, 1961; Sandberg *et al.*, 1971). In view of the fact that the humoral and the cellular antibodies have the same heavy and light chains it is reasonable to assume that activation of complement factors can take place when antigen aggregates surface immunoglobulin via cross-linking. It has indeed been suggested that antigens not requiring the thymus cells as helper cells during humoral antibody formation can activate the B cells directly using complement activating processes (Dukor, in prep.).

Certain mitogens can be shown to activate B lymphocytes into high rate IgM synthesis (Andersson, 1972a; Andersson *et al.*, 1973). Although the induction processes here are equally unknown, as is the antigen-induced antibody formation, it would seem quite possible that there exist several ways of switching on a B lymphocyte into high rate antibody formation. In the case of antigen the switching will be selective, involving only B cells with appropriate antigen-binding surface receptors. In the case of B cell mitogens a large proportion of cells will be switched on, with each cell producing the immunoglobulin it has the "genetic" potential to produce (Andersson, 1972a; Andersson *et al.*, 1973). Several alternative ways exist to try to relate antigen-binding receptors with induction of high rate antibody synthesis. One approach is to continue the work on isolated membrane immunoglobulins, looking either for subclasses of immunoglobulin with special intracellular distribution patterns (Merler and Silberschmidt, 1972), or, alternatively, trying to further characterize the site of membrane attachment of cellular immunoglobulin (Cline and Warner, 1971; Klein *et al.*, 1970; Takahashi *et al.*, 1971), searching for possible physical linkage to enzymatic systems known to be involved in the induction of DNA, RNA, and protein synthesis.

Aggregation of immunoglobulin can be shown to lead to activation of complement either via the conventional pathways starting with C1 factor using sites at homology region CH2 (Kehoe and Fougereau, 1969) or activating via the alternative complement pathway using C3 (Götze and Müller-Eberhard, 1970) via aggregation at the Fab_2 region, presumably involving homology region CH1 (Sandberg *et al.*, 1971). The cellular antibodies would seem to freely express these homology regions. Demonstration of complement activation at the cell surface when antigen is binding to immunocompetent cells has already been claimed (Nishioka *et al.*, 1967), but further work is necessary (a) to confirm this finding, and then (b) to try to prove if complement activation on a cell surface will lead to induction of cellular processes in immunocompetent cells.

CELLULAR AND HUMORAL
ANTIBODIES PRODUCED BY T CELLS

There exists convincing evidence that thymus-derived lymphocytes are specific immunocompetent cells with the capacity to become immune activated and rendered specifically tolerant. They can be shown to display immunological memory (*Trans. Rev.*, 1969). It would thus seem safe to conclude that T cells should, like B cells, be endowed with specific antigen-binding receptors expressing their immune potential. Indeed, it has been possible to link the existence of such specific T cell receptors with function, either by selectively inactivating immune T cells using highly radioactive antigens (Basten *et al.*, 1971), or, with still more direct proof, by the demonstration of specific adsorption *and* elution of immune (Golstein *et al.*, 1971; Wekerle *et al.*, 1972) or normal (Wekerle *et al.*, 1972) T cells from histoincompatible cellular monolayers *in vitro*. However, other experimental systems known to be capable of physically fractionating B cells according to their specific immune capacity have failed to demonstrate any similar fractionation of functional T cells (Wigzell, 1970; Rubin and Wigzell, 1973). Several experimental systems have been presented where specific binding of antigen to T cells has been reported (Basten *et al.*, 1971; Hogg and Greaves, 1972*a,b*), but frequent claims have been made that such binding has not been to "true" T cells (Takahashi *et al.*, 1971; Hunter *et al.*, 1972; Russell *et al.*, 1972). Experiments studying purified T cells in the absence of B cells have frequently failed to demonstrate any specific, antigen-binding T lymphocytes (Rubin and Wigzell, 1973; Good, 1970). It would thus seem safe to conclude that T lymphocytes have specific receptors for antigen on their outer cell surface, but such receptors are distinctly more difficult to demonstrate than are receptors on B cells.

Equally conflicting views exist on the chemical nature of such T lymphocyte receptors for antigen. According to some workers the T cell receptor is an immunoglobulin of IgM and kappa light chain type (Mason and Warner, 1970; Hogg and Greaves, 1972*b*) as studied by the use of anti-immunoglobulin class specific sera as interfering agents for T cell function. However, there does not seem to exist any clear-cut correlation between the actual specific anti-IgM or antikappa activity of a given antiserum and its interfering capacity with T cell function (Rouse and Warner, 1972). Recently, articles have been published where the direct demonstration of immunoglobulin on the surface of T cells (Hämmerling and Rajewsky, 1971; Bankhurst *et al.*, 1971) and actual chemical isolation of 7-8S IgM-like molecules from such cells have been claimed (Marchalonis *et al.*, 1972*a,b*). Furthermore, in functional *in vitro* tests where T cells have been separated from B cells and macrophages by cell impermeable membranes, transfer through the membrane of an antikappa-reactive helper antibody from the T cells to the macrophages has been reported (Feldmann, 1972).

On the other extreme, there are several reports claiming the complete absence of any interference by anti-immunoglobulin antibodies on T cell function (see Crone *et al.*, 1972). No immunoglobulin could be demonstrated on the surface of thymus-derived lymphocytes by fractionation procedures on anti-immunoglobulin coated columns (Rubin and Wigzell, 1973; Crone *et al.*, 1972) or any direct staining tests (Lamelin *et al.*, 1972; Raff *et al.*, 1970; Kincade *et al.*, 1971). Furthermore, using similar approaches to isolate surface immunoglobulin from T as compared to B lymphocytes, no evidence was found of any immunoglobulin on T cells (Vitetta and Uhr, 1972*b*). Using a similar approach as was used when claiming that T and B cells had the same amount of surface immunoglobulin (Marchalonis *et al.*, 1972*a,b*) other workers were completely unable to confirm the existence on T cells of any more immunoglobulin than would be accounted for by uptake from the surrounding medium (Vitetta and Uhr, 1972*b;* Grey *et al.*, 1972).

Further experiments are thus needed to decide as to the chemical nature of the antigen-binding T cell receptor. Two candidates for such receptors would seem possible. The first and more trivial candidate would be an immunoglobulin, not necessarily identical to the "classical" B cell immunoglobulins but with certain antigenic similarities explaining the spurious effects of anti-immunoglobulin sera on T cell function (see Crone *et al.*, 1972). Experimental support for such a hypothesis comes from studies on human peripheral lymphocytes activated with PHA, where an increase in the percentage of cells being stained with certain antikappa sera will take place *in vitro* (Hellström *et al.*, 1971). Depletion of B cells from such populations by the use of anti-immunoglobulin coated columns will not reduce the number of cells being stained with these antisera (Hellström *et al.*, unpublished experiments). Analysis on the specificity of these antisera would suggest that the reactive molecule on the T cells does not carry the complete antigenic specificities of kappa light chains but might rather be a cross-reactive molecule (Perlmann, personal communication).

An alternative candidate is put forward by workers on the genetics of immune responsiveness against certain antigens where this can be shown to be intimately linked to genes determining the major histocompatibility antigens of the species (McDevitt and Benacerraf, 1969). Such immune response genes (IR-genes) can be demonstrated to be present between the two subloci determining the serological specificities linked to the histocompatibility loci (McDevitt and Chinitz, 1969; Lieberman *et al.*, 1972). The IR-locus can be shown to be polymorphic and crossover findings within the IR-locus suggest the existence of many IR-genes within such a locus (Lieberman *et al.*, 1972). Antibodies directed against the histocompatibility-linked serological specificities of the major transplantation antigens determined by one chromosome can be shown to selectively block the T cell reactivity against antigens determined by IR-genes on that particular chromosome (Shevach *et al.*, 1972). This would indicate a steric hindrance of IR-gene products on the surface of T cells by antihistocompatibility antibodies. One explanation would be that in fact such IR-gene surface products are indeed the antigen-binding receptors for T cells. Direct isolation of the receptor from specific, immune T cells would be required to solve the dilemma of the T cell receptor for antigen.

ACKNOWLEDGMENTS

This work was supported by the Swedish Cancer Society, the Karolinska Institutet, and Anders Otto Swärds Stiftelse.

REFERENCES

Ada, G. L., 1970. *Transpl. Rev.* **5**:105.
Andersson, B., in preparation.
Andersson, J., 1972*a*. Thesis, Karolinska Institutet.
Andersson, B., 1972*b*. *J. Exp. Med.* **135**:312.
Andersson, J., and Melchers, F., 1973. *Proc. Nat. Acad. Sci.*
Andersson, J., Sjöberg, O., and Möller, G., 1973. *Transpl. Rev.*
Ashman, R. F., and Metzger, H., 1971. *Immunochem.* **8**:643.
Ashman, R. F., Kaplan, A. P., and Metzger, H., 1971. *Immunochem.* **8**:627.
Askonas, B. A., and Parkhouse, R. M. E., 1969. *Biochem. J.* **1**:115.
Asofsky, R., Binaghi, R. A., Edelmann, G., Goodman, H. C., Heremans, J. F., Hood, L., Kabat, E. A., Rejnek, J., Rowe, D. S., Small, P. A., and Trnka, Z., 1969. *Bull. World Health Organ.* **41**:975.
Bankhurst, A. D., and Warner, N. L., 1971. *J. Immunol.* **107**:368.
Bankhurst, A. D., Warner, N. L., and Sprent, J., 1971. *J. Exp. Med.* **134**:1005.
Basten, A., Miller, J. F. A. P., Sprent, J., and Pye, J., 1972. *J. Exp. Med.* **135**:610.
Basten, A., Miller, J. F. A. P., Warner, N. L., and Pye, J., 1971. *Nature New Biol.* **231**:104.
Baur, S., Schenkein, I., and Uhr, J. W., 1972. *J. Immunol.* **108**:748.
Baur, S., Vitetta, E. S., Sherr, C. J., Schenkein, I., and Uhr, J. W., 1971. *J. Immunol.* **106**:1133.
Becker, E. L., and Austen, K. F., 1966. *J. Exp. Med.* **124**:379.
Blomgren, H., and Andersson, B., 1971. *J. Immunol.* **106**:831.
Cline, M. J., and Warner, N. L., 1971. *J. Immunol.* **108**:339.
Coombs, R., Gurner, B., McConnell, I., and Munro, A., 1971. *Intern. Arch. Allergy* **39**:280.
Cooper, M. D., Lawton, A. R., and Bockman, D. E., 1971. *Lancet* **2**:791.
Cooper, M. D., Peterson, R. D. A., South, M. A., and Good, R. A., 1966. *J. Exp. Med.* **123**:75.
Crone, M., Koch, K., and Simonsen, M., 1972. *Transpl. Rev.* **10**:36.
Davie, J. M., and Paul, W. E., 1972*a*. *J. Exp. Med.* **135**:660.
Davie, J. M., and Paul, W. E., 1972*b*. *J. Exp. Med.* **135**:643.
Davie, J., and Paul, W. E., 1971*a*. *J. Exp. Med.* **134**:495.
Davie, J., and Paul, W. E., 1971*b*. *J. Exp. Med.* **134**:517.
Davie, J. M., and Paul, W. E., 1970. *Cell. Immunol.* **1**:404.
Davie, J. M., Paul, W. E., Mage, R. G., and Goldman, M. B., 1971. *Proc. Nat. Acad. Sci.* **68**:430.

Dukor, P., and Hartmann, K. U., in preparation.
Edelmann, G. M., Rutishauser, U., and Millette, C. F., 1971. *Proc. Nat. Acad. Sci.* 68:2153.
Edelmann, G. M., Cunningham, B. A., Gall, P. D., Rutishauser, U., and Waxdal, M. J., 1969. *Proc. Nat. Acad. Sci.* 63:78.
Eisen, H. N., and Siskind, G. W., 1964. *Biochemistry* 3:996.
Fanger, M. W., Hart, D. A., Wells, J. V., and Nisonoff, A., 1970. *J. Immunol.* 105:1484.
Feldmann, M., 1972. *J. Exp. Med.* 136:737.
Fröland, S. S., and Natvig, J. B., 1972a. *Scand. J. Immunol.* 1:1.
Fröland, S. S., and Natvig, J. B., 1972b. *J. Exp. Med.* 136:409.
Fröland, S. S., Natvig, J. B., and Berdal, P., 1971. *Nature* 234:251.
Golstein, P., Svedmyr, E., and Wigzell, H., 1971. *J. Exp. Med.* 134:1385.
Good, R. A., 1970. In R. T. Smith and M. Landy (eds.), *Immune Surveillance,* Academic Press, New York, p. 123.
Götze, O., and Müller-Eberhard, H. J., 1970. *J. Exp. Med.* 132:898.
Greaves, M. F., 1971. *Eur. J. Immunol.* 1:186.
Grey, H. M., Kubo, R. T., and Cerottini, J. C., 1972. *J. Exp. Med.* 136:1323.
Hämmerling, U., and Rajewsky, K., 1971. *Eur. J. Immunol.* 1:447.
Harding, B., Pudifin, D. J., Gotch, F., and MacLennan, I. C. M., 1971. *Nature* 232:80.
Hellström, U., Perlmann, P., and Wigzell, H., unpublished experiments.
Hellström, U., Zeromski, J., and Perlmann, P., 1971. *Immunology* 6:1099.
Hogg, N. M., and Greaves, M. F., 1972a. *Immunology* 22:959.
Hogg, N. M., and Greaves, M. F., 1972b. *Immunology* 22:967.
Hornick, C. L., and Karush, F., 1969. *Israel J. Med. Sci.* 5:1963.
Howard, J. G., and Benacerraf, B., 1966. *Brit. J. Exp. Pathol.* 47:193.
Huber, H., and Fudenberg, H., 1968. *Intern. Arch. Allergy* 34:18.
Hunter, P., Munro, A., and McConnell, I., 1972. *Nature New Biol.* 236:52.
Ishizaka, K., and Ishizaka, T., 1968. *J. Allergy* 42:330.
Ishizaka, T., Ishizaka, K., and Borsos, T., 1961. *J. Immunol.* 87:433.
Jerne, N. K., 1955. *Proc. Nat. Acad. Sci.* 41:849.
Kehoe, J. M., and Fougereau, M., 1969. *Nature* 224:1272.
Kelus, A. S., and Gell, P. G. H., 1967. *Progr. Allergy* 11:141.
Kincade, P. W., and Cooper, M. D., 1971. *J. Immunol.* 106:371.
Kincade, P. W., Lawton, A. R., and Cooper, M. D., 1971. *J. Immunol.* 106:1421.
Kincade, P. W., Lawton, A. R., Bockman, D. E., and Cooper, M. D., 1970. *Proc. Nat. Acad. Sci.* 67:1918.
Klein, E., and Eskeland, T., 1971. In O. Mäkelä, A. Cross, and V. Kosunen (eds.), *Cell Interactions and Receptor Antibodies in Immune Responses,* Academic Press, New York, p. 91.
Klein, E., Eskeland, T., Inoue, M., Strom, R., and Johansson, B., 1970. *Exp. Cell Res.* 62:133.
Lamelin, J. P., Lisowska-Berlin, B., Matter, A., Ryser, J. E., and Vassali, P., 1972. *J. Exp. Med.* 136:984.
Lawton, A. R., Asofsky, R., Hylton, M. B., and Cooper, M. D., 1972. *J. Exp. Med.* 135:277.
Lerner, R. A., McConahey, P., Jansen, I., and Dixon, F., 1972. *J. Exp. Med.* 135:136.
Lieberman, R., Paul, W. E., Humphrey, W., and Stimpfling, J. H., 1972. *J. Exp. Med.* 136:1231.
LoBuglio, A. F., Cohan, R. S., and Jandl, J. H., 1967. *Science* 158:1582.
Lynch, R. G., Graff, R. J., Sirisinha, S., Simms, E. J., and Eisen, H. N., 1972. *Proc. Nat. Acad. Sci.* 69:1540.
Mäkelä, O., and Nossal, G. J. V., 1961. *J. Immunol.* 87:447.
Manning, D. D., and Jutila, J. W., 1972. *J. Exp. Med.* 135:1316.
Marchalonis, J. J., Atwell, J. L., and Cone, R. E., 1972a. *Nature New Biol.* 235:240.
Marchalonis, J. J., Cone, R. E., and Atwell, J. L., 1972b. *J. Exp. Med.* 135:956.
Marchalonis, J. J., Cone, R. E., and Sauter, V., 1971. *Biochem. J.* 124:921.
Mason, S., and Warner, N. L., 1970. *J. Immunol.* 104:762.

McConnell, I., 1971. *Nature New Biol.* **233**:177.
McDevitt, H. O., and Benacerraf, B., 1969. *Adv. Immunol.* **11**:31.
McDevitt, H. O., and Chinitz, A., 1969. *Science* **163**:1207.
Merler, E., and Silberschmidt, M., 1972. *Immunology* **22**:813.
Mitchison, N. A., 1971. *Eur. J. Immunol.* **1**:10.
Natvig, J. C., and Turner, M. W., 1971. *Clin. Exp. Immunol.* **8**:685.
Nishioka, K., Tachibana, T., and Stock, C. C., 1967. In *Subviral Carcinogenesis, 1st International Symposium on Tumor Viruses*, p. 253.
Nossal, G. J. V., Warner, N. L., and Lewis, H., 1971. *Cell Immunol.* **2**:41.
Parkhouse, R. M. E., 1971. *Biochem. J.,* **123**:635.
Parkhouse, R. M. E., Janossy, G., and Greaves, M. F., 1972. *Nature New Biol.* **235**:21.
Paul, W. E., Siskind, G. W., and Benacerraf, B., 1966. *J. Exp. Med.* **123**:689.
Penn, G. M., Kunkel, H. G., and Grey, H. M., 1970. *Proc. Soc. Exp. Biol. Med.* **135**:660.
Perlmann, P., Perlmann, H., and Wigzell, H., 1973. *Transpl. Rev.*
Perlmann, P., personal communication.
Pernis, B., Forni, L., and Amante, L., 1971. *Ann. N.Y. Acad. Sci.* **190**:420.
Pernis, B., Forni, L., and Amante, L., 1970. *J. Exp. Med.* **132**:1001.
Pierce, C. W., Solliday, S. M., and Asofsky, R., 1972. *J. Exp. Med.* **135**:698.
Phillips, D. R., and Mollison, M., 1971. *Biochem. Biophys. Res. Commun.* **40**:284.
Phillips-Quagliata, J. M., Levine, B. B., Quagliata, F., and Uhr, J. W., 1971. *J. Exp. Med.* **133**:589.
Preudhomme, J. L., Neuport-Sautes, C., Piat, S., Silvestre, D., and Kourilsky, F. M., 1972. *Eur. J. Immunol.* **2**:297.
Rabellino, E., and Grey, H. M., 1971. *J. Immunol.* **106**:1418.
Rabellino, E., Colon, S., Grey, H. M., and Unanue, E. R., 1971. *J. Exp. Med.* **133**:156.
Raff, M. C., and Wortis, H., 1970. *Immunology* **18**:931.
Raff, M. C., Steinberg, M., and Taylor, R. B., 1970. *Nature* **225**:553.
Reif, A. E., 1970. *Proc. Soc. Exp. Biol. Med.* **133**:744.
Roelants, G. E., 1972. *Nature New Biol.* **236**:252.
Rouse, B. T., and Warner, N. L., 1972. *Cell. Immunol.* **3**:470.
Rubin, B., and Wigzell, H., 1973. *J. Exp. Med.*
Russell, S. M., Ferrarini, M., Munro, A., and Lachmann, P. J., 1972. *Eur. J. Immunol.* **2**:456.
Rutishauser, U., Millette, C. F., and Edelmann, G. M., 1972. *Proc. Nat. Acad. Sci.* **69**:1596.
Sandberg, A. L., Oliviera, B., and Osler, A. G., 1971. *J. Immunol.* **106**:282.
Sell, S., 1970. *Transpl. Rev.* **5**:19.
Shevach, E. M., Paul, W. E., and Green, I., 1972. *J. Exp. Med.* **136**:1207.
Singhal, S. K., and Wigzell, H., 1971. *Progr. Allergy* **15**:188. Contains information in a review form on earlier findings.
Takahashi, T., Old, L. J., McIntire, R., and Boyse, E. A., 1971. *J. Exp. Med.* **134**:815.
Taylor, R. B., Duffus, W. P., Raff, M. C., and DePetris, S., 1971. *Nature* **233**:225.
Thorbecke, G. J., Warner, N. L., Hochwald, G. M., and Ohanian, S. H., 1968. *Immunology* **15**:123.
Toivanen, P., Toivanen, A., and Good, R. A., 1973. *J. Immunol.*
Truffa-Bachi, P., and Wofsy, L., 1970. *Proc. Nat. Acad. Sci.* **66**:685.
Transplant Review **1**, 1969.
Uhr, J. W., and Phillips, J. M., 1966. *Ann. N.Y. Acad. Sci.* **129**:792.
Unanue, E. R., Perkins, W. D., and Karnovsky, M. J., 1972. *J. Immunol.* **108**:569.
Unanue, E. R., Grey, H. M., Rabellino, E., Campbell, P., and Schmidtke, J., 1971. *J. Exp. Med.* **133**:1188.
Vitetta, E. S., and Uhr, J. W., 1972a. *J. Immunol.* **108**:577.
Vitetta, E. S., and Uhr, J. W., 1972b. *J. Exp. Med.* **136**:676.
Vitetta, E. S., Bauer, S., and Uhr, J. W., 1971. *J. Exp. Med.* **134**:242.
Walters, C. S., and Wigzell, H., 1970. *J. Exp. Med.* **132**:1233.
Wekerle, H., Lonai, P., and Feldmann, M., 1972. *Proc. Nat. Acad. Sci.* **69**:1620.

Wigzell, H. In preparation.
Wigzell, H., 1970. *Transpl. Rev.* **5**:76.
Wigzell, H., and Andersson, B., 1969. *J. Exp. Med.* **129**:23.
Wigzell, H., and Mäkelä, O., 1970. *J. Exp. Med.* **132**:110.
Wilson, J. D., and Nossal, G. J. V., 1971. *Lancet* **2**:788.

Chapter 4

T Cell Modification of B Cell Responses to Antigen in Mice

Graham F. Mitchell

Basel Institute for Immunology
Grenzacherstrasse
Basel, Switzerland

INTRODUCTION

The antigen-reactive cells[1] required for expression of cell-mediated and humoral immunities have been designated T cells[2] and B cells, respectively (Roitt *et al.*, 1969). The circulating pool of lymphocytes (Gowans and Mc-Gregor, 1965) is a mixture of T and B cells in mice (Sprent and Miller, 1972) and rats (Howard *et al.*, 1972; Strober, 1972), and, as a consequence, all peripheral lymphoid organs (e.g., spleen and lymph nodes), lymphatic channels such as the thoracic duct, "unorganized" lymphoid aggregates, and the blood stream must contain both cell types. Antigens presumably make contact with reactive cells in many if not all of these lymphoid sites, and popular belief is that B cells have the option of differentiating to antibody-secreting cells, such as plasma cells, whereas T cells do not. The spectrum of T cell immunological activities has been extended to include a regulatory role in humoral antibody production. T cells and B cells, both with specificity for antigenic determinants, collaborate in numerous antibody responses *in vivo* and *in vitro*. The purpose of this paper is to examine existing data on the antibody-producing activity of B cells responding to antigens under conditions of T cell insufficiency in mice. There are numerous reviews on this topic in the literature, and the approach here, at least initially, will be somewhat negative. This hopefully does not reflect my attitude to the problem; an attempt is made to simply highlight difficulties

---

[1] Antigen-reactive cell—antigen-sensitive cell; immunologically competent cell.
[2] T cell—thymus-influenced cell; see list of abbreviations at end of chapter.

of interpretation of several experimental findings as well as stating the positive conclusions which have been drawn.

EXPERIMENTAL T CELL DEFICIENCIES

Nonspecific

Peripheral lymphoid organs, or cell suspensions prepared from them, have been depleted of T cells by various means—neonatal thymectomy, adult thymectomy plus irradiation, treatment with heterologous and isologous antisera against T cell antigens such as the theta (θ) antigen, and chronic thoracic duct drainage. The most heroic procedure used to date to reduce T cell numbers is that of Feldmann and Basten (1971)—48 hr thoracic duct drainage of "B mice" (see below) followed by anti-θ serum treatment of the spleen cells. Neonatal thymectomy, like chronic thoracic duct drainage, is usually a most unsatisfactory way of achieving a T cell deficit unless facilitated by some other manipulation, stress, or unknown environmental factors. The following are several considerations on the other methods. (1) "B mice" (thymectomized as adults, lethally irradiated, and transplanted with a source of hemopoietic stem cells) contain θ positive cells as do neonatally thymectomized mice (Raff and Wortis, 1970), and at least some of these cells behave as functional T cells, e.g., spleen cells from neonatally thymectomized mice respond poorly to sheep erythrocytes (SRBC) in Mishell and Dutton cultures and this response can be further reduced by anti-θ serum treatment (Mitchell et al., 1971). Bone marrow has been used to repopulate thymectomized, irradiated mice and resident or blood-borne T cells are certain to be transferred, and in large numbers, if the number of marrow cells injected is high or if strains such as C57BL are used (Cerottini et al., 1970). Early (14 day) fetal liver cells or anti-θ-treated marrow cells (Janossy and Greaves, 1971) must be better sources of stem cells when producing "B mice." Nevertheless, one is still left with the problem of residual host T cells not eliminated by the particular dose of irradiation used. (2) Some strains of mice (e.g., BALB/c) may have a high incidence of ectopic thymuses, and complete thymectomy in all mice is thus impossible (Law et al., 1964). (3) Sham thymectomized mice, irradiated and protected with stem cells *months* previously (i.e., controls for "B" mice) respond poorly compared with normal mice to antigens such as SIII (Howard et al., 1971; Mitchell and Humphrey, 1973), ϕX174 bacteriophage (Tao-Wiedmann, unpublished observations), and NIP-BSA (Aird, 1971; Mitchell and Kontiainen, unpublished observations). Confining the emphasis to only the T cell lesion in "B mice" *vs.* their irradiated controls is not justified unless the latter mice, and appropriately age-matched normal mice, have similar responses to the antigen under test. (4) Most anti-T sera must directly affect immunologically relevant lymphoid (and nonlymphoid) cells besides T cells. Anti-Ig (Baird *et al.*, 1971), and autoantibodies (Greaves and Raff, 1971; Schlesinger, 1972) have been demonstrated in anti-θ sera. Unidentified antibodies in anti-T sera (other than the readily detected cytotoxic antithymocytes antibodies) could conceivably alter the "homing" behavior of relevant cells in adoptive immune responses. These antibodies would therefore affect the activities of treated cells in *in vivo* cell transfers but not necessarily in *in vitro* systems. Obviously, the effects of treatment with anti-T sera must remain in doubt if reconstitution with a source of T cells has not been achieved. (5) Finally, one of the major unknowns associated with any *in vivo* manipulation which reduces T cell numbers is the capacity of other organs to take over thymic function(s) in the face of a T cell deficiency. Perhaps the anti T sera now available will permit a search for *de novo* T cell production in organs of T cell deficient mice.

All T cell-deprived mice will contain T cells reactive to some antigenic determinants but not others if several assumptions are granted—each T cell has restricted specificity for antigenic determinants, antigens expand T cell numbers in peripheral lymphoid organs (if tolerance induction is prevented), and T cells have a finite life span and must be constantly replaced. Any of a number of possibilities can then be invoked to explain the response, or lack of it, in a T cell-deprived animal. For example: (1) if thymectomized mice respond poorly to the first injection of antigen and better to subsequent injections (Svet-Moldavsky *et al.*, 1964; Sinclair, 1967a) then T cells have been expanded from a small starting population; (2) if thymectomized mice respond to a first but not subsequent challenge with antigen (see below) then the few T cells present have been recruited but then exhausted by contact with this particular antigen; and (3) if thymectomized mice respond poorly to low doses of antigen, then antigen has been excreted or catabolized before the few T cells could make contact. Increasing the antigen dose (Aird, 1971; Mitchell *et al.*, 1971; Torrigiani, 1972; Taylor and Wortis, 1968; cf. Dresser, 1972) will increase the probability of recruiting these T cells. If increasing the antigen dose reduces the response of thymectomized mice, then T cell tolerance has been induced because of an unfavorable ratio between antigen:antigen reactive T cells! It is not surprising, therefore, that highly variable results will be obtained in systems designed to examine the immunological effects of procedures which limit, but do not eliminate, T cells.

In any state of T cell deficiency in which no reduction of an antibody response is noted, the presence of even low numbers of residual T cells poses difficulties in interpretation simply because we know very little of peripheral T cell regulation. Defects in numbers of T cells with a particular specificity may be rapidly overcome following contact with antigen via antigen ± adjuvant-induced proliferation (Davies *et al.*, 1966; Krüger and Gershon, 1972; Nossal *et al.*, 1968). Thymectomy does not result in increased lymphopoiesis in peripheral lymphoid organs (Metcalf, 1966). However, the extent of antigen-mediated cell multiplication required to increase specifically-reactive T cells by orders of magnitude would go unnoticed in thymidine labeling or chromosome marker experiments, especially in actively hemopoietic organs such as the spleen. There is no doubt that conclusions drawn from earlier studies on thymectomized mice will be altered by similar studies in the future using inbred congenitally athymic nu/nu nude mice. Similarly, conclusions drawn from experiments using C3H or CBA anti-θ^{AKR} sera will be modified when high titer anti-T sera, raised in congenic pairs of mice, become available and when more is known about the expression of T cell antigens in different anatomical sites or different stages of the T cell cycle or lineage.

In concluding this section on nonspecific T cell deficiencies, mention should be made of manipulations which in the future may be used to achieve transient deficiencies of T cells in certain organs. Pertussis vaccine (Morse, 1966), hydrocortisone (Claman, 1972; Cohen, 1972), and glycosidases (Gesner and Ginsburg, 1964) are known to affect the mobility and distribution of lymphocytes. It is conceivable that drugs will be used in the future to sequester T cells into immunologically irrelevant sites or to remove T cells from mixed populations of cells *in vitro*.

Specific (Antigen-Induced)

A selective defect in T cell function (and presumably a "blocking," if not a reduction in numbers, of specifically reactive T cells) can be induced with antigen. Chiller *et al.* (1970) and Taylor (1969) have depleted thymuses of cells reactive to foreign serum proteins. In these systems—parenteral injection of antigen and test for the cooperative activity of thymocytes and B cells in adoptive transfers—T cells with specificity for antigen could have been recruited out of the organ or tolerized. However, as discussed by Weigle *et al.* (1972), immunogenic inocula do not recruit T cells from the thymus. Recruitment has been the favored interpretation of the findings of Sprent *et al.* (1971) and Rowley *et al.* (1972) who showed that the thoracic duct lymph in mice and rats could be depleted of reactive T cells. However, the possibility exists that cells are not removed but are modified (activated) by antigen such that they do not home to appropriate sites in recipients used to test the immunological performance of the cells. In any case, the apparent or actual loss of T cells is specific for the antigen injected.

The evidence for T cell ("carrier determinant"-reactive or "helper" cell) defects in both high and low zone tolerant mice is compelling (Mitchison, 1972; Rajewsky *et al.*, 1972), and T cells binding antigen are reported to be reduced in high zone tolerant mice (Möller and Sjöberg, 1972). Specifically-reactive thymocytes can be inactivated by heavily radiolabeled antigen (Basten *et al.*, 1971) as can carrier-reactive cells (Roelants and Askonas, 1971). Mice injected with large doses of SRBC and cyclophosphamide are specifically tolerant of SRBC (Aisenberg, 1967; Dietrich and Dukor, 1967). At least one of the deficiencies in such mice is at the T cell level (Many and Schwarz, 1970; Miller and Mitchell, 1971). Specific deletion of reactive T cells has been achieved with monolayers of H-2 bearing cells (Brondz, 1972; Goldstein *et al.*, 1972) but not as yet with antigen-coated columns (Wigzell, 1970; c f. Davie and Paul, 1970). Julius *et al.* (1972) used a fluorescence cell sorter to achieve depleted and enriched cell suspensions of antigen-binding cells. Thus far, T cells have not been removed by this technique. The bulk of the available evidence points to a low antigen-binding capacity of T cells *vs.* B cells (e.g., Warner, 1972), and techniques dependent on this property *alone* for depletion of T cells cannot be expected to be highly efficient.

The time course of recovery of T cell responsiveness following induction of an antigen specific deficiency has been examined by Chiller *et al.* (1971). In situations of T + B cell tolerance, recovery of full T cell responsiveness in adoptive transfer experiments lags well behind recovery of B cell responsiveness. Observations in irradiated mice repopulated with hemopoietic cells can be interpreted in a similar fashion. In "B mice" the B cell population is able to interact very well with thoracic duct cells (and presumably with the T cells of this cell population) 2 weeks after irradiation and bone marrow repopulation. However, full immunological responsiveness (to SRBC) in sham thymectomized, irradiated mice does not reappear until at least 6 weeks after irradiation and marrow transfer (Miller and Mitchell, 1969). The system has not been studied further in terms of recovery of T cell functions *vs.* B cell functions.

This brief list of specific and nonspecific T cell deficiencies in mice or lymphoid cell suspensions serves to illustrate the point that numerous methods are now available which achieve this end. The emphasis has been on T cell *deficiency* rather than on T cell *absence*. Attaining the latter condition is obligatory before it is possible to remove the quotes from "T cell independent" responses discussed below.

"T CELL INDEPENDENT" RESPONSES OF B CELLS

Antibody production to a large number of antigens is increased by the presence of reactive T cells. Nevertheless, several antigens elicit "T cell independent" responses, and it follows that a proportion of B cells must be capable of responding to antigen by producing antibodies "independently" of any T cell influence. The intention in this section is to examine the class of antibody produced by B cells responding to antigen in the presence of low numbers, perhaps the absence, of T cells and the subsequent fate of these B cells—i.e., do they subsequently behave as a specifically primed, tolerized, or unchanged cell population? Furthermore, there are now some data on "T cell independent" responses to persisting antigens in mice, and this will also be examined.

Class of Antibody Produced

Several studies can be cited which show a marked effect of T cell depletion on secondary rather than on primary responses and on IgG rather than on IgM antibody production. (1) Athymic nu/nu mice injected with SRBC contain direct but very few, if any, indirect (developed with anti-IgG sera) PFC in their spleen and hemolysins but not hemagglutinins in their serum (Kindred, 1971; Pantalouris and Flisch, 1972; Wortis, 1971). (2) The anti-SRBC hemagglutinin, but not the hemolysin, response of germ-free neonatally thymectomized mice is markedly reduced when compared with responses in sham thymectomized controls (Miller *et al.*, 1967). (3) In aged neonatally thymectomized Swiss mice, 7S hemolysin titers to SRBC, but not 19S hemolysin titers, lag well behind these in controls (Sinclair, 1967*b*). (4) In "B mice" injected with large amounts of SRBC, γG_1 PFC are reduced rather than IgM (direct) PFC (Taylor and Wortis, 1968) and the γG_1 antibody response to KLH and BSA is reduced more than other (sub)classes in thymectomized mice (Torrigiani, 1972). (5) In the anti-BγG response of thymectomized rats, titers of mercaptoethanol (ME)-resistant antibodies are much lower than ME-sensitive antibody titers (Isaković *et al.*, 1965). (6) The secondary but not the primary anti-MS-2 coliphage antibody response is reduced in neonatally thymectomized mice (Basch, 1966). (7) In the tetanus toxoid system of Hess and Stoner (1966), 20% of neonatally-thymectomized pathogen-free mice show a decrease in secondary (and tertiary) but not primary antibody titers to fluid and alum precipitated tetanus toxoid, respectively. (8) "B mice" produce direct PFC to rabbit IgG fragments but not indirect PFC (Hunter and Munro, 1972). Finally, (9) the low primary IgM antibody titers to aqueous injections of the synthetic polypeptide (T,G)-A--L (Grumet, 1972; Warner, 1972) are not reduced in "B mice" (of high responder H-2 genotype) whereas IgG antibody production is abolished (Mitchell *et al.*, 1972*b*).

One study has not shown an impaired putative IgG antibody response in T cell-deprived mice. Andersson (1972) has detected indirect PFC in the spleens of "B mice" injected with PVP but the numbers are marginally above direct PFC numbers (3X above a direct PFC response of 100 per spleen). These indirect PFC, as in many other systems, have not yet been shown to be IgG secretors, and there is one instance where developing sera reveals the presence of more IgM-secreting PFC to antigen-coated SRBC (Baker and Stashak, 1969). Another study, that of Sinclair (1967*a*), is not in line with the general statement that primary responses are less T cell dependent than secondary responses. He observed a marked decrease in primary 19S and 7S hemolysin titers to SRBC, but no decrease in secondary titers, in young Swiss albino mice. However, thymectomized mice produced large amounts of 7S hemolysins (as determined by sucrose gradient analyses) late in the primary response. The data can be explained (and the notion of high T cell dependence of 7S antibody preserved) by postulating that reactive T cells are expanded by SRBC from a small pool left after thymectomy in this mouse strain (Miller and Osoba, 1967). Recently, Tao-Wiedmann (unpublished observations) has shown that nu/nu mice produce ME-resistant anti-ϕX174 bacteriophage antibodies which react with anti-γG_{2a} antisera. The early serum titer after a single injection of ϕX174 is not markedly reduced below that in normal mice but, as in the MS-2 coliphage system (Basch, 1966), titers after rechallenge with ϕX174 are much lower.

Although IgG *antibody* production is usually T cell dependent, IgG *immunoglobulin* levels are within the normal range in neonatally thymectomized mice (Arnason *et al.*, 1964, Fahey *et al.*, 1965; Humphrey *et al.*, 1964) and, more importantly, in nu/nu mice (Warner, 1972). However, Luzzati and Jacobson (1972) have reported a reduced amount of γG_1 in nu/nu mice. The generation of allotypically marked γG_{2a} immunoglobulin from fetal liver cells in irradiated mice is unaffected by the absence of the thymus (Tyan and Herzenberg, 1968). These observations in mice, with the possible exception of γG_1, complement studies in the chicken which have shown thymus independence (and bursa dependence) of Ig production (Cooper *et al.*, 1966; Warner *et al.*, 1969).

All this evidence for relative "T cell independence" of IgM antibody responses does not lead to the interpretation that IgM antibody production is insensitive to the presence of reactive T cells. In hapten-carrier systems, "carrier"-primed cells, presumably of the T type (Cheers *et al.*, 1971; Mitchison, 1971a; Raff, 1970), enhance IgG, but also IgM, antihapten responses (Dutton *et al.*, 1970; Katz *et al.*, 1970; Kontiainen, 1971; Schirrmacher and Rajewsky, 1970). In the SRBC system, production of direct PFC *in vivo* (Cunningham and Sercarz, 1971; Mitchell *et al.*, 1972a) and *in vitro* (Chan *et al.*, 1970; Schimpl and Wecker, 1970) is increased by primed or unprimed T cells. However, a series of antigens elicit levels of IgM antibody in "B mice" which are comparable to those in controls even though in some cases titers are not substained, e.g., SIII (Davies *et al.*, 1970; Howard *et al.*, 1971; Mitchell and Humphrey, 1973). LPS (Andersson and Blomgren, 1971; Möller and Michael, 1971), NIP_{High}-BSA (Aird, 1971), and NIP-MRBC (Munro, unpublished observations). D-amino acid synthetic polypeptides (Sela *et al.*, 1972) and levan (Miranda, unpublished observations) induce antibody responses in irradiated mice injected with bone marrow cells which are not increased by T cells. PVP elicits normal (Andersson and Blomgren, 1971) if not slightly elevated responses (Kerbel and Eidinger, 1972) in thymectomized mice. Many of these antigens have been shown to be highly persistent *in vivo* and there is evidence that IgG responses are readily inhibited by determinants on such antigens (see below).

Studies by Feldmann and Basten (1971) have clearly shown a lack of T cell dependence of the *in vitro* response to *Salmonella adelaide* polymerized flagellin (POL) and DNP-POL. Predominantly IgM antibodies are produced in this Marbrook culture system even by primed cells. Studies with POL *in vivo* have shown the adoptive secondary serum antibody response to be T cell dependent (Mitchell *et al.*, 1971).

As mentioned in a previous section, a high primary (involving predominantly IgM) and a low secondary (involving predominantly IgG) response in T cell deficient mice can be ascribed to low numbers of reactive T cells which are recruited at the time of initial antigen injection and then exhausted. Functional T cell activity in adult thymectomized mice can be diminished by injections of BSA (Cantor, 1972). Nevertheless, one is hard pressed to ascribe "T cell independent" antibody responses to sufficient numbers of specifically reactive T cells in such severe T cell deficiencies as exist in nu/nu mice, in children with no epithelial thymus rudiment (Good *et al.*, 1971), or in anti-θ-treated spleen cells from "B mice" (but see Cohn, 1972).

Normal primary responses and impaired secondary responses in thymectomized mice suggest that T cells are required for the generation of memory B cells. In the presence of only low numbers of T cells, B cells may "exhaustively differentiate" to antibody-secreting cells (Sterzl, 1966) without undergoing sufficient "self-renewal" or "nonexpressive differentiation" in preparation for a secondary response. In this speculative vein, it is further conceivable that, after antigen activation of T cells, cell surface products coded for by T cell genes such as Ir-1 (Benacerraf and McDevitt, 1972) may mediate this effect in B cells. However, Roelants and Askonas (1972) have demonstrated that B cells are primed in "B mice" after exposure to antigen in that they later respond in secondary fashion when T cells are injected. Because of the presence of many residual T cells in "B mice," this type of experiment needs to be repeated in nu/nu mice (see below).

In conclusion, a defect in IgG or secondary responsiveness in T cell deficient mice is more readily demonstrated than a defect in IgM or primary responsiveness. If an antigen is largely an IgM inducer, then it may well elicit a T cell independent response. However, IgM antibody production to many antigens is sensitive to the presence of reactive T cells. Moreover, γG_1 antibody is the most highly T cell dependent (sub)class, but it is not possible to say that reactive T cells are obligatory for IgG antibody production. Since no clear statement is possible on Ig class and "T cell independence," it is worthwhile considering another property of antibodies which often distinguishes IgM from IgG antibodies—i.e., intrinsic combining site affinity (Hornick and Karush, 1972; Mäkelä and Cross, 1970; Merler *et al.*, 1968; Metzger, 1970; Voss and Sigel, 1972) (see below).

Fate of B Cells

Immunological memory and tolerance have been demonstrated in B cell populations following injection of antigen into normal mice. What is the fate of B cells after contact with antigen in T cell deficient mice, in mice in which T cells have been rendered specifically tolerant, or in mice in which T cells are genetically unable to recognize (and/or respond to) the "carrier" determinants of the antigen? There is no evidence for an increased susceptibility of thymecto-mized mice to tolerance *induction* using T cell dependent foreign proteins (Mitchison, 1968). In fact, two studies have indicated that small numbers of T cells may facilitate the induction of partial tolerance to SRBC in "B mice" (Gershon and Kondo, 1970; Miller and Mitchell, 1970). In apparent contrast to these results, we have recently observed a reduction of SRBC responsiveness in nu/nu mice, but not "B mice," injected with a single high dose of SRBC. BALB/c nu/nu (derived from the third backcross generation, G. L. Bomholtgard Ltd., Ry, Denmark), when injected with SRBC, failed to respond to a later injection of SRBC given together with BALB/c nu/+ thymocytes. In previously untreated mice or mice injected with HRBC, T cells + SRBC effected good reconstitution of the anti-SRBC response (Table I). We have interpreted this tentatively as a demonstration of B cell susceptibility to tolerance induction in mice with a severe T cell deficiency. It is conceivable that when the time interval between injection of antigen and injection of T cells + antigen is increased that some B cell *priming* may be observed (Roelants and Askonas, 1972). Low amounts of residual antigen may sensitize B cells during the time when B cell

Table I. Inhibition of Anti-SRBC PFC Response in "BALB/c nu/nu" Mice

Pretreatment (day −7)	PFC per spleen 7 days after injection of T cells + 10^8 SRBC I.V.[1]	
	Direct	Indirect
10^9 SRBC I.V.	1,230	650
Zero or 10^9 HRBC I.V.	18,470	87,100

[1] Thymocytes from "BALB/c nu/+" mice (see text) injected with 1.5 mg hydrocortisone I.P. 2 days previously. Geometric mean responses of 3 and 5 mice per group. Developing sera as in Table II (Andersson and Mitchell, 1972).

unresponsiveness is being repaired. "Repair" in this case presumably involves either regeneration of B cells from their precursors in hemopoietic organs (Lafleur *et al.*, 1972) (bursa equivalent sites?) or a release from B cell blockade by antigen. Because of the "Mitchison and Weigle phenomenon" (Cohn, 1972)—antigen dose requirements for the maintenance of tolerance—the appropriate residual antigen may well be "in certain anatomical sites" rather than simply "in low amounts."

Chiller *et al.* (1971), Mitchison (1971*b*), and Rajewsky *et al.* (1972) have shown that T cell tolerance is induced prior to B cell tolerance when using large numbers of low dosages (→ low zone tolerance) or low numbers of high dosages of antigen (→ high zone tolerance). A requirement for reactive T cells for tolerance induction of B cells (Gershon and Kondo, 1970) thus seems most unlikely (Weigle *et al.*, 1972). B cells are known to recover more rapidly than T cells and thus T cell tolerance will be easier to detect than B cell tolerance (Miller *et al.*, 1971; Mitchison, 1971*c;* Rajewsky *et al.*, 1972). In terms of antibody affinity it has been shown that high affinity antibodies are more susceptible to tolerance induction than are low affinity antibodies (Werblin and Siskind, 1972), and in keeping with this, IgG antibodies are more sensitive than IgM antibodies (Weber and Kolsch, 1972).

Impaired B cell responsiveness may follow the injection of hapten-carrier antigens in which the *in vivo* T cell response to the carrier is presumed or shown to be defective. Such antigens include DNP-D-GL in guinea pigs (Katz *et al.*,

Table II. Inhibition of Indirect Anti-DNP PFC Response with DNP-lys-SIII In C3H Mice

Pretreatment (day −7)	PFC per spleen 7 days after injection of DNP-FγG[1]			
	Anti-DNP		Anti-FγG	
	Direct	Indirect	Direct	Indirect
180μg DNP-lys-SIII I.V.	2370	0	1520	27,700
-	1740	10,260	1890	42,100

[1] 200μg alum precipitated DNP$_3$-FγG plus 10^9 B. pertussis organisms I.P. Anti-DNP and anti-FγG PFC determined using DNP-Fab of rabbit anti SRBC and FγG anti-SRBC antibodies to coat SRBC. Indirect PFC developed with a rabbit anti-mouse IgG serum absorbed with Fab on sepharose (Mitchell *et al.*, 1972*c*). Geometric mean responses of 5 mice per group (Hamilton *et al.*, 1972).

1971a; Davie et al., 1972), DNP-lys-SIII (Mitchell et al., 1972c; Mitchell and Humphrey, 1973), DNP-mouse globulins (Havas, 1969; Golan and Borel, 1971), TNP-MRBC (Naor et al., 1971), NIP-mouse γG_1 (Walters et al., 1972), picrylated autologous cells in guinea pigs (Battisto and Bloom, 1966), and NIP-MRBC (Hamilton, unpublished observations). IgG production to subsequently injected fully-immunogenic conjugates seems to be more sensitive to inhibition than IgM production (Table II). We have found DNP-lys-SIII to be highly inhibitory in low doses in adoptive secondary responses whereas much higher doses are required for inhibition of primary responses in intact mice. Many of these tolerogens themselves give rise to low IgM antihapten responses at certain doses and most are highly persistent in vivo. [Using N*IP-MRBC, 20% of the injected radioactivity is still present (with large amounts in cells of the blood) 6 days after injection at a time when whole body counts of mice injected with N*IP-SRBC have declined to <1% of the injected radioactivity (Mitchell and Hamilton, unpublished observations).] As discussed in the next section, it is likely that the impaired B cell activity, which in many of these systems often results in only a delayed response to the potent immunogenic conjugate (Mitchison, 1971c), is a function of antigen persistence.

Responses to Persisting Antigens

Persistent antigens such as SIII (e.g., Howard, 1972), PVP (Andersson, 1972), LPS (Britton et al., 1968), D-amino acid polypeptides (Janeway and Humphrey, 1968), and haptenated autologous erythrocytes induce "T cell independent" responses in vivo. NIP_High -BSA is a "T cell independent antigen" (Aird, 1971), and in mice injected with labeled foreign albumins and globulins heavily conjugated with NIP or DNP, whole body radioactivity may initially be lost more rapidly but then persists much longer than in mice injected with lightly haptenated proteins (Klaus et al., unpublished observations). Many of the antigens mentioned above elicit prominent macroglobulin responses and are tolerogens in high doses. It now seems, however, that IgG (or at least ME-resistant or 7S) antibodies may be produced to immunogenic doses (Andersson, 1972; Argyris and Askonas, 1968; Mitchell and Humphrey, 1973; Sela et al., 1972). Rabbits certainly produce large amounts of IgG anti-SIII antibodies (with restricted heterogeneity) when injected with pneumococci (Kimball et al., 1970).

No T cell reactivity to LPS (Sjöberg, 1971) or SIII (Parrot and DeSousa, 1966; Davies et al., 1970) has been found in mice, but it is unlikely that, by chance, all persisting antigens lack determinants capable of binding to T cells. [In systems designed to look at the sharing of specificities between "helper" cells (T cells) and B cells in mice, no differences in reactivity patterns have been detected. The antigens used have been foreign serum albumins (Rajewsky and Pohlit, 1971; Rajewsky et al., 1972). However, there are several observations which are interpretable as a preferential binding of antigenic determinants to B cells rather than to T cells—i.e., a pre-emption of determinants by B cells and exclusion of T cells (Taylor and Iverson, 1971). The "carrier effect," using haptenated proteins, suggests that T cells compete rather poorly for many haptens such as DNP in mice. Related antigens such as flagellin—acetoacetylated flagellin—and lysozyme—carboxymethylated lysozyme—do not cross-stimulate in antibody production, the antibodies do not crossreact, and yet in the elicitation of delayed hypersensitivity reactions they crossreact very well (Parish, 1971; Thompson et al., 1972). Conceivably, these pairs of antigens possess different haptenic determinants which bind avidly to specific B cells and leave sufficient unmodified "carrier" determinants (with low avidity for B cells) available for T cells. T cells are stimulated by small amounts of antigen (Cunningham and Sercarz, 1971; Falkoff and Kettman, 1972). In contrast to these antigen pairs, the synthetic polypeptides (T,G)-A--L and (H,G)-A--L, which do not cross-stimulate in antibody production, induce antibodies which crossreact extensively (McDevitt, 1968). These antigens presumably do not share sufficient numbers of T cell-stimulating "carrier determinants." In this latter system, H-2 linked surface products on T or B cells may profoundly affect the innate low "carrier"-binding capacity of T cells (discussed in McDevitt et al., 1971).] For some persisting antigens, there may be very few antigen-binding T cells *ab initio*, while for others the reactive T cells are readily tolerized. The preferential suppression of IgG rather than IgM anti-DNP responses using DNP-lys-SIII suggests that B^γ cells, reactive to determinants on persisting antigens, are more susceptible to tolerance induction than B^μ cells. This leads to a ranking of susceptibility to tolerance induction of T cell$\rightarrow$ B^γ cell $\rightarrow$ B^μ cell, and for the B cell at least this susceptibility may reflect the antigen-binding capacity of the cells (i.e., affinity, number, mobility of receptors).

A possible means by which T cells influence antigen-binding B cells is suggested by the observations that determinants on persistent antigens induce "T cell independent" IgM responses at certain doses and more readily inhibit IgG than IgM responses. Conceivably, activated T cells elaborate (or at least are associated with the production of) factors which influence mobility of phagocytes (e.g., David, 1968; Ramseier, 1969; Remold et al., 1971), and degradation of antigen by phagocytes (Mackaness, 1969). Phagocytes such as macrophages and granulocytes will remove antigen from the milieu of these T cells as well as from antigen-binding B cells in the same microenvironment. This removal of antigen reduces the tolerogenicity of the antigen for these cells. At the B cell level, the cells most vulnerable to tolerance induction will be those of high antigen binding capacity (e.g., high affinity B^γ cells). Antigens such as high molecular weight SIII, which is not excreted and is nondegradable, inhibit high affinity B cells regardless of T cell and phagocyte involvement. On the other hand, degradable foreign proteins will trigger rather than inhibit high affinity B cells only if T cells and phagocytes are recruited. Predictions are that high affinity *vs.* low affinity antibodies [often, but not always reflected in IgG *vs.* IgM (Hornick and Karush, 1972)] and high crossreactivity *vs.* low crossreactivity antibodies (Little and Eisen, 1969; Little *et al.*, 1969) will be T cell dependent (Gershon and Paul, 1971; Gershon and Kondo, 1972); tolerance of B cells with high antigen binding capacity will be facilitated by either a lack of reactive T cells, by antigen persistence, or a lack of phagocytes; antigens which are injected in doses high enough to engage B cells but which are rapidly catabolized or removed en masse from the B cell surface, will induce some high affinity antibody in T cell-deficient mice; and finally, low affinity IgM antiself antibodies may be rather common (Schlesinger, 1972).

The emphasis in this hypothesis is on the *number* and *duration* of antigen-mediated signals at the B cell surface rather than on an obligatory inductive "second signal" mediated by a T cell product (see Cohn, 1972). In this scheme, the "second signal" is a discontinuation of the "first signal" mediated by

Table III. Features of the Working Hypothesis on B cell Triggering Developed in this Article

Antigen binding Capacity (ABC) of B cell	Fate of B cell under conditions of:	
	Antigen persistence	Antigen removal
High[1]	Inhibition	Antibody production (high affinity)
Intermediate	Inhibition	Antibody production (average affinity)
Low	Antibody production (low affinity)	Not triggered

[1] B cells with high ABC of either B^μ or B^γ type give rise to IgG antibody-secreting progeny cells whereas B^μ and B^γ cells of lower ABC give rise to IgM and IgG secretors, respectively. By invoking a C_H gene switch in B^μ cells of high ABC, IgG antibody combining sites will have higher "intrinsic affinities" for determinant used for immunization, and greater crossreactivity for other determinants, than IgM antibodies. The B cell progeny of B^μ cells of high ABC will be B^γ cells, this switch being T cell independent but antigen dose dependent. However, the expression of high ABC B^γ cells (i.e., IgG antibody production) will be highly dependent upon antigen removal. If it is assumed that the net ABC of the B cell population is increased after priming, then the expression of primed B cells will again be highly dependent upon antigen removal; thus the T cell influence in the case of degradable antigens.

antigen. T cell products promote clearance and catabolism of antigen at the B cell surface by attracting and/or activating phagocytic cells. Procedures which limit the amount of antigen in "free solution" or on the B cell surface will facilitate the activity of T cells and phagocytes in protecting B cells from inhibition by excess antigen. Antibody (and complement?) dependent follicular localization, granuloma formation, and sequestration of antigen in the liver, as well as antigen characteristics such as low epitope density and *in vivo* instability, will prevent the binding of large amounts of antigen to B cells. Table III illustrates the points of this working hypothesis for which there is obviously scant evidence as yet.

CONCLUSIONS

An attempt has been made to evaluate existing methods of depleting mice or lymphoid cell suspensions of T cells. Under conditions of T cell insufficiency in mice, antibody production is usually of the IgM class and titers of IgG (and in particular γG_1) antibodies are usually very low. However, no universally valid statement can be made about different Ig classes and "T cell independence," and a more accurate association may be with combining site *affinity* of antibodies. An hypothesis is developed which relates "T cell independence," antigen persistence, and low affinity antibody production.

A role for antigen-reactive T cells in the expression of antigen-reactive B cells is now established. The nature of the interaction between T and B cells is unresolved although the literature bristles with possibilities (e.g., Burnet, 1968; Claman and Mosier, 1972; Cohn, 1972; Katz and Benacerraf, 1972; Miller *et al.*, 1971; Mitchison *et al.*, 1970). Two experimental approaches, now widely used, are likely to yield much information on the interaction(s) between T and B cells—(1) isolation of T cell products which directly or indirectly provide an inductive "second signal" to B cells, and (2) examination of the characteristics and behavior of antigens which elicit B cell responses in T cell deficient states and the subsequent fate of these B cells. We presently have much better assay systems than several years ago, e.g., athymic nu/nu mice replacing thymectomized mice, anti-θ sera raised in congenic mice replacing heterologous and C3H anti-θ^{AKR} isoantisera, H-2 linked genetic unresponsiveness in which the lesion may be at the T cell level, and Mishell and Dutton plus Marbrook culture systems replacing *in vivo* adoptive transfers.

Caution is required in the interpretation of *in vitro* studies. The organization of peripheral lymphoid organs (which is preserved despite extensive lymphocyte traffic through the organs) must play some role in the interaction between antigen, antigen-reactive cells, and ancillary cell types. For unknown reasons, IgG responses have been difficult to induce *in vitro* using spleen cells, and this is precisely the response which is highly T cell dependent *in vivo*. It is interesting that in situations where IgG (indirect PFC) antihapten responses are obtained, these responses are more sensitive to hapten inhibition than IgM (direct PFC) antihapten responses (Rittenberg and Bullock, 1972). If it evolves that T cells affect B cells directly, then there is little doubt that, in the characterization of the "second signal," *in vitro* approaches will supersede all *in vivo* systems.

In this paper emphasis has been given to the notion that antigen persistence results in T cell independent production of antibodies with low average intrinsic association constants (often IgM). One of the many assumptions made was that polyvalency of IgM [and thus increased "functional affinity" *vs.* "intrinsic affinity," c f., IgG (Hornick and Karush, 1972; Pike, 1967)] , plays no role in the triggering of B^μ cells. The possibility was considered that T cell products *in vivo* influence B cell activities *indirectly* by promoting phagocytosis of antigen and thereby removing tolerogenic amounts of antigen from the milieu of B cells with high antigen-binding capacity. Under most circumstances, the influence of T cells on B cell activity must be limited both in time and anatomically. However, there is evidence from *in vitro* systems (Dutton *et al.*, 1971; Feldmann and Basten, 1972; Hartmann, 1970; Schimpl and Wecker, 1971) and the *in vivo* "allogeneic effect" (Katz *et al.*, 1971*b;* Kreth and Williamson, 1972; McCullagh, 1970) for an "expanding" or "long-range" influence of T cells on B cells. In view of the above hypothesis, it will be interesting to determine whether these phenomena are mediated by activated phagocytes which remove antigen from B cells. Moreover, many "suppressor T cell" and "antigenic competition" phenomena could be explained by a hyperactive T cell + phagocyte axis which leads to a diversion of antigen from B cells.

As mentioned above, many possible mechanisms whereby T cells modify antibody production in the B cell lineage have been discussed in the literature. The next few years should see a clearing of the field as well as further extension of T–B cell phenomena into other aspects of immunobiology.

ABBREVIATIONS

B cell—bursa- (and in mammals, bursa equivalent-) influenced cell
B^μ cell—presumed immediate precursor of IgM secreting cells
B^γ cell—presumed immediate precursor of IgG secreting cells
SRBC—sheep red blood cells
MRBC—mouse red blood cells
HRBC—horse red blood cells
DNP—2,4-dinitrophenyl
TNP—2,4,6-trinitrophenyl
DNP-lys-SIII—2,4-dinitrophenyl lysine conjugated with CNBr to type III pneumococcal polysaccharide (SIII) from *Streptococci pneumoniae*
DNP-D-GL—2,4-dinitrophenyl conjugated to a copolymer of D-glutamic acid and D-lysine
NIP—3-iodo, 4-hydroxy, 5-nitrophenylacetyl
BSA—bovine serum albumin

NIP_{High} -BSA—BSA heavily conjugated with NIP

FγG—fowl gamma globulin

BγG—bovine gamma globulin

PVP—polyvinyl-pyrrolidone

LPS—*Escherichia coli* lipopolysaccharide

(T,G)-A--L and (H,G)-A--L, poly-L-(tyrosine, glutamic acid) or poly-L-(histidine, glutamic acid)-poly-DL-alanine--poly-L-lysine;
    KLH, keyhole limpet hemocyanin

POL—polymerized flagellin from *Salmonella adelaide.*

Ig—immunoglobulin

γG_1 and γG_{2a}—subclasses of IgG

PFC—plaque-forming or antibody-secreting cells

direct PFC—PFC developed with complement only

indirect PFC—PFC developed with anti-IgG sera and complement

ME—2-mercaptoethanol

θ—theta isoantigen of mice

"B mice"—mice thymectomized as adults, lethally irradiated, and transplanted
    with a source of hemopoietic stem cells

nu/nu and nu/+—gene designations in athymic nude and normal heterozygous mice

ABC—antigen-binding capacity

ACKNOWLEDGMENTS

I thank Drs. Tien-wen Tao-Wiedmann, Louis Lafleur, Russel Little, and John Hamilton in Basel and Drs. John Humphrey and Gerry Klaus in Mill Hill for helpful discussions and for use of unpublished data.

REFERENCES

Aird, J., 1971. *Immunology* 20:617.

Aisenberg, A. C., 1967. *J. Exp. Med.* 125:833.

Andersson, B., 1972. Doctorate Thesis, Tryckeri Balder AB., Stockholm.

Andersson, B., and Blomgren, H., 1971. *Cell. Immunol.* 2:411.

Andersson, K., and Mitchell, G. F., 1972, unpublished observations.

Argyris, B. F., and Askonas, B. A., 1968. *Immunology* 14:379.

Arnason, B. G., de Vaux St. Cyr, C., and Shaffner, J. B., 1964. *J. Immunol.* 93:915.

Baird, S., Santa, J., and Weissman, I., 1971. *Nature New Biol.* 232:56.

Baker, P. J., and Stashak, P. W., 1969. *J. Immunol.* 103:1342.

Basch, R. S., 1966. *Intern. Arch. Allergy* 30:105.

Basten, A., Miller, J. F. A. P., Warner, N. L., and Pye, J., 1971. *Nature New Biol.* 231:104.

Battisto, J. R., and Bloom, B. R., 1966. *Nature* 212:156.

Benacerraf, B., and McDevitt, H. O., 1972. *Science* 175:273.

Britton, S., Wepsic, T., and Möller, G., 1968. *Immunology* 14:491.

Brondz, B. D., 1972. *Transpl. Rev.* 10:112.

Burnet, F. M., 1968. *Nature* 218:426.

Cantor, H., 1972. In Silvestri, L. G. (ed.), *Cell Interactions, Proceedings of the 3rd Lepetit Colloquium,* North Holland Publishing Co., Amsterdam, p. 172.

Cerottini, J-C., Nordin, A. A., and Brunner, K. T., 1970. *Nature* 227:72.
Chan, E. L., Mishell, R. I., and Mitchell, G. F., 1970. *Science* 170:1215.
Cheers, C., Breitner, J. C. S., Little, M., and Miller, J. F. A. P., 1971. *Nature New Biol.* 232:248.
Chiller, J. M., Habicht, G. S., and Weigle, W. O., 1971. *Science* 171:813.
Chiller, J. M., Habicht, G. S., and Weigle, W. O., 1970. *Proc. Nat. Acad. Sci., U.S.* 65:551.
Claman, H. N., 1972. *New Engl. J. Med.* 287:388.
Claman, H. N., and Mosier, D. E., 1972. *Progr. Allergy* 16:40.
Cohen, J. J., 1972. *J. Immunol.* 107:841.
Cohn, M., 1972. *Cell. Immunol.* 5:1.
Cooper, M. D., Peterson, R. D. A., South, M. A., and Good, R. A., 1966. *J. Exp. Med.* 123:75.
Cunningham, A. J., and Sercarz, E. E., 1971. *Eur. J. Immunol.* 1:413.
David, J. R., 1968. *Fed. Proc.* 27:6.
Davie, J. M., and Paul, W. E., 1970. *Cell. Immunol.* 1:404.
Davie, J. M., Paul, W. E., Katz, D. H., and Benacerraf, B., 1972. *J. Exp. Med.* 134:426.
Davies, A. J. S., Carter, R. L., Leuchars, E., Wallis, V., and Dietrich, F. M., 1970. *Immunology* 19:945.
Davies, A. J. S., Leuchars, E., Wallis, V., and Koller, P. C., 1966. *Transplant* 4:438.
Dietrich, F. M., and Dukor, P., 1967. *Pathol. Microbiol.* 30:909.
Dresser, D., 1972. *Eur. J. Immunol.* 2:50.
Dutton, R. W., Falkoff, R., Hurst, J. A., Hoffmann, M., Kappler, J. W., Kettman, J. R., Lesley, J. F., and Vann, D., 1971. In B. Amos (ed.), *Progress in Immunology,* Academic Press, New York, p. 355.
Dutton, R. W., Campbell, P., Chan, E., Hurst, J., Hoffmann, M., Kettman, J., Lesley, J., McCarthy, M., Mishell, R. I., Raidt, D. J., and Vann, D., 1970. In S. Cohen, G. Cudkowicz, and R. T. McCluskey (eds.), *Cellular Interactions in the Immune Response,* S. Karger, Basel, p. 31.
Fahey, J. L., Barth, W. F., and Law, L. W., 1965. *J. Nat. Cancer Inst.* 35:663.
Falkoff, R., and Kettman, J., 1972. *J. Immunol.* 108:54.
Feldmann, M., and Basten, A., 1972. *Nature New Biol.* 237:13.
Feldmann, M., and Basten, A., 1971. *J. Exp. Med.* 134:103.
Gershon, R. K., and Kondo, K., 1972. *Immunology* 23:335.
Gershon, R. K., and Kondo, K., 1970. *Immunology* 18:723.
Gershon, R. K., and Paul, W. E., 1971. *J. Immunol.* 106:872.
Gesner, B. M., and Ginsburg, V., 1964. *Proc. Nat. Acad. Sci., U.S.* 52:750.
Golan, D. T., and Borel, Y., 1971. *J. Exp. Med.* 134:1046.
Goldstein, P., Svedmyr, E. A. J., and Blomgren, H., 1972. *Eur. J. Immunol.* 2:380.
Good, R. A., Biggar, W. D., and Park, B. H., 1971. In B. Amos (ed.), *Progress in Immunology,* Academic Press, New York, p. 700.
Gowans, J. L., and McGregor, D. D., 1965. *Progr. Allergy* 9:1.
Greaves, M. F., and Raff, M. C., 1971. *Nature New Biol.* 233:239.
Grumet, F. C., 1972. *J. Exp. Med.* 135:110.
Hamilton, J. A., unpublished observations.
Hamilton, J. A., Andersson, K., and Mitchell, G. F., 1972, unpublished observations.
Hartmann, K-U., 1970. *J. Exp. Med.* 132:1267.
Havas, H. F., 1969. *Immunology* 17:819.
Hess, M. W., and Stoner, R. D., 1966. *Intern. Arch. Allergy* 30:37.
Hornick, C. L., and Karush, F., 1972. *Immunochemistry* 9:325.
Howard, J. G., 1972. *Transpl. Rev.* 8:50.
Howard, J. C., Hunt, S. V., and Gowans, J. L., 1972. *J. Exp. Med.* 135:200.
Howard, J. G., Christie, G. H., Courtenay, B. M., Leuchers, E., and Davies, A. J. S., 1971. *Cell. Immunol.* 2:614.
Humphrey, J. H., Parrot, D. M. V., and East, J., 1964. *Immunology* 7:419.
Hunter, P., and Munro, A. J., 1972. *Immunology* 23:69.

Isaković, K., Smith, S. B., and Waksman, B. H., 1965. *J. Exp. Med.* **122**:1103.
Janeway, C. A., and Humphrey, J. H., 1968. *Immunology* **14**:225.
Janossy, G., and Greaves, M. F., 1971. *Clin. Exp. Immunol.* **9**:483.
Julius, M. H., Masuda, T., and Herzenberg, L. A., 1972. *Proc. Nat. Acad. Sci., U.S.* **69**:1934.
Katz, D. H., and Benacerraf, B., 1972. *Adv. Immunol.* **15**:1.
Katz, D. H., Davie, J. M., Paul, W. E., and Benacerraf, B., 1971a. *J. Exp. Med.* **134**:201.
Katz, D. H., Paul, W. E., Goidl, E. A., and Benacerraf, B., 1971b. *J. Exp. Med.* **133**:169.
Katz, D. H., Paul, W. E., Goidl, E. A., and Benacerraf, B., 1970. *J. Exp. Med.* **132**:261.
Kerbel and Eidinger, D., 1972. *Eur. J. Immunol.* **2**:114.
Kimball, J. W., Papenheimer, A. M., and Jaton, J-C., 1970. *J. Immunol.* **106**:1177.
Kindred, B., 1971. *Eur. J. Immunol.* **1**:59.
Klaus, G. G., Kontiainen, S., and Mitchell, G. F., unpublished observations.
Kontiainen, S., 1971. *Eur. J. Immunol.* **1**:276.
Kreth, H. W., and Williamson, A. R., 1972. *Nature* **234**:454.
Krüger, J., and Gershon, R. K., 1972. *J. Immunol.* **108**:581.
Lafleur, L., Miller, R. G., and Phillips, R. A., 1972. *J. Exp. Med.* **135**:1363.
Law, L. W., Dunn, T., Trainin, N., and Levey, R. H., 1964. In V. Defendi and D. Metcalf
    (eds.), *The Thymus,* Wistar Inst. Press, Philadelphia, p. 105.
Little, J. R., and Eisen, H. N., 1969. *J. Exp. Med.* **129**:247.
Little, J. R., Border, W., and Freidin, R., 1969. *J. Immunol.* **103**:809.
Luzzati, A. L., and Jacobson, E. B., 1972. *Eur. J. Immunol.* **2**:473.
Mackaness, G. B., 1969. *J. Exp. Med.* **129**:973.
Mäkelä, O., and Cross, A. M., 1970. *Progr. Allergy* **14**:145.
Many, A., and Schwarz, R. S., 1970. *Proc. Soc. Exp. Biol. Med.* **133**:754.
McCullagh, P. J., 1970. *J. Exp. Med.* **132**:916.
McDevitt, H. O., 1968. *J. Immunol.* **100**:485.
McDevitt, H. O., Bechtol, K. B., Grumet, F. C., Mitchell, G. F., and Wegmann, T. G., 1971.
    In B. Amos (ed.), *Progress in Immunology,* Academic Press, New York, p. 495.
Merler, E., Karlin, L., and Matsumoto, S., 1968. *J. Biol. Chem.* **243**:386.
Metcalf, D., 1966. *The Thymus,* Springer-Verlag, Berlin.
Metzger, H., 1970. *Adv. Immunol.* **12**:57.
Miller, J. F. A. P., and Mitchell, G. F., 1970. *J. Exp. Med.* **131**: 675.
Miller, J. F. A. P., and Mitchell, G. F., 1969. *Transpl. Rev.* **1**:3.
Miller, J. F. A. P., and Osoba, D., 1967. *Physiol. Rev.* **47**:437.
Miller, J. F. A. P., Basten, A., Sprent, J., and Cheers, C., 1971. *Cell. Immunol.* **2**:469.
Miller, J. F. A. P., Dukor, P., Grant, G., Sinclair, N. R. St. C., and Sacquet, E., 1967. *Clin.
    Exp. Immunol.* **2**:531.
Mitchell, G. F., and Hamilton, J. A., unpublished observations.
Mitchell, G. F., and Humphrey, J. H., 1973. In B. Janković (ed.), *Proceedings of the Fourth
    International Conference on Germinal Centers of Lymphatic Tissue,* Plenum Press,
    New York, p. 125.
Mitchell, G. F., and Kontiainen, S., unpublished observations.
Mitchell, G. F., Chan, E. L., Noble, M. S., Weissman, I. L., Mishell, R. I., and Herzenberg, L.
    A., 1972a. *J. Exp. Med.* **135**:165.
Mitchell, G. F., Grumet, F. C., and McDevitt, H. O., 1972b. *J. Exp. Med.* **135**:126.
Mitchell, G. F., Humphrey, J. H., and Williamson, A. R., 1972c. *Eur. J. Immunol.* **2**:460.
Mitchell, G. F., Mishell, R. I., and Herzenberg, L. A., 1971. In B. Amos (ed.), *Progress in
    Immunology,* Academic Press, New York, p. 324.
Miranda, J. J., unpublished observations.
Mitchison, N. A., 1972. In L. G. Silvestri (ed.), *Cell Interactions, Proceedings of the Third
    Lepetit Colloquium,* North Holland Publishing Co., Amsterdam, p. 112.
Mitchison, N. A., 1971a. *Eur. J. Immunol.* **1**:18.
Mitchison, N. A., 1971b. In O. Mäkelä, A. Cross, and T. V. Kosunen (eds.), *Cell Interactions
    and Receptor Antibodies in Immune Response,* Academic Press, London, p. 249.
Mitchison, N. A., 1971c. In N. W. Nisbet and M. W. Elves (eds.), *Immunological Tolerance
    to Tissue Antigens,* Orthopaedic Hospital, Oswestry, England, p. 67.

Mitchison, N. A., 1968. *Immunology* 15:509.
Mitchison, N. A., Rajewsky, K., and Taylor, R. B., 1970. In J. Sterzl and I. Riha (eds.), *Developmental Aspects of Antibody Formation and Structure.* Academia, Prague, p. 547.
Möller, E., and Sjöberg, O., 1972. *Transpl. Rev.* 8:26.
Möller, G., and Michael, G., 1971. *Cell. Immunol.* 2:309.
Morse, S., 1966. *J. Exp. Med.* 123:283.
Munro, A. J., unpublished observations.
Naor, D., Mishell, R. I., and Wofsy, L., 1971. *J. Immunol.* 105:1322.
Nossal, G. J. V., Cunningham, A., Mitchell, G. F., and Miller, J. F. A. P., 1968. *J. Exp. Med.* 128:839.
Pantalouris, E. M., and Flisch, P. A., 1972. *Eur. J. Immunol.* 2:236.
Parish, C. R., 1971. *J. Exp. Med.* 134:21.
Parrot, D. M. V., and DeSousa, M. A. B., 1966. *Nature* 212:1316.
Pike, R. M., 1967. *Bacteriol. Rev.* 31:157.
Raff, M. C., 1970. *Nature* 226:1257.
Raff, M. C., and Wortis, H. H., 1970. *Immunology* 18:931.
Rajewsky, K., and Pohlit, H., 1971. In B. Amos (ed.), *Progress in Immunology,* Academic Press, New York, p. 337.
Rajewsky, K., Brenig, C., and Melchers, I., 1972. In L. G. Silvestri (ed.), *Cell Interactions, Proceedings of the Third Lepetit Colloquium,* North Holland Publishing Co., Amsterdam, p. 196.
Ramseier, H., 1969. *J. Exp. Med.* 130:1279.
Remold, H. G., Ward, P. A., and David, J. R., 1971. In O. Mäkelä, A. Cross, and T. V. Kosunen (eds.), *Cell Interactions and Receptor Antibodies in Immune Responses,* Academic Press, London, p. 411.
Rittenberg, M. B., and Bullock, W. W., 1972. *Immunochemistry* 9:491.
Roelants, G. E., and Askonas, B. A., 1972. *Nature New Biol.* 239:63.
Roelants, G. E., and Askonas, B. A., 1971. *Eur. J. Immunol.* 1:151.
Roitt, I. M., Greaves, M. F., Torrigiani, G., Brostoff, J., and Playfair, J. H. L., 1969. *Lancet* 2:367.
Rowley, D. A., Gowans, J. L., Atkins, R. C., Ford, W. L., and Smith, M. E., 1972. *J. Exp. Med.* 136:499.
Schimpl, A., and Wecker, E., 1971. *Eur. J. Immunol.* 1:304.
Schimpl, A., and Wecker, E., 1970. *Nature* 226:1258.
Schirrmacher, V., and Rajewsky, K., 1970. *J. Exp. Med.* 132:1019.
Schlesinger, M., 1972. *Progr. Allergy* 16:214.
Sela, M., Mozes, E., and Shearer, G. M., 1972. *Proc. Nat. Acad. Sci., U.S.* 69:2696.
Sinclair, N. R. St. C., 1967a. *Immunology* 12:549.
Sinclair, N. R. St. C., 1967b. *Clin. Exp. Immunol.* 2:701.
Sjöberg, O., 1971. *J. Exp. Med.* 133:1015.
Sprent, J., and Miller, J. F. A. P., 1972. *Eur. J. Immunol.* 2:384.
Sprent, J., Miller, J. F. A. P., and Mitchell, G. F., 1971. *Cell. Immunol.* 2:171.
Sterzl, J., 1966. *Nature* 209:416.
Strober, S., 1972. *Nature New Biol.* 237:247.
Svet-Moldavsky, G. J., Zinzar, S. N., and Spector, N. M., 1964. *Nature* 202:353.
Tao-Wiedmann, T. W., unpublished observations.
Taylor, R. B., 1969. *Transpl. Rev.* 1:114.
Taylor, R. B., and Iverson, G. M., 1971. *Proc. Roy. Soc. Ser. B.* 176:393.
Taylor, R. B., and Wortis, H. H., 1968. *Nature* 220:927.
Thompson, K., Harris, M., Benjamini, E., Mitchell, G., and Noble, M., 1972. *Nature New Biol.* 238:20.
Torrigiani, G., 1972. *J. Immunol.* 108:161.
Tyan, M. L., and Herzenberg, L. A., 1968. *J. Immunol.* 101:446.
Voss, E. W., Jr., and Sigel, M. M., 1972. *J. Immunol.* 109:665.
Walters, C. S., Moorhead, J. W., and Claman, H. N., 1972. *J. Exp. Med.* 136:546.

Warner, N. L., 1972. In M. G. Hanna, Jr., (ed.), *Contemporary Topics in Immunobiology,*
    Vol. I, Plenum Press, New York, p. 87.
Warner, N. L., Uhr, J. W., Thorbecke, G. J., and Ovary, Z., 1969. *J. Immunol.* 103:1317.
Weber, G., and Kolsch, E., 1972. *Eur. J. Immunol.* 2:191.
Werblin, T. P., and Siskind, G. W., 1972. *Transpl. Rev.* 8:104.
Weigle, W. O., Chiller, J. M., and Habicht, G. S., 1972. *Transpl. Rev.* 8:3.
Wigzell, H., 1970. *Transpl. Rev.* 5:76.
Wortis, H. H., 1971. *Clin. Exp. Immunol.* 8:305.

Chapter 5

Genetic Control of Antibody Responses to Myeloma Proteins of Mice

Rose Lieberman and William E. Paul

Laboratory of Immunology
National Institute of Allergy and Infectious Diseases
National Institutes of Health
Bethesda, Maryland

INTRODUCTION

Immunoglobulins of the mouse are polymorphic and the polymorphism is ascribable in part to allelism of the structural genes for the immunoglobulin heavy chain constant regions (C_H genes). The existence of allotypic forms of mouse immunoglobulin has permitted the establishment of the genetic relationship between the C_H genes for different classes of immunoglobulins (Potter and Lieberman, 1967a,b) and also the determination of the linkage between C_H genes and the genes controlling the variable regions of immunoglobulin heavy chains (V_H genes) (Blomberg et al., 1972; Sher and Cohn, 1972; Eichmann, 1972; Pawlak et al., 1973). More recently, it has become clear that the immunoglobulins constitute a set of antigens that are of particular value in the identification and linkage analysis of genes controlling immune responses (Lieberman and Humphrey, 1971, 1972; Lieberman et al., 1972). The latter genes are referred to as immune response (Ir) genes.

The usefulness of the immunoglobulins as antigens stems from the limited ways in which immunoglobulin of one allotype differs from immunoglobulins of the same class, but of a different allotype. In this respect, immunoglobulins effectively represent "simple" antigens when mice, whose own immunoglobulins are of a different allotypic form than that of the antigen, are immunized. It is the purpose of this communication to briefly review the current information on mouse immunoglobulin allotypes and then to discuss the genetic control of the immune response to these antigens.

As an introduction, we initially outline the allotype system and the Ir genes thus far identified and then treat in more detail each of the major classes in terms of the allotypic forms existing and the evidence for genetic control of the immune response to immunoglobulins of that class.

Allotypic determinants or specificities controlled by C_H genes have been identified serologically for four of the six known mouse immunoglobulin classes (Potter and Lieberman, 1967a,b; Herzenberg *et al.*, 1968). Thus, IgA, IgF (γ_1), IgG (γ_{2a}), and IgH (γ_{2b}) allotypes are known; as yet no allotypic specificities for the IgM (μ) or IgG$_3$ (ι) classes have been demonstrated. The C_H genes constitute a series of closely linked loci in a single chromosome region. The immunoglobulin region is not associated with any of the known linkage groups, nor has the chromosome on which it exists been identified.

Antiallotype antisera are prepared by immunizing appropriate strains of mice with normal immunoglobulins or with myeloma proteins. When myeloma proteins are used, the antisera also identify a specific determinant (idiotype) present on the Fab region of the protein. In general, the myeloma proteins used in this laboratory are derived from BALB/c mice as plasmacytomas can be induced relatively easily in this strain but only infrequently in most other strains (Potter, 1972). NZB mice are also susceptible to plasmacytoma induction (Warner, 1971). One strategy which has been employed to obtain myeloma proteins of different allotype than BALB/c mice is to produce mice congenic to BALB/c with a BALB/c genetic background and an immunoglobulin C_H genetic region derived from a different strain. Using this approach, myeloma proteins with allotypes of C57BL and AL, respectively, have been derived from C.BL Ig C_H and C.AL Ig C_H mice (Potter and Lieberman, 1967a,b; Potter, 1972).

It has been known for some time that antibody responses to myeloma proteins are rarely obtained unless the strain which has been immunized possesses immunoglobulin of a different allotypic form than that of the myeloma protein used for immunization. When allotype differences do not exist, neither anti-idiotype nor antiallotype antibody is formed in most instances (Lieberman and Humphrey, 1971). In a few exceptional cases, low concentrations of anti-idiotype antibody have been produced by mice not differing at the allotype locus (Sirisinha and Eisen, 1971). Thus, immune responsiveness to immunoglobulins is controlled by genes coding for immunoglobulin H chains.

More recently, it has become apparent that many strains of mice which differ from BALB/c at the C_H locus make either no or meager anti-idiotype or antiallotype antibody responses to a given BALB/c myeloma protein. It has now been shown that capacity to produce large amounts of antibody to myeloma proteins of a given class depends, in addition to an appropriate C_H genotype, upon the possession of immune response genes which are located within the major histocompatibility (H-2) gene complex of the mouse. Thus far Ir genes controlling antibody responses to IgA and IgG (γ_{2a}) myeloma proteins of

BALB/c origin have been described and mapped (Lieberman and Humphrey, 1971, 1972; Lieberman et al., 1972). Recent studies indicate that Ir genes for BALB/c IgH (γ_{2b}) proteins also exist.

The Ir-IgA and Ir-IgG genes reported thus far and the Ir-IgH genes described in this review are all based on studies of the immune response to IgA, IgG, and IgH myeloma proteins of BALB/c origin. At this point in our continuing studies of Ir-Ig genes it has become apparent that different Ir genes are involved when myeloma proteins are derived from strains with different Ig genomes than BALB/c. For example, the immune response to IgH myeloma proteins from C.AL Ig C_H congenic strains having the AL allotype involves Ir genes that are different from those controlling the immune response to IgH myeloma proteins of BALB/c origin. In addition, there is the real possibility that Ir genes exist which control recognition of idiotypic determinants of myeloma proteins. In order to distinguish among these genes we shall designate the Ir gene not only by class of immunoglobulin but also by the specific protein used to elicit the response. Ir-IgA shall be designated Ir-IgA (M467) since the majority of the strains were immunized with MOPC 467 of BALB/c origin (Lieberman and Humphrey, 1971). Ir-IgG shall be designated Ir-IgG (M173) since MOPC 173 of BALB/c origin was used in these studies (Lieberman and Humphrey, 1972; Lieberman et al., 1972). In this chapter, studies identifying two Ir-IgH genes were based on the immune response to MOPC 195 and UPC-120 of BALB/c origin. These genes are designated Ir-IgH (M195) and Ir-IgH (UPC-120).

One feature of particular interest which has emerged from the study of the Ir genes for IgA [Ir-IgA (M467)] and IgG [Ir-IgG (M173)] proteins is the existence of at least two Ir loci in the H-2 region. McDevitt and his colleagues have shown that Ir-1, a gene controlling immune responses to a series of branch chain synthetic polypeptides, is linked to H-2 and is localized to the region between the H-2K gene and the gene(s) controlling serum substance [the Ss-Slp gene(s)] (McDevitt and Chinitz, 1969; McDevitt et al., 1972). Our studies of Ir-IgA (M467) and Ir-IgG (M173) reveal that they are both in the same general region as Ir-1. Ir-IgG (M173) is clearly at a different locus within that region than Ir-IgA (M467) and Ir-1.

IMMUNOGLOBULIN ALLOTYPES OF THE MOUSE

A large battery of serologic reagents (homologous antisera) have been prepared which identify immunoglobulin allotypes of the mouse. Most of these have been developed using myeloma proteins as antigens although normal immunoglobulins are also employed. Antisera prepared with normal immunoglobulins often exhibit specificity for determinants on more than one immunoglobulin class and require absorption before they may be used as typing reagents.

Two general nomenclature systems are currently in use to designate the allotypic determinants and the allelic forms of the genes controlling the C_H regions (Table I). In one system (Potter and Lieberman 1967a,b), the determinants are designated with an upper case letter indicating the immunoglobulin class and an arabic superscript indicating the specific determinant (e.g., G^1). In some instances, the class on which a determinant appears has not yet been established. Such determinants are referred to as unassigned and appear as superscripts without any class designation (e.g., 2). An italicized upper case letter indicates the genetic locus and is the same letter as that used to indicate the immunoglobulin class. The allele at that locus is designated by the upper case letter together with arabic superscripts showing *all* of the known determinants on the C_H region controlled by that allele (e.g., $G^{1,6,7,8}$) (Table II). In the other system (Herzenberg *et al.*, 1968), the determinants are designated by a numerical code (e.g., 1.1) in which the number before the decimal point indicates the class

Table I. List of Determinants Assigned to Specific IgC$_H$: Alignment of Determinants Identified by Different Investigators [a]

	Immunoglobulin class			
G	H	F	A	Unassigned
G^1 (1.10)	H^9 (3.4)	F^{19} (4.1)	A^{12} (2.2)	2
G^3 (1.3)	H^{11} (3.2)	F^- (4.2)	A^{13} (2.3)	10
G^5 (1.11)	H^{16} (3.9)	F^8	A^{14} (2.4)	18
G^4	H^4		A^{15}	20
G^6 (1.12)	H^{22}		A^{17}	21
G^7 (1.1)	H^{23}		(2.1)	24
G^8	(3.1)			
G^{35}	(3.3)			
(1.2)	(3.7)			
(1.4)	(3.8)			
(1.5)				
(1.6)				
(1.7)				
(1.8)				

[a] The allotypic determinants on various classes of mouse immunoglobulin are designated both by Potter–Lieberman and Herzenberg nomenclatures. Potter–Lieberman notation for a given determinant is shown with the Herzenberg notation for the same determinant appearing next to it in parentheses. Unassigned specificities are those for which the immunoglobulin class is not yet established.

Table II. Listing of Alleles of I g C_H Genes. Alignment of Alleles Identified by Different Investigators[a]

Prototype strain	Potter and Lieberman (1967a-b) Allele	Herzenberg et al. (1968) Allele	Herzenberg et al. (1968) Determinant
BALB/c	$G^{1,6,7,8}$	1^a	1,2,6,7,8,10,12
C57BL/6	G^-	1^b	4,7
DBA/2	$G^{3,8}$	1^c	2,3,7
AKR/J	$G^{4,6,7,8}$	1^d	1,2,5,7,12
A/J	$G^{4,6,7,8}$	1^e	1,2,5,6,7,8,12
CE/J	$G^{5,7,8}$	1^f	1,2,8,11
RIII/J	$G^{3,8}$	1^g	2,3
SEA/J	$G^{1,6,7,8}$	1^h	1,2,6,7,10,12
Kitty-Hawk (wild)	$G^{35,8}$	--	
Kitty-Hawk (wild)	$G^{35,7,8}$	--	
BALB/c, SEA	$A^{12,13,14}$	$2^{a,h}$	2,3,4
C57BL/6	A^{15}	2^b	--
DBA/2, RIII	--	$2^{c,g}$	1
AKR, A/J	$A^{13,17}$	$2^{d,e}$	3
CE	A^{14}	2^f	4
BALB/c, DBA/2, SEA	$H^{9,11,22}$	$3^{a,c,h}$	1,2,4,7,8
C57B1/6	$H^{9,16,22}$	3^b	4,7,8,9
AKR/J	$H^{4,23}$	3^d	1,3,7,8
A/J	$H^{4,23}$	3^e	1,3,7
CE/J	$H^{9,11}$	3^f	1,2,3,4
RIII/J	$H^{9,11}$	3^g	1,2,4(?)
All others	$F^{8,19}$ (fast)	$4^{a,c,d,e,f,g,h}$	
C57BL/6	F^- (slow)	4^b	
	Unassigned		
DD	10	--	
C57BL/6	2	--	
AKR, AL	18	--	
DBA/2	20	--	
RIII	21	--	
BL	24	--	

[a] See legend of Table I.

of H chain and the number after the decimal point indicates the determinant or specificity. The allele is shown by an arabic number representing the locus and a lower case superscript indicating the allele at that locus (e.g., *Ig-1*[a]). Tables I and II align the two nomenclature systems. Although many of the same determinants are identified in both systems, there are also determinants which are different for each system. One important difference between the two systems is that the Potter–Lieberman (1967*a,b*) system uses consecutive numbers to identify determinants regardless of the class on which that determinant appears. Consequently, a determinant which is on two different classes is given the same number. Thus, G^4 and H^4 refer to a specificity, 4, which is found on both IgG and IgH proteins (Table I). The Herzenberg (Herzenberg *et al.,* 1968) system starts with determinant 1 for each class and then uses consecutive numbers to designate additional determinants of that class. For example, specificities 1.1 and 2.1 are unrelated. In the remainder of this paper we will use the Potter–Lieberman system exclusively.

The distribution of determinants among the sera of different strains has been determined mainly by testing the capacity of specific antiallotype reagents to precipitate with such sera. Alternatively, when passive hemagglutination systems are used, the ability of sera to inhibit hemagglutination indicates the

Table III. Immunoglobulin Heavy Chain (IgC$_H$) Linkage Groups

$G^{1,6,7,8} H^{9,11,22} A^{12,13,14} F^{8,19}$	BALB/c, BDP, BRSUNT, CBA, C3H, C57BR, C57L, C58, MA, PL, ST, STR, 129
$^{10}G^{1,6,7,8} H^{9,11,22} A^{12,13,14} F^{8,19}$	DD
$^{2}G^{-} H^{9,16,22} A^{15} F^{-}$	C57BL/10, C57BL/6, C57BL, NBL, HR, LP, SJL, SM, STR/1
$^{21}G^{3,8} H^{9,11} A^{-} F^{8,19}$	RIII, SWR
$^{20}G^{3,8} H^{9,11,22} A^{-} F^{8,19}$	DBA/1, DBA/2, I, RF, STOLI, YBR
$^{10}G^{4,6,7,8} H^{4,23} A^{13,17} F^{8,19}$	A/J, NZB, NZW
$^{10,18}G^{4,6,7,8} H^{4,23} A^{13,17} F^{8,19}$	AL, AKR
$^{10,24}G^{4,6,7,8} H^{4,23} A^{13,17} F^{8,19}$	BL
$G^{5,7,8} H^{9,11} A^{14} F^{8,19}$	CE, DE, NH

Table IV. Immune Response to IgA Myeloma Proteins of BALB/c Origin[a]

IgA C_H H-2 determinant		Strains	No. of mice	HA (log 2)	
				Immunogen	Allotype
d	$A^{12,13,14}$	BALB/c	10	0	0
k		C₃H,C58,ST, C57BR,MA	44	0	0
u		PL	10	0	0
?		BRSUNT,STR,DD	28	0	0
a	$A^{13,17}$	A,AL	16	12.7,11.4	7.4,8.1
b		A.By	10	3.0	0.1
d		NZB,NZW	20	5.0,1.6	0.1,0
k		AKR	15	11.8	6.2
s		A.SW	10	9.7	6.1
k	A^{14}	CE	7	> 12.0	9.2
?		DE,NH	20	>12.0,9.2	7.6,4.2
d	A^-	DBA/2	10	0.4	0.4
k		RF	6	> 12.0	9.1
q		SWR,DBA/1	6	0.1,0	0,0
r		RIII	10	9.7	4.0
b	A^{15}	C57BL/6,LP	20	1.7,1.0	0.1,0
s		SJL	10	8.6	5.1
d		NBL	10	1.2	0.2
v		SM	5	0.6	0.0

[a] Notes:
   (1) Antisera reacted to IgA immunogen identify both allotypes and idiotypes.
   (2) Antisera reacted to IgA myeloma protein not used for immunization identify only allotype.
   low response arbitrarily chosen as < 3.0 (log 2).
   medium response arbitrarily chosen as 3.1-6.0 (log 2).
   high response arbitrarily chosen as >6.1 (log 2).
   NT—not tested
   (3) The same immunization procedures were used for the 20 different BALB/c IgA myeloma protein immunogens used here and were previously described by Lieberman and Humphrey (1971).
   (4) IgA myeloma proteins of BALB/c carry $A^{12,13,14}$ allotypic determinants.

Table V. Immune Response to BALB/c IgA Myeloma Protein (MOPC 467) of
B10 Congenic and Recombinant Mice[a]

Strain	Chromosome symbol	K	Ss-Slp	D	No. of mice	M467	M406
B10.A	a	k	d	d	8	10.8	2.0
B10	b	b	b	b	10	2.4	0.1
B10.129 (6M)	bc	bc	bc	bc	8	1.8	0
B10.D2	d	d	d	d	8	0.9	0
B10.BR	k	k	k	k	8	9.0	0.5
B10.P	p	p	p	p	6	6.3	2.0
B10.F	n	n	n	n	4	5.3	2.3
B10.A(2R)	hc	k	d	b	10	9.5	2.0
B10.A(4R)	hd	k	b	b	6	7.8	3.2
B10.A(5R)	ic	b	d	d	10	0.3	0.0
B10.AKM	m	k	k	q	8	5.3	0.1

The table above has a spanning header "Origin of H-2 Region" over columns Chromosome symbol, K, Ss-Slp, D; and "HA (log 2)" over M467, M406.

[a] Antibody reacting with M467 immunogen identifies both allotypes and idiotypes. Antibody reacting to M406 only identify allotype. None of these strains share any IgA-C_H allotypic determinants with those present on the BALB/c IgA myeloma protein M467 used for immunization. MOPC 467 (M467) and MOPC 406 (M406) are γA myeloma proteins of BALB/c origin. The lower case letters under the genes K, Ss-Slp, and D represent the alleles at those loci present in the strain indicated.

presence in that serum of a given determinant. By testing backcross and F_2 generations, it has been shown that the loci controlling the C_H genes for IgG, H, A, and F are linked and that at least nine different C_H linkage groups exist. These are shown in Table III.

GENETIC CONTROL OF THE IMMUNE RESPONSE
TO BALB/c IgA MYELOMA PROTEINS

A large number of inbred, H-2 congenic, and recombinant strains have been immunized with IgA myeloma proteins derived from BALB/c mice. The antibody response, which is shown in Tables IV and V, was determined by a passive hemagglutination technique (Gold and Fudenberg, 1967) using antisera absorbed with sheep erythrocytes. In each instance, sera were titered with erythrocytes coated with the IgA myeloma protein used for immunization and with another, unrelated, IgA protein. The hemagglutination titer against the latter cells represents the activity of antiallotype antibody while the titer obtained with cells coated with the immunizing protein reflects both antiallotype and anti-idiotype antibody.

Table IV demonstrates that mice possessing the same IgA C_H genes as BALB/c ($A^{12,13,14}$) make no measurable antiallotype or anti-idiotype response to BALB/c IgA proteins. On the other hand, some strains of mice possessing $A^{13,17}$, A^{14}, A^-, and A^{15} IgA C_H genes produce high titers of antibody while other mice with similar IgA C_H genes make very meager responses. Inspection of Table IV shows that mice of the H-2 types a,k,r, and s generally make strong antibody responses to IgA proteins whereas mice of the H-2 types b,d,q, and v usually produce little or no anti-IgA antibody.

These data confirm the previous findings that no anti-idiotype response (or antiallotype response) is obtained unless the immunized animals differ at the IgA C_H locus from the animal which was the donor of the myeloma protein. In addition, the results suggest that genetic factors associated with H-2 may have an important role in determining responsiveness to BALB/c IgA myeloma proteins. That responsiveness to the IgA myeloma protein MOPC 467 is a dominant trait is demonstrated by the high response of progeny of a cross between A mice (high responder to IgA, Ig-C_H type $A^{13,17}$, H-2^a) and C57BL/6 mice (low responder to IgA, Ig-C_H type A^{15}, H-2^b).

The importance of the H-2 region in these responses is demonstrated by the pattern of responsiveness of congenic mice of the B10 series. These mice are virtually identical, genetically, to C57BL/10 mice with the exception of the genetic region in which the H-2 complex is located. This series of mice is of particular usefulness in the analysis of the genetic basis of the response to IgA myeloma proteins as they are of the A^{15} genotype and thus share none of the allotypic determinants which BALB/c IgA proteins display.

The B10·A (H-2^a), B10·BR (H-2^k), B10·P (H-2^p), and B10·F (H-2^n) make considerable responses to IgA myeloma proteins whereas the B10 (H-2^b), B10·129 (6M) (H-2^{bc}), and B10·D2 (H-2^d) make meager responses (Table V). Thus, there is a clear association of H-2 type and immune responsiveness to IgA myeloma proteins. We have termed the gene controlling this response, the Ir-IgA $(M467)$ gene. Before considering the data which allow us to more precisely locate Ir-IgA $(M467)$ within the H-2 complex, a very brief statement of the current view of the structure of the H-2 region is given (Klein and Shreffler, 1972; Klein, 1973). The H-2 region is located within the IX linkage group and is now known to be on the seventeenth chromosome. The H-2 region itself consists of a series of genes of which three are of main importance in dividing H-2 into regions. These are the K gene, which controls certain of the H-2 serological specificities, the Ss-Slp gene(s), which control serum substance and sex limited protein, and the D gene which controls the remaining H-2 serological specificities. The order of these genes on the chromosome is as follows: centromere.....K..Ss-Slp...D.... Thus K is spoken of as on the "left" side of the H-2 complex and D as on the "right" side. There is considerable genetic material between K and D (recombination frequency $\sim$ 0.5%) (Shreffler, 1970) and between K and Ss-Slp and Ss-Slp and D. One potentially confusing aspect of nomenclature is that the upper case letters K and D designate genes within H-2 while the lower case letters k and d denote H-2 types.

The region within the H-2 complex in which the *Ir-IgA (M467)* gene is located is suggested by the responses of B10·A, B10·D2, and B10·BR mice (Table V). The B10·A (H-2^a) and B10·BR (H-2^k) both make considerable responses to IgA proteins while the B10·D2 (H-2^d) makes a meager response. The H-2^a histocompatibility complex appears to have been derived from a recombination between the H-2^k and H-2^d chromosomes in which the K gene derived from the H-2^k chromosome type and the Ss-Slp and D genes derived from the H-2^d chromosome type. Thus, the responsiveness of the B10·A and B10·BR suggests that *Ir-IgA (M467)* is closely linked to the allele of the K gene associated with the H-2^k chromosome type.

Further evidence of linkage between the *H-2K* and *Ir-IgA (M467)* genes is shown by the antibody responses of B10 congenic mice in which the H-2 regions were generated from known recombinations. Three different strains derived from recombinations between H-2^a and H-2^b and one strain derived from an H-2^k/H-2^q recombination have been studied. In each case, the pattern of response is similar to that of the parental strain which donated the *H-2K* gene. In particular, the response of the B10·A(4R) and B10·A(5R) strains indicates that *Ir-IgA (M467)* is located to the "left" of Ss-Slp. The data do not establish whether *Ir-IgA (M467)* is between the *H-2K* gene and Ss-Slp or alternatively to the "left" of *H-2K*. Indeed, the genetic information now at hand does not exclude the possibility that *Ir-IgA (M467)* is the *H-2K* gene. We will consider the relationship of *Ir-IgA (M467)* to other *H-2* linked *Ir* genes under Mapping of Ir Genes in the H-2 Complex.

GENETIC CONTROL OF THE IMMUNE RESPONSE TO BALB/c IgG MYELOMA PROTEINS

The immune response of various inbred strains of mice to the BALB/c IgG myeloma protein MOPC 173 is shown in Table VI. The hemagglutinin titer to erythrocytes coated with the MOPC 173 protein represents both anti-idiotype and antiallotype antibody, while the titer against erythrocytes coated with the IgG myeloma protein LPC-1 reflects antiallotype activity only.

Mice of the same Ig-C_H linkage group as BALB/c fail to make a detectable anti-idiotype or antiallotype response as anticipated. Among mice of the $G^{4,6,7,8}$, $G^{5,7,8}$, $G^{3,8}$, and G^- IgG C_H genotypes, all of which differ from that

Table VI. Immune Response to BALB/c IgG (γ_{2a}) Myeloma Protein (MOPC 173)[a]

H-2	C_H determinants	Strain	No. of mice	HA (log 2)	
				M173 immunogen	LPC1 allotype
b	$G^{1,6,7,8}$	129/SN	20	0	0
d		BALB/c	20	0	0
k		C57BR/cd	20	0	0
a	$G^{4,6,7,8}$	A/J	10	1.1	0.6
a		A/He	16	0.8	0.5
b		A.By	14	13.0	1.30
d		NZW	5	0.5	0.3
k		AKR	10	1.7	1.4
s		A.SW	10	14.2	3.6
k	$G^{5,7,8}$	CE	8	0	0
?		DE	8	0	0
b	$G^{3,8}$	D1.LP	17	8.40	6.50
d		DBA/2	9	0.66	0.33
k		RF	8	0	0
q		DBA/1	18	0	0
q		SWR	9	2.9	0.77
r		RIII	8	7.8	8.37
b	G^-	C57BL/6	18	6.5	5.12
b		C57BL/Ka	10	3.60	3.40
h		LP	19	12.83	10.0
d		NBL	8	2.87	2.87
r		LP.RIII	15	9.00	8.50
s		SJL	8	10.87	10.25
v		SM	5	8.83	8.16

[a] Antibodies reacted to M173 identify both allotypic and idiotypic determinants. Antibodies reacted to LPC-1 only identify allotypic determinants. BALB/c IgG myeloma proteins carry IgC_H $G^{1,6,7,8}$ determinants.

Table VII. Immune Response to BALB/c IgG (γ_{2a}) Myeloma Protein (MOPC 173) of B10 Congenic and Recombinant Mice[a]

Strain	Origin of H-2 region				HA (log 2)		
	Chromosome symbol	K	Ss-Slp	D	No. of animals	M173	LPC-1
B10·A	a	k	d	d	9	2.9	2.8
B10	b	b	b	b	15	7.3	6.8
B10·129 (6M)	bc	bc	bc	bc	10	9.1	9.6
B10·D2	d	d	d	d	10	1.2	1.2
B10·BR	k	k	k	k	8	2.0	2.0
B10·P	p	p	p	p	6	11.3	8.7
B10·F	n	n	n	n	4	>12.0	9.3
B10 · A(1R)	hb	k	d	b	9	1.6	0
B10·A(2R)	hc	k	d	b	6	2.7	0
B10·A(4R)	hd	k	b	b	6	8.3	1.6
B10·A(3R)	ib	b	d	d	10	9.8	5.3
B10·A(5R)	ic	b	d	d	10	9.3	2.1

[a] Notes:
  (1) Antisera reacting to the immunogen MOPC 173 identify both allotype and idiotype.
  (2) Antisera reacting to LPC-1 identify only allotype.
  (3) MOPC 173 and LPC-1 carry $G^{1,6,7,8}$ allotypic determinants. IgG proteins of B10 origin are of G^- type.

of the BALB/c, responsiveness to MOPC 173 is associated with H-2 type. Mice of the H-2 types b, r, s, and v generally make vigorous antibody responses to MOPC 173 while mice of the H-2 types a, d, k, and q produce meager or undetectable quantities of antibody.

That responsiveness to MOPC 173 is a dominant trait is shown by the finding that the offspring of a cross between a highly responsive strain of IgG-C_H type G^- and a poorly responsive strain of the same IgG-C_H genotype are good responders. Thus, the progeny of B10·A mice (*H-2*[a]; poor responders to IgG proteins) and LP mice (H-2[b]; good responders to IgG proteins) make an excellent antibody response to MOPC 173.

On the basis of the pattern of responsiveness of congenic strains, an H-2 linked immune response gene for BALB/c IgG myeloma proteins is demonstrated. This gene termed *Ir-IgG (M173)* is associated in the B10 recombinant series (Table VII) with H-2 types b, bc, p, and n, while mice of H-2 types a, d, and k lack the allele at the *Ir-IgG (M173)* locus which permits a vigorous response. An examination of the B10 congenic mice with recombinant H-2 regions derived from H-2^a and H-2^b chromosome types allows us to more precisely determine the H-2 region in which Ir-IgG $(M173)$ is located.

In the B10·A (1R), 2R, and 4R strains, the K gene of the H-2 complex derives from the B10·A parent and is of H-2^a type, while the D gene derives from the B10 parent and is of H-2^b type. In the 1R and 2R strains, the Ss-Slp genes are of H-2^a type, and thus the recombination event generating these chromosomes, which are termed H-2^{hb} and H-2^{hc}, occurred between the Ss-Slp genes and the D gene. In the 4R, on the other hand, the recombination event occurred between the K gene and the Ss-Slp genes. B10·A (1R) and 2R are poorly responsive to MOPC 173 proteins, and B10·A (4R) is a good responder. Thus, the 1R and 2R respond in a manner similar to the B10·A, which donated K and Ss-Slp while the 4R resembles B10 which, in its case, donated Ss-Slp and D. One can conclude on the basis of these three recombinant strains (1R, 2R, and 4R) that Ir-IgG $(M173)$ is to the "right" of K and to the "left" of D.

A more precise localization comes from the examination of the response of B10·A (3R) and 5R. In both these strains the K gene derives from the B10 and the Ss-Slp and D genes from B10·A. Both of these strains are highly responsive to MOPC 173 indicating that the Ir-IgG $(M173)$ gene is to the "left" of Ss-Slp. Thus, on the basis of the response of all five of these recombinant strains we can locate Ir-IgG $(M173)$ to the "right" of K and to the left of Ss-Slp. A more complete discussion of the location of Ir-IgG $(M173)$ in relationship to other Ir genes will be found under the heading Mapping of Ir Genes in the H-2 Complex. It should be pointed out at this time, however, that the pattern of response to the IgA and IgG myeloma proteins exhibited by these recombinant strains indicates that Ir-IgA $(M467)$ and Ir-IgG $(M173)$ are at separate loci in the H-2 complex. This conclusion is derived from the fact that the recombination event generating the B10·A (4R) chromosome (the H-2^{hd} chromosome type) occurred to the "right" of Ir-IgA $(M467)$ and to the "left" of Ir-IgG $(M173)$.

GENETIC CONTROL OF THE IMMUNE RESPONSE
TO BALB/c IgH (γ_{2b}) MYELOMA PROTEINS

The antibody response to the BALB/c IgH myeloma protein MOPC 195 was tested in many of the inbred and H-2 congenic and recombinant strains previously discussed. As was the case with myeloma proteins of other classes, the response was evaluated with erythrocytes coated with MOPC 195 protein and with erythrocytes coated with another IgH myeloma protein, MOPC 141. Antibodies to the former identify both idiotype and allotype; antibodies to the latter only identify allotype.

Several interesting points are revealed from an examination of the response to MOPC 195 (Table VIII). First, two strains of mice of apparently the same

Table VIII. Immune Response to IgH (γ_{2b}) Myeloma Protein (MOPC 195) of BALB/c Origin[a]

H-2	IgH C_H determinant	Strains	No. of mice	HA (log 2)	
				M 195	M141
d	$H^{9,11,22}$	BALB/c	8	0	0
k	$H^{9,11,22}$	C57BRr	8	0	0
d	$H^{9,11,22}$	DBA/2	7	1.3	0.2
k	$H^{9,11,22}$	RF	8	>12.0	0.1
q	$H^{9,11,22}$	DBA/1	8	>12.0	0.4
r	$H^{9,11}$	RIII	4	>12.0	>12.0
k	$H^{9,11}$	CE	8	3.0	0
f	$H^{9,11}$	NH	5	2.4	0
q	H^9	AQR	10	9.9	6.2
a	$H^{23,4}$	AL	8	3.8	3.6
a	$H^{23,4}$	A	8	6.4	5.4
f	$H^{23,4}$	A.Ca	10	6.8	2.8
s	$H^{23,4}$	A.Sw	5	>12.0	>12.0
k	$H^{23,4}$	AKR	5	6.4	0.4
m	$H^{23,4}$	AKR.M	8	0	0

[a] Notes:
  (1) Several strains carrying the same IgH C_H determinants are from different Ig heavy chain linkage groups (see Table III).
  (2) BALB/c IgH (γ_{2b}) myeloma proteins M195 and M141 carry $H^{9,11,22}$ determinants.
  (3) Antisera reacted to the immunogen M195 identify both allotypic determinants and idiotypic determinants; to M141 identify only allotypic determinants.

IgH-C_H type as BALB/c ($H^{9,11,22}$) make a substantial anti-idiotype response to MOPC 195. These strains, RF and DBA/1, although not now distinguishable from BALB/c at the IgH-C_H locus, do not possess the same Ig-C_H linkage group that the BALB/c possesses (Table III). Thus, the BALB/c Ig-C_H genotype is $G^{1,6,7,8} H^{9,11,22} A^{12,13,14} F^{8,19}$ while the DBA/1 and RF genotype is $G^{3,8} H^{9,11,22} A^- F^{8,19}$. Thus, it is possible that unrecognized allotype differences between BALB/c and DBA/1 and RF exist in IgH proteins. Alternatively, the response of these mice may represent an exception from the general rule that anti-idiotype responses are not formed unless the responding strain possesses immunoglobulin of a different allotype than that of the immunizing protein. In addition, the evaluation of immune response to MOPC 195 has allowed the identification of a new allotype specificity (H^{22}) on the basis of antisera prepared in RIII mice to MOPC 195.

Among mice of different IgH C_H types than BALB/c, responses are observed in those of H-2 types a, k, q, r and s while one strain of H-2^m type (AKR.M) fails to respond. This unresponsive strain is of particular importance because it is congenic to the AKR strain, which responds to MOPC-195.

Our analysis of the response of the B10 congenic and recombinant strains is still in progress and is too preliminary to be discussed here. Thus, we cannot, at this time, precisely map the Ir-IgH gene(s) within the H-2 region, although the data in the AKR congenic strains clearly indicates linkage to H-2. Indeed, the fact that AKR mice respond to MOPC-195 and AKR.M mice do not suggests the possibility that an Ir-IgH $(M$-$195)$ gene may be to the right of the Ss-Slp gene. This is so because the AKR.M (H-2^m) histocompatibility type is identical to the AKR (H-2^k) at the K and Ss-Slp genes but differs at the D gene. If this finding can be confirmed, it will be the first demonstration of an Ir-gene associated with the D region gene.

A further point of interest is that H-2 linked genetic control has also been observed in the response of mice to a different BALB/c IgH myeloma protein, UPC-120. Here, however, the pattern of responsiveness is quite different from that to MOPC-195. This suggests that Ir gene products may distinguish between different proteins of the same immunoglobulin class and thus may, under some conditions, recognize idiotypic determinants.

MAPPING OF Ir GENES IN THE H-2 COMPLEX

In this review we have demonstrated the existence of a series of Ir genes which control responses to myeloma proteins of BALB/c origin. We will now indicate the most likely alignment of these genes and their relationship to the genes at the Ir-1 locus (or loci). Figure 1 presents the ordering of these genes in relation to each other and to the three marker genes (K, Ss-Slp, D) of the H-2 complex which at present best explains our results. The support for this ordering of the Ir genes is as follows:

1. The Ir-1 locus is located between the K gene and the Ss-Slp gene(s) on the basis of the extensive studies of McDevitt et al. (1972) on responsiveness of recombinant strains to the branched chains polymers (T,G)-A--L, (H,G)-A--L, and (Phe,G)-A--L. Furthermore, the fact that B10.A (4R) mice resemble B10.A

mice in their responsiveness to the branched chain polymers indicates that *Ir-1* is located to the "left" of the site at which the recombination event generating the H-2 region of the B10.A (4R) occurred.

2. The *Ir-IgA (M467)* locus is also located on the centromeric side of both the *Ss-Slp* genes and the site of the recombination event generating the H-2 region of B10.A (4R) mouse. No information exists to establish whether this gene is to the "right" of the *K* gene, equivalent to the *K* gene, or to the "left" of *K*. It seems likely, moreover, that the *Ir-IgA (M467)* and *Ir-1* are not identical. This is mainly based on the finding that the pattern of responsiveness to IgA and to (H,G)-A-L, although similar in mice of *H-2ᵃ*, *H-2ᵈ*, and *H-2ᵏ* types, is quite different in *H-2ˢ* mice. Two *H-2ˢ* strains (A.Sw and SJL) respond to IgA but not to (H,G)-A-L. This finding, although suggestive, does not establish that the loci are separate. To do that will require a recombinant mouse in which responsiveness to one antigen can be separated from responsiveness to the other antigen.

3. The *Ir-IgG (M173)* locus is placed to the "right" of the *K locus* and of the *Ir-IgA (M467)* and the *Ir-1* loci and to the "left" of the *Ss-Slp* locus principally on the basis of the response of the B10.A (4R) and B10.A (5R) mice. The (4R) derives its *K* gene from the B10.A and its *Ss-Slp* and *D* genes from the B10. It responds to *(T,G)-A-L*, *(H,G)-A-L*, and the IgA myeloma protein M467 like the B10.A, but it responds to the IgG myeloma protein M173 like the B10. Thus, *Ir-IgG (M173)* must be to the right of *Ir-1* and *Ir-IgA (M467)*. In the case of the B10.A (5R) and *K* gene derives from the B10 and the *Ss-Slp* and *D* genes from the B10.A. The B10.A (5R) resembles the B10 in its response to the IgG protein M173 and thus *Ir-IgG (M173)* can be placed to the left of the *Ss-Slp* genes.

4. The *Ir-IgH (M195)* locus (loci) has not yet been mapped. As indicated under Genetic Control of the Immune Response to a BALB/c IgH (γ_{2b}) Myeloma Protein, the relative responsiveness of AKR and AKR.M mice suggest the possibility that this gene is to the "right" of *Ss-Slp*.

Our order for the Ir genes controlling responses to the various myeloma proteins must be regarded as tentative, as the number of recombinations which are relevant are still very small and we have not as yet excluded double crossovers. Nonetheless, this ordering is the simplest, which adequately explains the available data. On the basis of our findings and those of McDevitt *et al.*

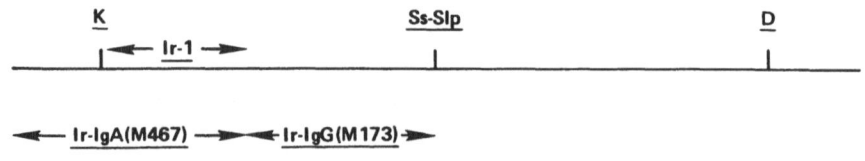

Figure 1

(1972), at least two independent Ir loci in the H-2 complex exist. It seems very possible, moreover, that *Ir-1* and *Ir-IgA (M467)* are separate, and the site of *Ir-IgH (M195)* is still uncertain. On the basis of the study of a small number of antigens at least two and possibly four independent Ir loci within H-2 have already been demonstrated. Moreover, additional examples of H-2 linked genetic control of immune responses have been described (Vaz and Levine, 1970; Vaz *et al.*, 1970; Gasser and Silvers, 1971; Martin *et al.*, 1971; Merryman and Maurer, 1972; Merryman *et al.*, 1972), and although these genes have not yet been formally mapped it seems likely that the number of Ir genes within the H-2 complex will prove to be quite large.

FUNCTION OF Ir GENE PRODUCTS

The genetic control of the immune response of mice to myeloma proteins of BALB/c origin is particularly interesting as it provides a series of related antigens which identify discrete Ir loci. Furthermore, the genetic control is more complex than is true for the branch chain polyaminoacids in mice or for both synthetic and natural antigens in guinea pigs. In order for a mouse to mount a vigorous anti-idiotype antibody response to a given myeloma protein, two requirements must be met. First, the immunizing protein must bear allotypic determinants which the immunoglobulins of the immunized strain lack. Second, the mouse must possess a "responder" form of the Ir gene dealing with that class of immunoglobulin. Both these levels of genetic control appear to concern themselves primarily with *allotypic* determinants of the myeloma protein. Thus, the immune response to several BALB/c IgA myeloma proteins, each with its distinct idiotype, appears to depend upon the same Ig C_H and the appropriate Ir genes. Similar results have been obtained for BALB/c IgG proteins. Nonetheless, the antibody response is principally directed at idiotypic determinants. This is very reminiscent of the situation existing for hapten-carrier conjugates in which the genetic control seems to be specific for the carrier moiety and much of the antibody response is directed at the hapten (Benacerraf *et al.*, 1967). Indeed, we would propose that immune responses to myeloma proteins are classical thymus dependent responses in which the thymus-derived (T) lymphocytes are primarily specific for allotypic determinants, whereas B lymphocytes specific for allotypic and idiotypic determinants exist. Thus, in the absence of T lymphocytes specific for the allotypic determinants on the myeloma protein, responses are rarely obtained even if B cells specific for the relevant idiotypic determinants exist.

In animals whose own immunoglobulins bear the same allotypic determinants as that of the immunizing myeloma protein, the T cell pool would be tolerant in regard to these determinants and no antibody response would ensue even if the myeloma protein bore idiotypic determinants for which host B cells were specific. Furthermore, as *Ir* genes linked to the major histocompatibility complex (MHC) appear to function in T cells (Benacerraf and McDevitt, 1972; Grumet, 1972; Mitchell *et al.*, 1972), animals lacking the appropriate form of a given *Ir-Ig* gene would be deficient in T cells capable of responding to myeloma proteins of a given allotype and would not produce antibody when immunized with that myeloma protein. This formulation is probably somewhat oversimplified, as some recent experiments indicate that the response to different IgH proteins may involve distinct *Ir* genes, suggesting that in some cases Ir genes controlling responses to idiotypic determinants may exist.

How do *Ir* genes and their products control the responsiveness of T lymphocytes to antigens? As an initial point it is clear that *Ir* genes in some way function in the process of antigen recognition as they have a considerable degree of specificity. That is, the *Ir* gene controlling the response to γA proteins is different from that controlling the response to γG proteins. In the guinea pig different *Ir* genes are involved in the immune response to hapten conjugates of bovine serum albumin and of guinea pig albumin (Green and Benacerraf, 1971; Green *et al.*, 1972).

Two general and contrasting mechanisms by which this recognition function is mediated may be considered. The first, for which the evidence appears strongest, is that Ir gene products are recognition structures, probably located on T cell surfaces, which are important in cell activation by antigen. We will consider this possibility at greater length. The second possibility is that *Ir* genes or their products have a regulatory or controlling function which serves in the emergence of specific antigen binding receptors. This type of view holds that the gene in some way controls the receptors which are expressed but that the gene does not directly code for the receptor. The most obvious mechanism of this type is one in which the Ir gene specifies the antigen, or a substance highly cross reactive with the antigen, so that the animal becomes tolerant and does not make a response to that antigen. Although several examples of such genetic control of the immune response exist (Cinader *et al.*, 1964), including the situation for *Ig* C_H genes described here, this mechanism seems excluded for Ir genes linked to the MHC such as those considered in this review. Among the most cogent pieces of evidence against this explanation is the genetics of the *Ir-Ig* systems. In these cases, responses to allotypic proteins which are specified at a locus not linked to *H-2* are controlled by genes mapping within the *H-2* complex. Furthermore, in these instances, as in most other instances of MHC linked *Ir* genes, responsiveness is a dominant trait, which would hardly be expected from a tolerance mechanism. Finally, chimeric animals, such as allophenic mice derived from both responder and nonresponder parents are frequently responders (Bechtol *et al.*, 1972).

A more imaginative proposal is the thesis which Jerne (1971) has advanced to explain the "generation of diversity" in immunologic systems. Jerne suggested that the only recognition structures specified by germ line genes were antibodies specific for determinants coded for by the MHC of the animal, and that each individual member of a species has genes for antibodies specific for all of the possible alternative antigens specified by the MHC genes extant in the species. The individual has, of course, only two of the MHC of the species, one specified by each member of the relevant chromosome pair. Cells bearing receptors specific for antigens specified by the MHCs which the individual possesses are stimulated to divide, and, if mutations in the gene controlling their receptors do not occur, these cells are destroyed. Thus, a selection pressure for mutants at the receptor locus is developed, and these mutants provide the immunologic diversity of the individual. As the starting genes in this generation of diversity are selected by the MHCs of the individual, some relation between MHC and immune response could be anticipated. Against this concept is the very precise linkage between discrete, *independent* loci within the MHC and response to given antigens. This would imply that the number of germ line antibody genes would have to be sufficiently great to code for antibodies specific for products of all the alternatives at each of the *Ir* loci. As the latter is apt to be a very large number, the germ line antibody genes would have to be very numerous, so that much of the simplification inherent in the Jerne hypothesis is vitiated. In addition, the mechanisms allowing the generation from different precursors of genes whose products are capable of the relatively precise discriminations which are observed in genetic control of immune responses are quite obscure. Moreover, there now seems relatively strong evidence suggesting that a "direct action" type hypothesis for Ir gene product function is likely to be correct.

The most cogent evidence for direct involvement of Ir gene products in antigen recognition comes from studies of the effect of alloantisera on genetically controlled immune responses *in vitro*. A series of MHC-linked *Ir* genes exist in strain 2 and strain 13 inbred guinea pigs (Bluestein *et al.*, 1971). Alloantisera specific for strain 2 MHC determinants prevent activation of lymphocytes from immune $(2 \times 13)F_1$ guinea pigs by antigens, the response to which is controlled by an *Ir* gene contained within the strain 2 MHC. Responses controlled by Ir genes linked to the strain 13 MHC, although not blocked by anti-2 sera, are inhibited by anti-13 alloantisera (Shevach *et al.*, 1972). This implies that the Ir gene product directly functions in antigen recognition, and if it is blocked specific activation does not occur.

If the Ir gene product is an antigen-recognition structure, the question of its chemical nature becomes of paramount importance. The main immunologic recognition molecule which we know is immunoglobulin. Can immunoglobulin be the Ir gene product? There is indirect genetic evidence which suggests that "conventional" immunoglobulin is not the product of Ir genes. Mouse C_H genes for G,A,H, and F are not within the MHC (Potter and Lieberman, 1967a), and evidence indicates that V_H genes are linked to C_H genes (Blomberg *et al.*, 1972; Pawlak *et al.*, 1973). This demonstrates that the genes coding for V_H regions of serum immunoglobulin are not within the MHC. However, other sets of immuno-globulin variable region genes might be within the MHC. Study of the phenotype of T lymphocytes has not settled this issue. The question of surface immuno-globulin on T lymphocytes is unresolved (Vitetta *et al.*, 1972; Marchalonis *et al.*, 1972) and the capacity of anti-immunoglobulin sera to block activation of T lymphocytes is not established (Greaves *et al.*, 1969; Mason and Warner, 1970; Basten *et al.*, 1971; Crone *et al.*, 1972). Thus the possibility remains open that a nonimmunoglobulin molecule may function as the T cell receptor and may be the Ir gene product.

In addition, the possibility that Ir gene products, although important in antigen recognition by T lymphocytes, are not the sole or even the main antigen recognition structures of T lymphocytes must be seriously considered. Although speculation on these issues could be carried much further, it seems that progress in this area will require identification of Ir gene products and direct chemical and functional study of these molecules.

One final area which requires comment is the relationship between reactiv-ity in mixed lymphocyte cultures (MLC) and differences at *Ir* loci. Bach and his colleagues (1972) have recently demonstrated that congenic strains of mice possessing the same *K* and *D* genes may nonetheless express reactivity in MLC, strongly suggesting that other genes in the MHC have an important role in the control of the stimulating and/or responding structures on the cell surface. In particular, their studies indicated that differences including the genetic region between the *K* and *Ss-Slp* genes were particularly important in MLC responses. As all the *Ir* genes which have been mapped may be located in this genetic region, it is possible that *Ir* genes are especially important in MLC responses.

The relationship could be that only surface structures coded for by the MHC are important determinants in MLC responses and that Ir gene products are a major (perhaps the most important) set of these structures. Thus, Ir differences and MHC responses would correlate. Indeed, some genetic differences mapping into the region between (and including) *Ss-Slp* and *D* lead to MLC responses and preliminary evidence, discussed under Genetic Control of the Immune Response to a BALB/c IgH (γ_{2b}) Myeloma Protein, suggests the existence of an Ir gene in this general region. Nevertheless, more complex possibilities, such as the identity of Ir genes and genes controlling recognition in MLC responses, can be envi-sioned, but the clarification of these issues requires analysis of the product of these genes.

The study of *Ir* gene systems promises to lead to a major advance in our understanding of the antigen-recognition mechanisms of T lymphocytes. As so many of the immune responses which are of importance in resistance to pathogenic microorganisms and in immune responses to tumor and transplanta-tion antigens are mediated by T lymphocytes, this information should allow much more intelligent efforts to manipulate these crucial immune responses.

ACKNOWLEDGMENT

We are grateful to Dr. Michael Potter for his generous gifts of myeloma proteins and to Drs. J. H. Stimpfling and J. Klein for the many congenic and recombinant mouse stains. Mr. W. Humphrey, Jr., has provided superb technical assistance.

REFERENCES

Bach, F. H., Widmer, M. B., Bach, M. L., and Klein, J., 1972. Serologically defined components of the major histocompatibility complex of the mouse. *J. Exp. Med.* 136:1430.

Basten, A., Miller, J. F. A. P., Warner, N. L., and Pye, J., 1971. Specific inactivation of thymus-derived (T) and non-thymus-derived (B) lymphocytes by [125] I-labelled antigen. *Nature New Biol.* 231:105.

Bechtol, K. B., Herzenberg, L. A., and McDevitt, H. O., 1972. Genetic origin of antibody to (T,G)-A--L in tetraparental mice. *Fed. Proc.* 3163.

Benacerraf, B., and McDevitt, H. O., 1972. Histocompatibility-linked immune response genes. *Science (Washington, D.C.)* 172:273.

Benacerraf, B., Green, I., and Paul, W. E., 1967. The immune response of guinea pigs to hapten-poly-L-lysine conjugates as an example of the genetic control of the recognition of antigenicity. *Cold Spring Harbor Symp.* XXXII:569.

Blomberg, B., Geckler, W. R., and Weigert, M., 1972. Genetics of the antibody response to dextran in mice. *Science (Washington, D.C.)* 177:178.

Bluestein, H. G., Green, I., and Benacerraf, B., 1971. Specific immune response genes of the guinea pig. I. Dominant genetic control of immune responsiveness to copolymers of L-glutamic acid and L-alanine and L-glutamic acid and L-tyrosine. *J. Exp. Med.* 134:458.

Cinader, B., Dubiski, S., and Wardlaw, A. C., 1964. Distribution, inheritance and properties of an antigen, MUB1 and its relation to hemolytic complement. *J. Exp. Med.* 120:897.

Crone, M., Koch, C., and Simonsen, M., 1972. The elusive T cell receptor. *Transpl. Rev.* 10:35.

Eichmann, K., 1972. Idiotypic identity of antibodies to streptococcal carbohydrate in mice. *Eur. J. Immunol.* 2:301.

Gasser, D. L., and Silvers, W. K., 1971. Genetic control of the immune response in mice. III. An association between H-2 type and reaction to H-Y. *J. Immunol.* 106:875.

Gold, E. R., and Fudenberg, H. H., 1967. Chromic chloride: a coupling reagent for passive hemagglutinating reactions. *J. Immunol.* 99:859.

Greaves, M. F., Torrigiani, G., and Roitt, I. M., 1969. Blocking of the lymphocyte receptor site for cell mediated hypersensitivity and transplantation reactions by anti-light chain sera. *Nature* 222:885.

Green, I., and Benacerraf, B., 1971. Genetic control of immune responsiveness to limiting doses of proteins and hapten conjugates in guinea pigs. *J. Immunol.* 107:374.

Green, I., Paul, W. E., and Benacerraf, B., 1972. Histocompatibility-linked genetic control of the immune response to hapten guinea pig albumin conjugates in inbred guinea pigs. *J. Immunol.* 109:457.

Grumet, F. C., 1972. Genetic control of the immune response. A selective defect in immunologic (IgG) memory in nonresponder mice. *J. Exp. Med.* 135:110.

Herzenberg, L. A., McDevitt, H. O., and Herzenberg, L. A., 1968. Genetics of antibodies. *Ann. Rev. Genet.* 2:209.

Jerne, N. K., 1971. The somatic generation of immune recognition. *Eur. J. Immunol.* 1:1.

Klein, J., 1973. H-2 system: past and present. *Transpl. Proc.* (in press).

Klein, J., and Shreffler, D. C., 1972. Evidence supporting a two-gene model for the H-2 histocompatibility system of the mouse. *J. Exp. Med.* 135:924.

Lieberman, R., and Humphrey, W., Jr., 1972. Association of H-2 types with genetic control of immune responsiveness to IgG (γ2a) allotypes in the mouse. *J. Exp. Med.* 136:1222.

Lieberman, R., and Humphrey, W., Jr., 1971. Association of H-2 types with genetic control of immune responsiveness to IgA allotypes in the mouse. *Proc. Nat. Acad. Sci., U.S.A.* 68:2510.

Lieberman, R., Paul, W. E., Humphrey, W., Jr., and Stimpfling, J. H., 1972. H-2 linked immune response (Ir) genes. Independent loci for Ir-IgG and Ir-IgA genes. *J. Exp. Med.* 136:1231.

Marchalonis, J. J., Cone, R. E., and Atwell, J. L., 1972. Isolation and partial characterization of lymphocyte surface immunoglobulins. *J. Exp. Med.* 135:956.

Martin, W. J., Maurer, P. H., and Benacerraf, B., 1971. Genetic control of immune responsiveness to glutamic acid, alanine, tyrosine copolymers in mice. I. Linkage of responsiveness to H-2 genotype. *J. Immunol.* 107:715.

Mason, S., and Warner, N. L., 1970. The immunoglobulin nature of the antigen recognition site on cells mediating transplantation immunity and delayed hypersensitivity. *J. Immunol.* 104:762.

McDevitt, H. O., and Chinitz, A., 1969. Genetic control of antibody response: relationship between immune response and histocompatibility (H2) type. *Science (Washington, D.C.)* 163:1207.

McDevitt, H. O., Deak, B. D., Shreffler, D. C., Klein, J., Stimpfling, J. H., and Snell, G. D., 1972. Genetic control of the immune response. Mapping of the Ir-1 locus. *J. Exp. Med.* 135:1259.

Merryman, C. F., and Maurer, P. H., 1972. Genetic control of immune response to glutamic acid, alanine, tyrosine copolymers in mice. I. Association of responsiveness to H-2 genotype and specificity of the response. *J. Immunol.* 108:135.

Merryman, C. F., Maurer, P. H., and Bailey, D. W., 1972. Genetic control of immune response in mice to a glutamic acid lysine, phenylalanine copolymer. III. Use of recombinant inbred strains of mice to establish association of immune response genes with H-2 genotype. *J. Immunol.* 108:937.

Mitchell, G. F., Grumet, F. C., and McDevitt, H. O., 1972. Genetic control of the immune response. The effect of thymectomy on the primary and secondary antibody response of mice to poly-L-(Tyr,Glu)poly-D, L-Ala-poly-L-Lys. *J. Exp. Med.* 135:126.

Pawlak, L. L., Hart, D. A., Nisonoff, A., Mushinski, E. B., and Potter, M., 1973. Evidence for the linkage of the IgC$_H$ locus to a gene controlling the idiotypic specificity of anti-p-azophenylarsonate antibodies in strain A mice. *J. Exp. Med.* 137:22.

Potter, M., 1972. Immunoglobulin producing tumors and myeloma proteins of mice. *Physiol. Rev.* 52:631.

Potter, M., and Lieberman, R., 1967a. Genetic studies of immunoglobulin in mice. *Cold Spring Harbor Symp. Quant. Biol.* 22:187.

Potter, M., and Lieberman, R., 1967b. Genetics of immunoglobulins in the mouse. *Adv. Immunol.* 11:31.

Sher, A., and Cohn, M. O., 1972. Inheritance of an idiotype associated with the immune response of inbred mice with phosphorylcholine. *Eur. J. Immunol.* 2:326.

Shevach, E. M., Paul, W. E., and Green, I., 1972. Histocompatibility-linked immune response gene function in guinea pigs. *J. Exp. Med.* 136:1207.

Shreffler, D. C., 1970. Immunogenetics of the mouse H-2 system. In D. Aminoff (ed.), *Blood and Tissue Antigens,* Academic Press, New York, pp. 85–99.

Sirisinha, S., and Eisen, H. N., 1971. Autoimmune-like antibodies to the ligand binding sites of myeloma proteins. *Proc. Nat. Acad. Sci., U.S.A.* 68:3130.

Vaz, N. M., and Levine, B. B., 1970. Immune responses of inbred mice to low doses of antigen. Relationship to histocompatibility (H-2) type. *Science (Washington, D.C.)* 168:852.

Vaz, N. M., Vaz, E. M., and Levine, B. B., 1970. Relationship between histocompatibility (H2) genotype and immune responsiveness to low doses of ovalbumin in the mouse. *J. Immunol.* **104**:1572.

Vitetta, E., Bianco, C., Nussenzweig, V., and Uhr, J., 1972. Cell surface immunoglobulin. IV. Distribution among thymocytes, bone marrow cells and their deprived populations. *J. Exp. Med.* **136**:81.

Warner, N. L., 1971. Autoimmunity and the origin of plasma cell tumors (abstr.). *J. Immunol.* **107**:937.

Chapter 6

Histocompatibility Systems, Immune Response, and Disease in Man

Peter J. Morris*

Tissue Transplantation Laboratories and Department of Surgery
University of Melbourne, Royal Melbourne Hospital
Melbourne, Australia

INTRODUCTION

Over the last few years there has been an explosion of interest in the possible association of disease with the major histocompatibility system of man, HL-A. This interest arose first as a result of the demonstration of a linkage between susceptibility of mice to leukemia and H-2 (the major histocompatibility system in the mouse) and second as a result of the more recently demonstrated linkages between the genetic control of certain immune responses in mice and guinea pigs and the major histocompatibility systems of those two species. The human studies have been beset with difficulties attributable mainly to the serological difficulties associated with the determination of certain specificities of the HL-A system as well as the complex nature of many of the diseases investigated.

Nevertheless, many of the studies to be discussed in this review are strongly suggestive of an association between HL-A and certain diseases, but an interpretation of the nature of such associations can only be speculative at this time. As these speculations are based to a considerable extent on the work relating histocompatibility systems to leukemia in the mouse and to immune response genes in both the mouse and the guinea pig, these subjects will be briefly reviewed. However, the major section of the review will deal with the evidence for such an association in man.

This work has been supported in part by grants from the National Health and Medical Research Council of Australia, the Australian Kidney Foundation, and the Anti-Cancer Council of Victoria.
* Reader in Surgery, and Director.

HL-A AND H-2

HL-A is the major histocompatibility system in man, while H-2 is the major histocompatibility system in the mouse. These two systems appear to be homologous, and for this reason will be considered together. The recent developments in our knowledge of the genetic control of the H-2 region are relevant to HL-A and the subsequent discussions of HL-A and disease associations.

The HL-A system is an extremely complex one, and has been defined serologically on peripheral blood leukocytes and platelets. The specificities or "antigens" of this system can be divided into two series behaving as if they were determined by mutually exclusive alleles at each mutational site or locus (Table I). These loci are known as the first and second locus or the LA and Four locus. Over the last few years most of the undetected alleles have been determined in Caucasian populations, leaving a few low frequency specificities to be found in each series. The two loci are closely linked with a recombination frequency of

Table I. The HL-A System of Leukocyte Antigens with Caucasian Gene Frequences ($g = 1 - \sqrt{1-f}$ where f Is Antigen Frequency)[a]

First or LA locus antigens		Second or four locus antigens	
Antigen	Gene frequency	Antigen	Gene frequency
HL-A1	0.15	HL-A5	0.07
HL-A2	0.29	HL-A7	0.11
HL-A3	0.12	HL-A8	0.10
HL-A9	0.11	HL-A12	0.18
W23 (9.1)	0.02	HL-A13	0.03
W24 (9.2)	0.09	W5	0.09
HL-A10	0.06	W10	0.06
W25 (10.1)	0.02	W14	0.04
W26 (10.2)	0.03	W15	0.06
HL-A11	0.07	W16	0.04
W19	0.13	W17	0.04
W29 (19.1)	0.05	W18	0.05
W30 (19.3)	0.02	W21	0.03
W31 (19.4)	0.07	W22	0.03
W32 (19.5)	0.04	W27	0.04
W28	0.04		
TOTAL	0.93	TOTAL	0.97

[a] Some of the previously defined HL-A antigens have now been shown to comprise more than one component, e.g., HL-A9, and these components have been given a provisional W number.

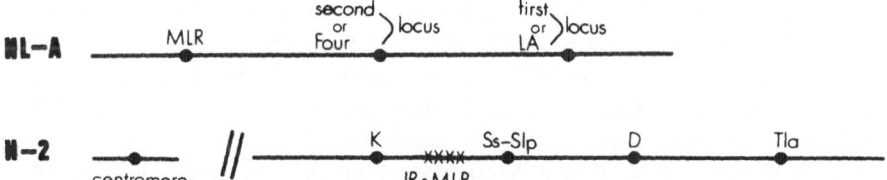

Figure 1. A comparison between the postulated genetic structure of the HL-A and H-2 histocompatibility systems (see text): MLR—mixed lymphocyte reaction locus; IR—immune response loci.

between 0.5% and 1% (Bodmer *et al.*, 1970; Svejgaard *et al.*, 1971). Several of the antigen combinations of the two series show a significant linkage disequilibrium in Caucasians, e.g., HL-A1 and HL-A8, which perhaps suggests the existence of some selective advantage for this haplotype.[1]

The definition of HL-A specificities has been difficult in that it has become increasingly apparent that there is an extreme degree of cross reactivity between the specificities within each series (but not across both series). This then has led to the further dissection of many of the more established HL-A specificities into narrower cross-reacting specificities included in the reactions of the original broader specificity. This, together with the fact that few truly identical antisera exist for most specificities has led to the suggestion that the presently defined serological specificities comprise a number of factors or determinants (Dausset *et al.*, 1965; Batchelor and Sanderson, 1970; Legrand and Dausett, 1973). Certainly much of the serological data from studies of different racial groups during the recent Fifth International Histocompatibility Workshop can only be explained satisfactorily on the basis of such a concept.

The stimulation of allogeneic lymphocytes in culture has been considered to be determined by incompatibility for the serologically determined HL-A specificities. However, a growing amount of evidence now suggests that the mixed lymphocyte reaction (MLR) is determined by a separate locus outside the first and second locus, and the MLR locus is as closely linked to the second locus as are the two serologically determined loci to each other (Yunis *et al.*, 1971; Dupont *et al.*, 1971; Gatti *et al.*, 1971; Eisjvoogel *et al.*, 1973; Sasportes *et al.*, 1972; Mempel *et al.*, 1972). Thus our concept of the HL-A system is now one of three mutational sites or loci, the products of two of these being determined serologically, while the products of the third can only be determined in a MLR (Fig. 1).

There has been a marked change in recent times in our concept of H-2, the

---

[1] A haplotype is the commonly used term in this field for the combination of an antigen of the first series and an antigen of the second series present on the same chromosome, e.g., HL-A1.8; HL-A3.7.

major histocompatibility system in the mouse, for it now appears that the genetic control of H-2 is very similar to that of HL-A, which does provide some considerable support for the speculations concerning the nature of the associations of HL-A with disease based on H-2 associations. The private specificities of H-2 can be arranged into two segregant series, just as in HL-A, these specificities again behaving as if they were determined by mutually exclusive alleles (Klein and Shreffler, 1971). These two loci are known as the D and K loci (with a recombination frequency of about 0.5%). In between these two serologically determined loci is a locus controlling quantitative and qualitative variation of a serum protein (Ss-Slp). This locus has nothing to do with histocompatibility but does provide an extremely useful marker for recombination in the H-2 area, allowing precise mapping of other genes in this H-2 complex.

The first of these of relevance to our discussion are the immune response genes (IR genes) which control the immune response to a number of antigens and will be discussed in more detail later. Let it suffice to say that at least one of these genes, IR1 [controlling the response to (T-G)-A--L], has been precisely mapped by McDevitt et al. (1972) between the K and Ss locus using appropriate recombinant strains. The response to immunoglobulin allotypes has also been mapped in the same area (Lieberman, 1973), so that one can envisage a linear arrangement of IR genes between the K and Ss locus.

The second locus is that controlling the MLR in the mouse. Again through the use of recombinant strains it has been possible to demonstrate that the MLR is not determined by serologically determined differences at the K and D loci predominantly, but by the products of a separate locus mapping between the K and the Ss locus, in the same general area as the IR genes (Shreffler, 1973; Bach and Klein, 1973). Until the gene products of the IR and MLR loci can be identified, it will not be possible to determine whether they are one and the same.

H-2 AND MURINE LEUKEMIA

Some well-defined but complex associations between H-2 and murine leukemias have been determined. Two such examples will be briefly discussed as they illustrate the potential difficulties of demonstrating associations between HL-A and disease in man.

The association between H-2 and Gross virus leukemogenesis was first described by Lilly et al. (1964) in studies of crosses between a susceptible strain of mice C3H(H-2^k) and a resistant strain C57BL(H-2^b). In the F1 hybrid (H-2^k/H-2^b), resistance proved to be dominant, and in segregating generations infected with the virus, the homozygotes (H-2^k/H-2^k) proved to be universally susceptible to the virus while the homozygotes (H-2^b/H-2^b) and heterozygotes (H-2^k/H-2^b) showed varying degrees of susceptibility (Table II). As further

Table II. Susceptibility to Gross Virus Leukemogenesis
and H-2 Type (Lilly, 1966)

Strain	H-2 type	% Developing leukemia	Mean latent period (days)
C3H	$H\text{-}2^k/H\text{-}2^k$	100%	69
C57BL	$H\text{-}2^b/H\text{-}2^b$	26%	191
(C3H×C57BL)	$H\text{-}2^k/H\text{-}2^b$	9%	258
	$H\text{-}2^k/H\text{-}2^k$	91%	86
F1×C3H			
	$H\text{-}2^k/H\text{-}2^b$	56%	90

strain combinations were studied it became apparent that at least two genes were involved in determining susceptibility to the Gross virus, one of which Lilly has named Rgv-1, which is closely linked to H-2. Rgv-1 has now been mapped at the K end of H-2 and might well be synonymous with the IR genes. A second gene, Rgv-2, was based on calculations of the number of independent segregating genes needed to explain the incidence of leukemia in the F1 backcross and F2 generations. Even more compelling evidence has been provided for the existence of genes other than Rgv-1 determining susceptibility to Gross leukemia virus more recently by Lilly (1971), when he showed that the F1 cross of two susceptible strains was in fact highly resistant to leukemia. This could only be explained on the basis of homozygosity for a recessive trait in both animals for more than one gene, not linked on the same chromosome. Thus the relationship between Gross virus leukemogenesis and H-2 is not an absolute one. Lilly has suggested that possibly the genes not linked to H-2 determine the ability of the virus to infect the host cells while the H-2 linked gene influences the progress of the disease to leukemia after infection has occurred. There is a marked delay in onset of leukemia in the resistant strains that develop the Gross leukemia compared to that in the susceptible strains.

An even more complex picture is seen in the case of the Friend murine leukemia virus which causes foci of neoplastic erythroid cells in the spleen of susceptible animals with subsequent development of leukemia. This is an excellent example of a disease in which susceptibility is controlled by many genes (Lilly, 1973). First, the virus itself is a complex, comprising SFFV (spleen focus-forming virus) which requires a helper virus for virion maturation and is specific for erythroid cells, and LLV (lymphatic leukemia virus) which acts as a helper virus for SFFV, induces leukemia, and is specific for a broad range of tissues. The genetic control of the disease is even more complex. First one gene, Fv-2, not linked to H-2, has an effect on the infectivity of SFFV, and here susceptibility is dominant, rather than resistance. This suggests that the effect of this gene is at the level of viral penetration. Further genes affecting erythroid differentiation (W, S1, F) also influence erythropoietic aspects of the Friend virus disease. Another gene, Fv-1, influences the helper activity of the LLV component of the Friend virus complex. None of these above-mentioned genes is linked to H-2. Finally, the gene Rgv-1, already discussed in relation to the Gross virus, and which is linked to H-2, probably affects the course of disease by influencing the immune response to virus-associated antigens. It seems likely that Rgv-1 influences susceptibility to most leukemia viruses as well as the mammary tumor virus (Lilly, 1973).

These two examples of associations between H-2 and susceptibility to leukemia in mice show that the genetic control of leukemia in mice is complex, and that the linkage with H-2 is only one of many genetic influences affecting the course of the disease. However, these examples serve to illustrate the potential problems of demonstrating significant associations between HL-A and disease in man, bearing in mind that one is also dealing with an outbred population, which complicates the genetic picture even further.

IMMUNE RESPONSE GENES

During the past decade the immune response to a rapidly growing number of antigens of restricted heterogeneity has been found to be genetically controlled. This genetic control in many instances has been shown to be linked to the major histocompatibility systems of mice, guinea pigs, and rats. As these developments have been extensively reviewed in a series of papers (McDevitt and Benaceraff, 1969; Benaceraff and McDevitt, 1972; McDevitt et al., 1972; Grumet and McDevitt, 1973) it is not proposed here to do more than summarize the current status of knowledge of the IR genes.

The antigens used for the demonstration of IR genes have needed to be of highly restricted heterogeneity and specificity and are of three types:

1. Synthetic polypeptides with limited numbers of different L-amino acids and their hapten conjugates, e.g., linear polymers—poly-L-lysine (PLL), dinitrophenyl poly-L-lysine (DNP-PLL); branched chain copolymers—poly-L-lysine backbone with poly-L-alanine side chains and terminal groups of glutamic acid with tyrosine [(T,G)-A--L] or histidene [(H,G)-A--L];
2. Weak native antigens, e.g., Ea-1[a] antigen on wild mice erythrocytes; mouse male (Y) histocompatibility antigen;
3. Limiting doses of strong native protein antigens, e.g., bovine serum albumin (BSA), hen albumin.

In most instances the genetic control of the immune response to these antigens has been shown to be closely linked to the major histocompatibility system of the species under investigation. For example, in the guinea pig, the gene controlling the response to PLL is so closely linked to the strain 2 histocompatibility gene that it has not been possible to differentiate it from the histocompatibility gene even in random-bred animals (Martin *et al.*, 1970). In the mouse, where much more precise knowledge of the genetic control of H-2 is available, it has proved possible to map the gene controlling the immune response to (T,G)-A--L between the K end of H-2 and the Ss locus, as described previously (McDevitt *et al.*, 1972). Thus the immune response genes are closely linked to the major histocompatibility systems in these species, and the immune response gene products may in fact be histocompatibility antigens. Although in the mouse the gene product is separate to the serologically detected products of the K and D loci, this does not mean that it cannot act as a histocompatibility antigen.

The immune response genes are autosomal dominant genes, and hence the hybrid offspring of a high responder and a low responder strain will be high responders. High responder strains exhibit both an IgM and IgG antibody response and delayed hypersensitivity after antigenic challenge, while a low responding strain exhibits only an IgM response. The ability to respond may be transferred to irradiated nonresponders with spleen, lymph node, or bone marrow cells, demonstrating that this genetic control is a function of immunocompetent cells.

A nonresponder animal will produce an IgG response similar to that of a responder (but not delayed hypersensitivity) if the antigen is attached to a carrier, thus suggesting that B cells can recognize the antigen but need to be triggered appropriately by T cell activation. It has also been shown recently that B cells in both high and low responder strains bind similar amounts of (T,G)-A--L although more cells bind antigen in the high responder strain after immunization (Hämmerling *et al.*, 1973). Furthermore, either neonatal thymectomy or adult thymectomy plus irradiation and bone marrow reconstitution will convert the immune response of a high responder to that of a low responder, i.e., an IgM response only (Mitchell *et al.*, 1972). Thus T cells are necessary for the expression of the immune response gene and seem to be involved at the stage of conversion of the IgM response to IgG. In the absence of activated T cells the switch over to IgG does not occur. As shown recently by Ordal and Grumet (1972) T cells can be activated by means other than a carrier by the induction of a graft versus host (GVH) reaction in the low responding F1 offspring of two low responder strains. The GVH reaction has to be induced at the time of antigenic challenge, to produce the switch over from IgM to IgG production.

Thus the immune response gene products appear to be expressed on T cells, and appear to be concerned in antigen recognition so that these cells are activated to trigger B cells and so switch the IgM response over to an IgG response in those B cells. However, it is not known whether the immune response gene products are expressed on B cells as well as T cells. Recent investigations of the response to (T,G)-A--L in allophenic mice suggest that they are not (Freed *et al.*, 1973). In these investigations allophenic mice were produced by fusing the mouse embryos of two congenic strains, one being a high responder and the other a low responder. The two strains differed not only in their H-2 genotype but also in their immunoglobulin allotype. If the immune response gene product is expressed only on T cells, then it could be expected that the high responder T cells would activate the B cells of both high and low responder origin, resulting in IgG antibody of both strain allotypes. If expressed on B cells too, then one would expect antibody only of the high responder strain allotype. The results of these investigations favor the former hypothesis, namely that the immune response gene product is present only on T cells, although these findings are not clear cut. In addition, the possibility of nonspecific stimulation of B cells by allogeneic interaction in these allophenic mice cannot be excluded.

The nature of the immune response gene product is not known. Although immunoglobulins have been demonstrated on T cells (Marchalonis *et al.*, 1972; Marchalonis and Cone, 1973), it is difficult to accept that the immune response gene product is an immunoglobulin, for there is no linkage between the genes controlling the constant and variable regions of the immunoglobulin heavy chains and either H-2 or HL-A. Thus one would have to postulate a new immunoglobulin receptor specific for T cells or the existence of another structural gene for heavy chains linked to the histocompatibility genes. Although possible, these alternatives do not seem as attractive as postulating the existence of a new antigen recognition system, acting either alone or in collaboration with immunoglobulin receptors.

The demonstration of immune response genes linked to histocompatibility genes in three species with 25 different antigens in a relatively short space of time suggests that these immune response genes play an important role in controlling immune responses to a wide variety of antigenic stimuli. They may therefore have considerable significance in influencing susceptibility to disease through their effect on the immune response to infectious agents, such as oncogenic viruses.

HL-A AND DISEASE

With the impetus of the investigations linking H-2 and leukemia in mice and more recently IR genes with histocompatibility systems in mice and guinea pigs, there has been a tremendous surge of studies of HL-A in disease, limited only by the relative paucity of HL-A typing laboratories. With the information now available, it should be possible to make some valid assessment of the existence of associations between HL-A and disease. Before discussing the different disease groups in more detail, the problems of establishing significant associations between various diseases and HL-A should be considered.

Serological Inadequacy in the Definition of HL-A Specificities

Some mention has already been made of this, but it should be borne in mind that many of the W specificities, in particular (Table I), are not well defined. This problem is perhaps more important in the comparison of studies from different laboratories.

The Definition of the Disease Itself

Obviously to group leukemias or lymphomas together in such studies would be incorrect as they are unlikely to have common etiologies, be they viral or otherwise. But even the different types of leukemia, as presently defined, may in fact represent more than one type of leukemia. For example, it would appear that chronic lymphatic leukemia may be divided into two subclasses based on whether it is a B cell leukemia or not (Wilson and Nossal, 1971). Thus failure to recognize such difficulties may obscure any association with HL-A that exists. Hodgkin's disease provides another such problem, in that it is unlikely that all cases labeled as Hodgkin's represent a disease with a common etiology. Thus studies of large groups of Hodgkin's may obscure associations with particular subgroups of the disease. Awareness of the above two problems assists in the interpretation of results, but there is no ready solution of these difficulties in many instances at this time.

Statistical Evaluation of an Association Between an HL-A Specificity and a Disease

The frequency of a particular antigen may be significantly altered from the normal, with a p value of less than 0.05. However, it must be remembered that the chances of finding such a significant association increase with the number of comparisons being made (Bodmer, 1971). For example, if the frequencies of 20 HL-A specificities are being compared in a disease population and in a normal population, there is a 1 in 20 chance of one of these comparisons being significantly altered at the 5% level. This can be corrected by multiplying the calculated p value by the number of HL-A specificities that have been compared. These corrected values have been given in Tables III-VI. The corrected p values have been taken from the original report, or have been calculated from the data in the report, if adequate. It can be noted that the majority of significant altered frequencies of HL-A reported in the following tables become insignificant after the application of a correction factor. This problem can also be solved without the application of a correction factor by mounting a pilot study of a particular disease. If an altered frequency of an HL-A specificity is found to be significant, a second prospective study is commenced, and if the same change is observed, then this is highly significant.

LEUKEMIAS (Table III)

Acute lymphatic leukemia in children has been the most intensively studied leukemia, since Walford's first description of a possible association between the

Table III. Studies of HL-A in Leukemias[a]

Disease	Reference[b]	Patients	Antigens showing an altered frequency ($p<0.05$)	Significance after correction factor
Acute lymphatic	(1)	28	↑HL-A2.12 haplotype	n.s.[c]
leukemia	(2)	34	↓HL-A11	n.s.
	(3)	102	-	-
	(4)	50	↑HL-A2	0.002
	(5)	58	-	-
	(6)	17	-	-
	(7)	16	↓HL-A1; ↑HL-A12	n.s.; <0.05
	(8)	10	-	-
	(9)	98	↑HL-A2; ↑HL-A8; ↑HL-A12; ↓HL-A9 (↑HL-A2.12 haplotype)	<0.002; n.s.; <0.002 n.s.
	(10)	20	-	-
	(11)	24	-	-
Chronic	(12)	44	-	-
lymphatic	(7)	21	↑W27	0.0005
leukemia	(13)	28	-	-
Chronic				
myeloid	(2)	15	↑HL-A1	n.s.
leukemia	(12)	47	↑HL-A3; ↓HL-A12	n.s.; n.s.
Acute myeloid				
leukemia	(2)	33	↑HL-A2	n.s.

[a] Only significant alterations in the distribution of HL-A are listed, both with and without a correction factor (see text).

[b] (1) Thorsby et al. (1971); (2) Jeannet and Magnin (1972); (3) Kourilsky et al. (1967); (4) Rogentine et al. (1972); (5) Lawler et al. (1971a); (6) Batchelor et al. (1971); (7) Walford et al. (1971); (8) Singal et al. (1971); (9) Sanderson et al. (1973); (10) Harris and Viza (1971); (11) Waters et al. (1973); (12) Degos et al. (1971); (13) Jeannet and Alberto (1972).

[c] n.s.—not significant at the 5% level.

disease and an increase in HL-A2 and HL-A12 as a haplotype (Walford *et al.*, 1970). Later studies by Walford *et al.* (1971) showed that only HL-A12 was significantly increased after the application of a correction factor. A possible increase of the HL-A2.12 haplotype has been seen in two other series, but in most studies no altered frequency of HL-A has been observed. The most thorough studies of this disease recently have been those of Lawler *et al.* (1971*b*) from the United Kingdom and Rogentine *et al.* (1972) from the United States, where quite large numbers of patients together with their families were studied. The U.K. study revealed no abnormal distribution of antigens or of antigen segregation in the families. However, the American study demonstrated a marked increase in the frequency of HL-A2. This study is of particular interest, for Negroes in the U.S. have a much lower frequency of HL-A2 than Caucasians (29% *vs.* 42% in this study), and also a much lower frequency of acute lymphatic leukemia than Caucasians (1.44 per 100,000 *vs.* 2.11 per 100,000).

At present, therefore, no firmly established association between HL-A and leukemia exists, although the study of Rogentine *et al.* (1972) mentioned above is very convincing. It is also of note that an increase in HL-A2 is seen in most of the other studies reported, although only reaching significance in the studies of Rogentine *et al.* (1972) and Sanderson *et al.* (1973).

The recent reports of Jeannet and Alberto (1972) and Walford *et al.* (1973) that certain HL-A antisera give an increased frequency with chronic lymphatic leukemia cells, not related to HL-A, emphasize the need for caution in attributing increased reactivity of anti HL-A antisera to increased frequency of HL-A antigens in the disease under study. It is suggested that this increased reactivity reflects the detection of leukemia specific antigens. For this reason family studies are particularly important to exclude the possibility that the increased reactivity of an anti-HL-A serum in a disease is due to the presence of an antibody to a disease specific antigen, for in this case segregation of the antigen would not occur in the family.

LYMPHOMAS (Table IV)

Hodgkin's disease is the most intensively studied with respect to HL-A of any so far. The first report of a disease association with HL-A was that of Amiel (1967), who found a significantly increased frequency of a specificity known as 4c at that time. This was confirmed by Forbes and Morris (1971) sometime later. But in addition they found that in their series, the increase in the frequency of 4c was due almost entirely to an increased frequency of W5, a specificity included in 4c. As was mentioned earlier, there is an extreme degree of cross reactivity existing in the HL-A system, and 4c represents one such example. 4c includes three cross-reacting antigens, HL-A5, W5, and W18, and in addition W15 crossreacts with these antigens to a greater or lesser extent. This then is relevant to the studies noted in Table IV, where it can be seen that one of this cross-reacting group of antigens was significantly increased in frequency in

Table IV. Studies of HL-A in Malignant Lymphomas[a]

Disease	Reference[b]	No. of patients	Antigen showing an altered frequency ($p<0.05$)	Significance after correction factor
Hodgkin's	(1)	41	↑4c	ns.[c]
	(2)	78	↑4c	<0.05
	(3)	127	↑HL-A11; ↑W5; ↑HL-A7	n.s.; <.006; n.s.
	(4)	112	↑HL-A1; ↑A5;	n.s.; n.s.
			↑HL-A8	n.s.
	(5)	98	↑W5; ↑5a	<0.05; <0.05
	(6)	82	↑HL-A10; ↑W18	n.s.; <0.05
	(7)	27	↑HL-A5	n.s.
	(8)	50	↑HL-A1; ↑HL-A8;	n.s.; n.s.
			↑W18	n.s.
	(9)	44	↑HL-A2; ↓HL-A3	n.s.; n.s.
	(10	33	↑W15	n.s.
	(11)	39	↑HL-A11	n.s.
	(12)	321	↑HL-A5; ↑W18;	n.s.; n.s.
			↓HL-A8	n.s.
	(13)	477	↑HL-A1; ↑W18;	n.s.; n.s.
			↑HL-A8; ↓HL-A12;	n.s.; n.s.
			↓HL-A13	n.s.
	(16)	20	↑HL-A5	n.s.
Follicular	(14)	56	↑HL-A12	<0.001
lymphoma	(12)	51	↑W5	n.s.
Reticulum cell sarcoma	(14)	28	-	-
Lymphosarcoma	(14)	50	↑HL-A7	n.s.
	(12)	39	↑W28	n.s.
Lymphomas (excluding	(10)	21	↑W28	n.s.
Hodgkin's)	(15)	39	↑HL-A12	<0.05
Myeloma	(6)	40	↑W18	<.002
	(10)	14	-	-

[a] Only significant alterations in the distribution of HL-A are listed, both with and without a correction factor (see text).

[b] (1) Amiel (1967); (2) Amiel (1971); (3) Morris and Forbes (1971a); (4) Falk and Osoba (1971); (5) van Rood and van Leeuwen (1971); (6) Bertrams et al. (1972a); (7) Zervas et al. (1970); (8) Kissmeyer-Nielsen et al. (1971a); (9) Coukell et al. (1971); (10) Jeannet and Magnin (1972); (11) Thorsby et al. (1971); (12) Takasugi et al. (1973); (13) Morris et al. (1973b); (14) Morris and Forbes (1971b); (15) Dick et al. (1972); (16) Roege et al. (1972).

[c] n.s.—not significant at the 5% level.

11 of these 13 studies, thus suggesting that there was an overall increase in the 4c/W15 group of cross-reacting antigens in Hodgkin's disease. That this was not attributable to the disease process itself was adequately excluded by Forbes and Morris (1972) in a large family study, which failed to show any abnormal segregation of HL-A, in particular in relation to the 4c antigens.

As a result of these studies it was decided to conduct an international collaborative study of HL-A and Hodgkin's disease as part of the Fifth International Histocompatibility Workshop, with a view to firmly establishing an association of this disease with HL-A. Eleven laboratories were involved, all using a common panel of antisera. As much of the histology as possible was reviewed by a panel of pathologists headed by H. Rappaport (Chelloul *et al.*, 1973). A total of 477 patients were included in the study, and the individual reports are included in *Histocompatibility Testing 1972* (Dausset and Bodmer, 1973). However, the report of the collaborative study (Morris *et al.,* 1973) showed increased frequencies of HL-A1, HL-A8, and W18, only the latter belonging to the 4c group of antigens. The increase in HL-A1 and HL-A8 had been noted in a previous study by Kissmeyer-Nielsen *et al.* (1971a).

Attempts to study smaller subgroups based on histology and age failed to reveal any striking changes other than that HL-A10 was increased in the older age group (over 45 years of age) of Hodgkin's patients, which may well be considered a different disease. However, the collaborative study did point out some of the difficulties of such projects. For example, some 10% of the histological sections submitted as Hodgkin's disease were not, in fact, so. Again, there were considerable discrepancies in the reactivity of certain antisera in different centres, both in the control and in Hodgkin's populations. In addition, because of the time factor, the studies were not prospective, and this may have led to a selection bias.

Thus it is still not possible to state that a definite association with HL-A has been established, although the weight of evidence does suggest that it exists. Further careful prospective studies will need to continue, and indeed a number of these are in progress. However, Hodgkin's disease may be an unrewarding one for such studies because of the heterogeneity of the disease itself.

With respect to the other lymphomas, there is a suggestion that the frequency of HL-A12 may be significantly increased, while a very significant increase in W18 in myeloma has been noted by Bertrams *et al.* (1972a).

IMMUNOPATHIC DISEASES (Table V)

In this group of diseases are included not only the well-defined autoimmune diseases but also diseases which are possibly autoimmune in origin or represent an abnormal sensitivity to an allergen. It is in this group that some of the most clear-cut associations between HL-A and disease are appearing.

Table V. Studies of HL-A in Immunopathic Diseases[a]

Disease	Reference[b]	No. of patients	Antigen showing an altered frequency ($p<0.05$)	Significance after correction factor
Systemic	(1)	24	↑W15	n.s.[c]
lupus	(2)	40	↑HL-A8; ↑W15	<0.02; n.s.
erythematosus	(3)	31	↑HL-A8	<0.001
Active chronic hepatitis	(4)	40	↑HL-A1; ↑HL-A8	<0.02; < .001
Myasthenia gravis	(5)	60	↑HL-A1; ↑HL-A8; ↑HL-A12	n.s.; <0.001 n.s.
Adult coeliac	(6)	49	↑HL-A1; ↑HL-A8	<0.02; <0.02
disease	(7)	24	↑HL-A8	<0.05
Ragweed hyper-sensitivity	(8)	46 (in 7 families)	Association with several HL-A haplotypes ($p<.01$)	
Childhood asthma	(9)	35	↑HL-A1 (↑HL-A1.8 haplotype)	n.s.
Multiple sclerosis	(10)	393	↑HL-A3; ↓HL-A9; ↓HL-A12; ↓HL-A13; ↑W5	n.s.; n.s. n.s.; n.s.; <0.01
	(11)	94	↑HL-A3; ↑W18; ↓HL-A2	<0.02; n.s.; n.s.
	(12)	56	↑HL-A3; ↑HL-A7	n.s.; n.s.
	(19)	135	↑HL-A3; ↑HL-A7	n.s.; n.s.
Dermatitis herpetiformis	(20)	35	↑HL-A1; ↑HL-A8	n.s.; n.s.
Rheumatoid	(13)	104	-	-
arthritis	(3)	34	-	-
Juvenile diabetes	(14)	44	-	-
Thyrogastric	(15)	33	-	-
autoimmunity	(21)	48	↑HL-A8	-
Rheumatic fever	(16)	76	↓HL-A3	n.s.
Glomerulo-nephritis	(17)	707	↑HL-A2	?
Regional enteritis	(18)	19	-	-

The most striking alterations found in autoimmune diseases are the increased frequency of HL-A1 and/or HL-A8 in systemic lupus erythematosus (SLE), active chronic hepatitis, myasthenia gravis, and W15 in SLE (Waters *et al.*, 1971; Grumet *et al.*, 1971; Mackay and Morris, 1972; Morris and Mackay, in prep.; Engelfriet *et al.*, in prep.). Again, in adult coeliac disease, which probably represents a hypersensitivity to gluten, a highly significant increase in HL-A8 appeared in two studies, from the U.S. and the U.K., respectively (Stokes *et al.*, 1972; Falchuk *et al.*, 1972). HL-A1 was also significantly increased in the U.K. study. It is also of interest that HL-A1 and/or HL-A8 may be associated with childhood asthma (Thorsby and Lie, 1971), augmented renal allograft rejection (Kissmeyer-Nielsen *et al.*, 1971b; Mickey *et al.*, 1971), and dermatitis lerpetiformis, another probable immunapathic disorder (White *et al.*, 1973). A recent report (Levine *et al.*, 1972) of an association between HL-A and ragweed hypersensitivity is exciting. In seven families, ragweed hypersensitivity segregated with HL-A, but with a different haplotype in each family. Certainly it is striking at this time how often HL-A1 and HL-A8 have shown an increased frequency in this group of diseases.

The autoimmune diseases showing the increased frequency of HL-A8 (and HL-A1 less often) belong to the multisystem cluster as described by Mackay (1969). These include SLE, dermatomyositis, scleroderma, active chronic hepatitis, myasthenia gravis, and Sjögren's disease. While in the thyrogastric cluster, which includes autoimmune thyroid disease, pernicious anemia, Addison's disease, hypoparathyroidism, and possible diabetes mellitus, no abnormal distribution of HL-A has been demonstrated, possible with the exception of thyrotoxicosis although it must be remembered that few studies have been reported. Thus it is possible that the association with HL-A might be found with a certain group of autoimmune disorders.

In four studies of multiple sclerosis, a neurological disorder in which both viral and autoimmune etiologies have been suggested, there is a significant increase in HL-A3 in all studies, while HL-A7 and the cross-reacting antigens W5 and W18 are increased in two of the studies. Thus here, too, there is a quite strong suggestion of an association with HL-A (Bertrams *et al.*, 1972b; Naito *et al.*, 1972; Arnason *et al.*, 1973; Jersild *et al.*, 1973).

---

[a] Only significant alterations in the distribution of HL-A are listed, both with and without a correction factor (see text).

[b] (1) Waters *et al.* (1971); (2) Grumet *et al.* (1971); (3) Morris and Mackay (1973); (4) Mackay and Morris (1972); (5) Engelfriet *et al.* (1973); (6) Stokes *et al.* (1972); (7) Falchuk *et al.* (1972); (8) Levine *et al.* (1972); (9) Thorsby and Lie (1971); (10) Bertrams *et al.* (1972b); (11) Naito *et al.* (1972); (12) Arnason *et al.* (1973); (13) Kueppers *et al.* (1973); (14) Finkelstein *et al.* (1972); (15) Whittingham *et al.* (1973); (16) Falk *et al.* (1973); (17) Mickey *et al.* (1970); (18) Thorsby and Lie (1971); (19) Jersild *et al.* (1973); (20) White *et al.* (1973); (21) Grumet *et al.* (1973).

[c] n.s.—not significant at the 5% level.

Table VI. Studies of HL-A in Genetic Disorders[a]

Disease	Reference[b]	No. of patients	Antigen showing an altered frequency ($p<0.05$)	Significance after correction factor
Psoriasis	(1)	66	↑HL-A13; ↑W17	<0.002; n.s.[c]
	(2)	156	↑HL-A13; ↑W17; ↓HL-A12	<0.01; <0.02 <0.0001
	(3)	86	↑HL-A13; ↑W17	n.s.; <0.001
	(5)	44	↑HL-A13; ↑W17	n.s.; <0.0001
Retinoblastoma	(4)	122	↑W5*; ↓HL-A12 (* hereditary form only)	<0.02; <0.02

[a] Only significant alterations in the distribution of HL-A are listed, both with and without a correction factor (see text).

[b] (1) Russell et al. (1972); (2) White et al. (1972); (3) Grumet (1973); (4) Bertrams et al. (1973); (5) Svejgaard et al. (1973).

[c] n.s.—not significant at the 5% level.

GENETIC DISEASES (Table VI)[1]

Psoriasis, a common dermatological disease with a strong genetic influence, has perhaps shown the most consistent findings in relation to HL-A, in that in three quite large studies the frequencies of both HL-A13 and W17 were found to be increased, and in most instances these altered frequencies were still significant after the application of a correction factor (Russel et al., 1972; White et al., 1972; Grumet, 1973; Svejgaard et al., 1973).

Retinoblastoma is included in this group, although it is a childhood cancer, for it does have a strong genetic influence in its etiology. A very significant increase of W5 was found in the hereditary form of the disease only, while HL-A12 was decreased in both forms of the disease (Bertrams et al., 1973).

CANCER (OTHER THAN LYMPHOMAS) (Table VII)

A wide variety of solid tumors have been studied, mainly from Terasaki's group, but no striking associations have appeared with the exception of retinoblastoma, mentioned above, and nasopharyngeal carcinoma in Chinese (Simons et. al., 1973).

[1] Ankylosing spondylitis, another disease which might be included in this group, has recently been shown to have a striking association with W27 in two separate studies (Caffrey and James, 1973, Schlosstein et al., 1973). The frequency of W27, namely, 95% and 88% respectively, in patients in these two studies compared with around 8% in normal Caucasians represents the most significant association between HL-A and a disease yet described.

Table VII. Studies of HL-A in Cancer (Other Than Lymphomas)[a]

Cancer	Reference[b]	No. of patients	Antigen showing an altered frequency ($p<0.05$)	Significance after correction factor
Melanoma	(1)	101	↓W18	=0.05
	(2)	50	-	-
Nasopharyngeal Ca	(3)	144	↑HL-A2; ↓HL-A11 ↓HL-A13; ↓W10; ↓W18	<0.05; n.s.; <0.05; n.s.; n.s.
Bladder	(2)	139	↓W5	n.s.
Breast	(2)	384	↑HL-A1	n.s.
Prostate	(2)	214	-	-
Lung	(2)	250	↓W5	n.s.
	(4)	146	↑HL-A8; ↓W14; ↓W15; ↓W27	n.s.; n.s.; n.s. n.s.
Colon	(2)	121	↓W5	n.s.
Cervix	(2)	142	↑HL-A1; ↓HL-A9; ↑HL-A12	n.s.; n.s. n.s.
Rectum	(2)	55	↑HL-A9	n.s.
Stomach	(2)	63	-	-
Endometrium	(2)	68	-	-
Ovary	(2)	69	-	-

[a] Only significant alterations in the distribution of HL-A are listed, both with and without a correction factor (see text).

[b] (1) Kueppers *et al.* (1973); (2) Takasugi *et al.* (1973); (3) Simons *et al.* (1973); (4) Pietsch and Morris, (1973*a*).

[c] n.s.—not significant at the 5% level.

The HL-A and nasopharyngeal cancer study in the Chinese population of Singapore and Hong Kong is of particular interest in that this tumor may well have a viral etiology. It has indeed a marked predilection for Chinese originating from Southern China.

INFECTIOUS DISEASES (Table VIII)

This group of diseases should be of particular interest, especially those that have been significant in the form of epidemics in man's history. Unfortunately

Table VIII. Studies of HL-A in Infectious Diseases[a]

Disease	Reference[b]	Patients	Antigen showing an altered frequency ($p<0.05$)	Significance after correction factor
Tuberculosis	(1)	119	-	-
Haemophilus influenzae	(2)	25	↓HL-A8*; ↑W28* (* in epiglottis form only)	n.s.; n.s.[c]
Infectious mononucleosis	(3)	110	↑4c	n.s.
Poliomyelitis	(4)	111	↑HL-A3; ↑HL-A7	$<0.02; <0.02$
Australia antigen carriers	(5)	48	↑HL-A3; ↑W19	?; ?
Sarcoidosis	(6)	132	-	-

[a] Only significant alterations in the distribution of HL-A are listed, both with and without a correction factor (see text).

[b] (1) Rosenthal et al. (1973); (2) Whisnant et al. (1971); (3) Ting et al. (1972); (4) Pietsch and Morris (1973a); (5) Vermylen et al. (1972); (6) Kueppers et al. (1973).

[c] n.s.—not significant at the 5% level.

there are no data available for such infectious diseases which might have influenced man's evolution. The most impressive results to date are the increased frequency of HL-A3 and HL-A7 in people who had previously suffered paralytic poliomyelitis before the introduction of the Salk vaccine [Pietsch and Morris, 1973a (a)]. Insufficient data were available regarding the virus type causing the disease, as this may have enabled even more precise definition of the HL-A association with poliomyelitis, as the types 1, 2, and 3 poliomyelitis viral antigens do not crossreact to any great extent.

The increase of the 4c group of antigens in infectious mononucleosis (Ting et al., 1973) is of interest in view of the possible relationship between Hodgkin's disease and this infection (Lukes et al., 1969; English, 1970), remembering that the 4c group of antigens is probably associated with Hodgkin's disease. However, until further studies are carried out, this can only be regarded as an interesting possible linkage between the two conditions.

HL-A AND IMMUNE RESPONSES

There is little information available in man concerned with the study of associations between HL-A and immune responses. The most striking report to date is that describing a strong association between ragweed hypersensitivity and HL-A. In the first study (Levine *et al.*, 1972) seven families were studied, and IgE antibody production segregated with HL-A, but with different haplotypes in each family. In the second study (Marsh *et al.*, 1973) a strong association between HL-A7 and reaginic skin sensitivity to a minor ragweed pollen allergen was demonstrated.

My group has examined the HL-A phenotypes of the high and low responders to immunization with salmonella Adelaide flagellin. This group had been previously studied in relation to Gm allotypes and in fact it seemed that a high response to flagellin was associated with Gm a,g (Wells *et al.*, 1971). As might be expected, bearing in mind that there is no association between Gm allotypes and HL-A, no altered frequency of HL-A antigens has been found in the two groups. This does emphasize that genes other than histocompatibility linked immune response genes can influence the immune response to antigens, as also illustrated by the response of mice to Dextran (Blomberg *et al.*, 1972).

A search for possible associations between HL-A and skin test reactions to mumps, candida, trichophyton, varidase, and tuberculin is being carried out by my group. To date a significant increase in HL-A1 and HL-A8 has appeared with reactivity to trichophyton. These two antigens also show an increased frequency, but not significantly so, in people giving a positive response to mumps antigen.

A significant association has been shown between the production of anti-HL-A antisera in response to transfusions, pregnancy, or renal allografting and the HL-A phenotype of the serum producer (Morris and Dumble, 1972). However, this is probably due to the absence of any cross reactivity between the molecular configuration of the immunizing HL-A antigens and those of the recipient resulting in a vigorous response to certain antigens, rather than an association between an immune response gene controlling the response to HL-A antigens and HL-A.

There is need for a great deal of further investigation in this area. One of the problems that investigators are faced with is the ethical one of immunizing volunteers with antigens of limited heterogeneity, as used in the mouse, with the possible risk of inducing undesirable crossreacting immune responses. However, it should be possible to do much of this work in *in vitro* systems which would enable one to bypass these ethical considerations of immunizing human volunteers.

NATURE OF ASSOCIATION BETWEEN HL-A AND DISEASE

The HL-A system of histocompatibility antigens is a complex polymorphic system, and it seems reasonable to attribute a major biological role to such a polymorphic system of cell surface antigens. The major histocompatibility systems of all other species also exhibit a similar degree of polymorphism, and presumably have a similar role. The mechanism by which this genetic polymorphism is maintained is unknown, and has been discussed in detail by Bodmer (1972). Let it suffice to say that in general a balanced polymorphism is maintained by some selective advantage for the heterozygote over the homozygote. This does not necessarily imply that every polymorphism is maintained in this way, for a selective pressure on one genetic system would induce a balanced polymorphism in a closely linked neutral system.

The marked differences in HL-A patterns in different racial groups lend support to evolution of the HL-A system in Caucasians by selective pressure. The most likely agent of this selective pressure over the ages would be infection. For example, the HL-A pattern of the New Guinea Highlanders (Morris *et al.*, 1971) reveals a very restricted degree of polymorphism with a high degree of homozygosity. As this is not found for other polymorphisms in this area, it suggests that this population may not have been exposed to the selective pressures leading to the extreme degree of polymorphism found in Caucasians. This is perhaps indirect evidence in favor of the maintenance of the HL-A polymorphism by some selective advantage for the heterozygote.

Perhaps more direct evidence is provided by the study of Piazza *et al.* (1973) of HL-A patterns in populations of common origin in Sardinia, both in the lowlands where malaria was endemic until recently, and in the highlands where malaria has not existed. There was a much greater frequency of the two red cell abnormalities, thalassaemia and G-6-P-D deficiency, in the lowlands, as compared to the highlands. It is now commonly accepted that thalassaemia, G-6-P-D deficiency, and sickle-cell anaemia are balanced polymorphisms maintained through the selective advantage of the heterozygote over the homozygote toward plasmodial infection. In the Sardinian studies there was also a significant difference between the frequencies of the second locus HL-A antigens of the highlands and the lowlands, which did not exist for 22 other genetic markers, suggesting that differential selection, through the agency of malaria, was responsible for these differences in HL-A. As malaria has been the most significant disease in mankind's history in terms of human wastage, it could certainly be expected to have exerted the greatest selective pressure on any polymorphism where the heterozygote received some advantage. Malaria would explain similar differences in HL-A between the populations of the New Guinea Highlands and coastal areas (Morris *et al.*, 1973a), but in this case the picture is not so clear, due to the different origins, at least in time, of the two populations.

If, then, the HL-A polymorphism is maintained by selective pressures, one might expect to find an association between HL-A and certain diseases that could exert such a pressure. A more direct stimulus to such studies was provided both by the demonstration of the association of susceptibility to murine leukemias and H-2 and the linkage between immune response genes and the major histocompatibility systems of mice and guinea pigs. However, the experimental data does point out the difficulties that are to be expected in studies of disease and HL-A in man. First, leukemia susceptibility in mice is under the control of several genes in all models studied, which complicates the search for associations in the outbred population. Second, immune response genes have been demonstrated with antigens of very restricted heterogeneity, and many of these are not suitable for use in man. Nevertheless, considerable progress has been made in the studies relating HL-A and disease, as described earlier.

At this stage it can be said that there are some fairly definite associations between HL-A and certain disease states. With respect to cancer, it seems likely that an association exists with Hodgkin's disease, although this is not clearly established, and possibly there is an association with acute lymphatic leukemia in children and with nasopharyngeal cancer in Chinese. A strong association with myeloma and with retinoblastoma in single studies needs to be confirmed. A common factor in these cancers, with the exception of retinoblastoma, is the distinct possibility that they might be due to a virus (Hehlmann et al., 1972a,b). In the case of retinoblastoma of children there is a strong genetic influence in its etiology.

There is little evidence in other cancers, where a viral etiology is less likely, to suggest that an association with HL-A may exist. Of the predominantly genetic disorders, psoriasis is the only one studied in depth, and here there is a striking concordance between the results of separate studies suggesting a very real association between HL-A and psoriasis. The immunopathic disorders represent another group of diseases where some very convincing data exist suggesting an association with HL-A. The most striking feature of this group of conditions is that the antigen showing an increased frequency was generally HL-A8, with or without a similar alteration in the frequency of HL-A1. Finally, a limited number of infectious diseases have been investigated, and here a strong association with poliomyelitis has been demonstrated in one study.

Thus the data available to date might be said (if I am allowed to take some liberties) to show an association between HL-A and tumors of viral etiology, certain immunopathic disorders, certain genetic disorders, and possibly viral infections if the poliomyelitis study is considered to be valid. What then could be the nature of such associations, and can any mechanism of association common to all the above disease groups be proposed?

One possibility that must be excluded in any consideration of an association between HL-A and disease is that it represents the detection of a non-HL-A antigen, say a tumor specific antigen, by an antibody present in the HL-A antisera. That such can occur has been demonstrated in chronic lymphatic leukemia (Jeannet and Magnin, 1972; Walford et al., 1973). However, the family studies in the diseases in question allow this possibility to be excluded, and a number of such studies have been done, as for example in Hodgkin's (Forbes and Morris, 1972) and acute lymphatic leukemia (Rogentine et al., 1972). In all cases the HL-A antigen in question has shown a normal segregation within the family. Thus this possible explanation can be excluded from consideration.

The second possible explanation for an association between HL-A and disease is that particular HL-A antigens act as a receptor site for a virus causing the disease, facilitating cell penetration. There are some data hinting at this possibility, as for example the previously discussed Fv-2 locus affecting susceptibility of mice to the SSFV component of the Friend virus. Here, susceptibility is dominant over resistance, which is recessive, suggesting that this locus exerts its influence at a stage of viral penetration. However, this locus is not linked to a known histocompatibility system. Again, Crittenden and Briles (1971) have demonstrated an association between susceptibility to the subgroup B Rous sarcoma virus in chickens and the erythrocyte antigen, R1. As susceptibility of chick embryo fibroblasts to these viruses *in vitro* can be shown to be genetically controlled, and thus dominant over resistance (Crittenden, 1968), it again suggests an effect at a cell surface level. It has not yet proved possible to demonstrate the presence of R1 on these chick embryo fibroblasts used in the latter experiments, which would firmly relate the presence of an erythrocyte isoantigen on the cell surface to viral penetration, but this might be due to technical difficulties. Dausset *et al.* (1972) have studied the susceptibility of fibroblasts in culture, established from members of HL-A phenotyped families, to infection with a number of DNA and RNA viruses. Other genetic markers were also noted. No evidence for an effect of HL-A or of the other genetic markers on susceptibility to any of the viruses could be demonstrated. But although histocompatibility antigens have not been shown to be involved in viral adsorption and penetration, it is certainly a distinct possibility.

One of the problems about postulating such a mechanism is that it would mean that the heterozygote would be susceptible to the virus. Theoretically, then, this would remove any selective advantage the heterozygote had over the homozygote in the maintenance of the HL-A polymorphism. However, as susceptibility or resistance is certain to prove a polygenic effect, as illustrated by the mouse leukemia models, and the possible viral tumors that may be associated with HL-A are relatively uncommon, I do not find this possibility unacceptable.

The third explanation has been termed by Snell (1968) "molecular mimicry." This hypothesis states that the viral antigens are so similar to the cell surface histocompatibility antigens that an initial immune response against the virus is not initiated, the organism recognizing the virus as self. This mechanism might also act at the level of viral expression at the cell surface after infection when either the viral antigens or resulting tumor antigens fail to stimulate an immune response because of their similarity to the host's own histocompatibility antigens. The report by Tennant (1968) that appropriate H-2 antisera neutralize the B/T-L leukemia virus supports such a concept, as does the cross reactivity between HL-A antigens and streptococcal M protein shown by Hirata *et al.* (1970) although this finding could not be confirmed by Fox and Peterson (1970). Here again the argument against this hypothesis is the same as for the previous suggestion, namely that in such a case susceptibility would be dominant in the heterozygote, thus not giving the heterozygote any selective advantage in evolution.

The fourth explanation would propose a linkage between immune response genes and HL-A as the reason for HL-A and disease associations. As discussed earlier, the immune response gene effect is dominant over susceptibility, and this then makes it less attractive as a mechanism for linking viral infections or tumors to HL-A, unless it is postulated that in such cases, as for example Hodgkin's disease, the linked immune response gene is defective, resulting in a deficient immune response to either the causative virus or the tumor antigen. There is no evidence in the human that the HL-A associations in these diseases are associated with the homozygous expression of a particular HL-A antigen, which would be compatible with the recessive homozygosity of susceptibility. However, it is possible that in these instances it is not the linkage between HL-A and a defective immune response gene that determines susceptibility, but a linkage between HL-A and another gene determining susceptibility to the disease in a way not yet known.

In the case of the immunopathic diseases, a linkage with an immune response gene is most attractive in concept. However, it does not appear that this can be an immune response gene in the conventional sense, where a relatively high degree of specificity appears to exist, as the antigens which are appearing as disease-associated in this group are for the most part HL-A8 with or without HL-A1. As the immunogenic stimuli in these disorders, ranging from active chronic hepatitis to gluten enteropathy, seem unlikely to have anything in common, this means that one must postulate a gene linked to HL-A8 (or possibly the HL-A1.8 haplotype) which can affect immune responsiveness in general. On the other hand, it should be remembered that the association between ragweed hypersensitivity and HL-A demonstrated in families by Levine *et al.* (1972) was not with a particular antigen or haplotype, but with several. This could be due presumably to the existence of several very specific IR genes to ragweed antigens, or to a rather loose linkage between the ragweed antigen IR gene and HL-A, such that there is a high degree of recombination between the two. However, the family data described in their report do not favor this latter suggestion.

Thus, more information is needed about immune responses to a variety of antigens in the human, as this may elucidate this point. However, the very strong association of HL-A8 with a number of autoimmune and allergic disorders makes the former hypothesis worthy of consideration, and perhaps suggests that there is more than one mechanism of control of immune responsiveness associated with HL-A in man. Such a mechanism could have a marked selective advantage in that the presence of HL-A8, or possibly the HL-A1.8 haplotype in the child would provide an increased resistance to infection. The slight disadvantage given by a greater propensity to develop autoimmune disorders would not outweigh the above, in that these would not become evident until later on in the reproductive life. Such a selective advantage for HL-A1.8 might explain the present linkage disequilibrium that exists between these two antigens in Caucasians.

It is worthy of note that in general the reported associations of HL-A and disease are with second locus antigens. As the MLR locus appears to be at the second locus end of HL-A, and as the immune response genes in the mouse have been mapped in the same area of H-2 as the locus determining MLR, this might be considered as indirect evidence that immune response genes are involved in the association between HL-A and disease.

In the case of the genetic disorders, such as psoriasis, it is possible that the gene determining psoriasis is linked to HL-A. However, it could also be postulated that there are fewer genes influencing the development of this common dermatological condition, and hence the association between an immune response gene linked to HL-A and the disease is not obscured to such an extent as in other HL-A associated conditions. However, no etiological agent has been described for psoriasis for which an immune response gene might be involved.

The evolution of HL-A as an extremely complex polymorphism does suggest an important biological role for this system of cell surface antigens, other than its role in stimulating graft rejection, as does the apparent maintenance of this polymorphism in Caucasians. The possible association between HL-A and disease does allow rational hypotheses, based on animal models, to be formed concerning the maintenance of such a polymorphism. However, the nature of these possible associations between HL-A and disease is not clear. It is possible that more than one of the possible mechanisms described above could be involved in different circumstances. Some more recent data in the immunopathic disorders suggest involvement of an immune response gene linked to HL-A, which appears to be extremely broad in its specificity, in contradistinction to the IR genes described in the mouse and guinea pig which have a relatively restricted specificity. But in the case of the leukemias and lymphomas, as well as in the genetic disorders, there is little evidence which favors primarily any of the possible mechanisms discussed already for the association between HL-A and disease.

REFERENCES

Amiel, J. L., 1971. Hodgkin's disease and HL-A. *Transpl. Proc.* 3:1277.

Amiel, J. L., 1967. Study of the leucocyte phenotypes in Hodgkin's disease. In E. S. Curtoni, P. L. Mattiuz, and M. R. Tosi (eds.), *Histocompatibility Testing 1967,* Munksgaard, Copenhagen, pp. 79–81.

Arnason, B. G., Fuller, T. C., Lehrich, J. R., and Winn, J. H., 1972. Leukocyte antigens (HL-A) in multiple sclerosis. *Proceedings of the Transplantation Society Congress.* p. 8. (abstract).

Bach, F., and Klein, J., 1973. In M. Landy and H. McDevitt (eds.), *Genetic Control of Immune Responsiveness,* Academic Press, New York.

Batchelor, J. R., Edwards, J. H., Stuart, J., 1971. HL-A and Acute Lymphocytic Leukemia. *Lancet* 1:699.

Batchelor, J. R., and Sanderson, A. R., 1970. Implications of cross-reactivity in the HL-A system. *Transpl. Proc.* 2:133.

Benaceraff, B., and McDevitt, H., 1972. Histocompatibility-linked immune response genes. *Science* 175:273.

Bertrams, J., Schildberg, P., Hopping, W., Böhme, U., and Albert, E., 1973. HL-A antigens in retinoblastoma. *Tissue Antigens* 3:78.

Bertrams, J., Kuvert, E., Böhme, U., Reis, H. E., Gallmeier, W. M., Wetter, O., and Schmidt, C. G., 1972a. HL-A antigens in Hodgkin's disease and multiple myeloma. *Tissue Antigens* 2:41.

Bertrams, J., Kuwert, E., and Liedtke, U., 1972b. HL-A antigens and multiple sclerosis. *Tissue Antigens* 2:405.

Blomberg, B., Geckeler, W. R., and Weigert, M., 1972. Genetics of the antibody response to Dextran in mice. *Science* 177:178.

Bodmer, W. F., 1971. In discussion. *Transpl. Proc.* 3:1294.

Bodmer, W. F., 1972. Evolutionary significance of the HL-A system. *Nature* 237:139.

Bodmer, W. F., Bodmer, J. G., and Tripp, M., 1970. Recombination between the LA and 4 loci of the HL-A system. In P. Terasaki (ed.), *Histocompatibility Testing 1970*, Munksgaard, Copenhagen, pp. 187–191.

Caffrey, M. F., and James, D. C., 1973. Human lymphocyte Antigen Association in Ankylosing Spondylitis, *Nature* 242:121.

Chelloul, N., Burke, J., Motteram, R., Capon, J. Le, and Rappaport, H., 1973. HL-A antigens and Hodgkin's disease (ii) Report on the histological analysis. In J. Dausett and W. Bodmer (eds.), *Histocompatibility Testing 1972*, Munksgaard, Copenhagen. pp. 769-771.

Coukell, A., Bodmer, J. G., and Bodmer, W. F., 1971. HL-A types of 44 Hodgkin's patients. *Transpl. Proc.* 3:1291.

Crittenden, L. B., 1968. Observations on the nature of a genetic cellular resistance to Avian tumor viruses. *J. Nat. Cancer Inst.* 41:145.

Crittenden, L. B., and Briles, W. E., 1971. Genetic resistance to infection and oncogenesis by Avian RNA tumor viruses. *Transpl. Proc.* 3:1259.

Dausset, J., and Bodmer, W. (eds.), 1973. *Histocompatibility Testing 1972*, Munksgaard, Copenhagen.

Dausset, J., Florman, A. L., Bachvaroff, R., Kanra, G. Y., Sasportes, M., and Rapaport, F. T., 1972. *In vitro* approach to a correlation of cell susceptibility to viral infection with HL-A genotypes and other biological markers. *Proc. Soc. Exp. Biol. (N.Y.)* 140:1344.

Dausset, J., Ivanyi, P., and Ivanyi, D., 1965. Tissue alloantigens in humans: identification of a complex system (Hu 1). In J. Dausset and W. Bodmer (eds.), *Histocompatibility Testing 1965*, Munksgaard, Copenhagen, pp. 51–62.

Degos, L., Drolet, Y., and Dausset, J., 1971. HL-A antigens in chronic myeloid leukemia (CML) and chronic lymphoid leukemia (CLL). *Transpl. Proc.* 3:1309.

Dick, F. R., Fortuny, I., Theologides, A., Greally, J., Wood, N., and Yunis, E. B., 1972. HL-A and lymphoid tumors. *Cancer Res.* 32:2608.

Dupont, B., Staub Nielsen, L., and Svejgaard, A., 1971. Relative importance of Four and LA loci in determining mixed lymphocyte reaction. *Lancet* 2:1336.

Eijsvoogel, V. P., du Bois, M. J., Melief, C. J. M., de Groot-Kooy, M. L., Koning, C., van Rood, J. J., van Leeuwen, A., du Toit, E., and Schellekens, P., 1973. Position of a locus determining mixed lymphocyte reaction (MLR), distinct from the known HL-A loci, and its relation to cell mediated lympholysis (CML). In J. Dausset and W. Bodmer (eds.), *Histocompatibility Testing 1972*, Munksgaard, Copenhagen. pp. 501-508.

Engelfriet, C. P., Feltkamp, Th. E. W., Nijenhuis, L. E., Galama, S. M. D., Rijn, A. van, Loghem, E. van, Berg-Loonen, E. van den, Possum, A. van, and Loghem, J. van. HL-A phenotype and haplotype frequencies in patients with myasthenia gravis, in preparation.

English, J. M., 1970. Infectious mononucleosis followed by Hodgkin's disease. *Lancet* 1:948.

Falchuk, Z. M., Rogentine, G. N., and Strober, W., 1972. Predominance of histocompatibility antigen HL-A8 in patients with gluten-sensitive enteropathy. *J. Clin. Invest.* 51:1601.

Falk, J., and Osoba, D., 1971. HL-A antigens and survival in Hodgkin's disease. *Lancet* 2:1118.

Falk, J. A., Fleischman, J. L., Zabriskje, J. B., and Falk, R. E., 1973. A study of HL-A antigen phenotype in rheumatic fever and rheumatic heart disease patients. *Tissue Antigens* 3:173.

Finkelstein, S., Zeller, E., and Walford, R. L., 1972. No relation between HL-A and juvenile diabetes. *Tissue Antigens* 2:74.

Forbes, J. R., and Morris, P. J., 1972. Analysis of HL-A antigens in patients with Hodgkin's disease and their families. *J. Clin. Invest.* 51:1156.

Forbes, J. F., and Morris, P. J., 1970. Leucocyte antigens in Hodgkin's disease. *Lancet* 2:849.

Fox, E. N., and Peterson, R. D., 1970. Streptococcal M protein vaccines, rheumatic fever and human histocompatibility antigens. *J. Immunol.* 105:1031.

Freed, J. H., Bechtol, K. B., Herzenberg, L. A., and McDevitt, H. O., 1973. Analysis of anti-(T,G)-A–L antibody in tetraparental mice. *Transpl. Proc.* 5:167.

Gatti, R. A., Meuwissen, J. H., Terasaki, P. I., and Good, R. A., 1971. Recombination within the HL-A locus. *Tissue Antigens* 1:239.

Grumet, F. C., 1972. Preliminary HL-A typing of 86 psoriasis patients and 100 control patients, personal communication.

Grumet, F. C., Coukell, A., Bodmer, J. G., Bodmer, W. F., and McDevitt, H. O., 1971. Histocompatibility antigens associated with systemic lupus erythematosus. *New Engl. J. Med.* 285:193.

Grumet, F. C., Konishi, J., Payne, R. D., and Kriss, J. P., 1973*b*. Association of Graves' Disease with HL-A8. Personal communication.

Grumet, F. C., and McDevitt, H. O., 1973*a*. The nature of the responding organism: responders and non-responders. In A. J. S. Davies and R. L. Carter (eds.), *Current Topics in Immunobiology*, Vol. 2, Plenum Press, New York.

Hämmerling, G. J., Masuda, T., and McDevitt, H. O., 1973. Genetic control of the immune response: frequency and characteristics of antigen binding cells in high and low responder mice. *J. Exp. Med.* 137:1180.

Harris, R., and Viza, D., 1971. HL-A leukaemia, and leukaemia-associated antigens. *Lancet* 1:1134.

Hehlmann, R., Kufe, D., and Spiegelman, S., 1972*a*. RNA in human leukemic cells related to the RNA of a mouse leukemia virus. *Proc. Nat. Acad. Sci.* 69:435.

Hehlmann, R., Kufe, D., and Spiegelman, S., 1972*b*, Viral-related RNA in Hodgkin's disease and other human lymphomas. *Proc. Nat. Acad. Sci.* 69:1727.

Hirata, A. A., Armstrong, A. S., Kay, J. W. D., and Terasaki, P. I., 1970. Specificity of inhibition of HL-A antisera by streptococcal M proteins. In P. I. Terasaki (ed.), *Histocompatibility Testing 1970*, Munksgaard, Copenhagen, pp. 475–481.

Jeannet, M., and Alberro, P., 1972. HL-A antigens in chronic lymphocytic leukemia: preliminary evidence for the existence of "leukemia specific" antigens. *Schweiz. Med. Wschr.* 102:1172.

Jeannet, M., and Magnin, C., 1972. HL-A antigens in haematological malignant diseases. *Eur. J. Clin. Invest.* 2:39.

Jersild, C., Svejgaard, A., Fog, T., and Ammitzbøll, T., 1973. HL-A antigens and diseases. (ii) Multiple sclerosis. *Tissue Antigens* (in press).

Kissmeyer-Nielsen, F., Jensen, K. B., Ferrara, G. B., Kjerbye, K. E., and Svejgaard, A., 1971*a*. HL-A phenotypes in Hodgkin's disease. Preliminary report. *Transpl. Proc.* 3:1287.

Kissmeyer-Nielsen, F., Jensen, K. B., Ferrara, G. B., Kjerbye, K. C., and Svejgaard, A., 1971*b*. Scandiatransplant: preliminary report of a kidney exchange program. *Transpl. Proc.* 3:1019.

Klein, J., and Shreffler, D. C., 1971. The H-2 model for the major histocompatibility systems. *Transpl. Rev.* 6:3.

Kourilsky, F. M., Dausset, J., Feingold, N., Dupuy, J. M., and Bernard, J., 1967. Etude de la repartition des antigènes leucocytaires chez des malades atteint de leucémie aigue en remission. In J. Dausset, G. Mathé, and J. Hamburger (eds.), *Advance in Transplantation,* Munksgaard, Copenhagen, pp. 515–522.

Kueppers, F., Rosenthal, I., Scholz, S., Klimmek, R., and Albert, E., 1973. HL-A antigens and haplotypes in patients with melanoma. *Z. Immun.-Forsch.* (in press).

Kueppers, F., Brackertz, D., and Mueller-Eckhardt, C. L., 1972. HL-A antigens in sarcoidosis and rheumatoid arthritis. *Lancet* 2:1425.

Lawler, S., Hardesty, R. M., Batchelor, J. R., Edwards, J. H., and Stuart, J., 1971a. Histocompatibility and acute lymphatic leukaemia. *Lancet* 1:699.

Lawler, S. D., Klouda, P. T., Hardesty, R. M., and Till, M. M., 1971b. The HL-A system in lymphoblastic leukaemia. A study of patients and their families. *Brit. J. Haemat.* 21:595.

Legrand, L., and Dausset, J., 1973. Serological evidence of the existence of several antigenic determinants (or factors) on the HL-A gene products. In J. Dausset and W. Bodmer (eds.), *Histocompatibility Testing 1972,* Munksgaard, Copenhagen.

Levine, B., Stember, R., and Fotino, M., 1972. Ragweed Hay Fever: genetic control and linkage to HL-A haplotypes. *Science* 178:1201.

Lieberman, R., 1973. In M. Landy and H. McDevitt (eds.), *Genetic Control of Immune Responsiveness,* Academic Press, New York. pp. 117–122.

Lilly, F., 1973. In M. Landy and H. McDevitt (eds.), *Genetic Control of Immune Responsiveness,* Academic Press, New York. pp. 279–288.

Lilly, F., 1971. The influence of H-2 type on gross virus leukemogenesis in mice. *Transpl. Proc.* 3:1239.

Lilly, F., 1966. The histocompatibility-2 locus and susceptibility to tumor induction. In *Murine Leukemia,* Nat. Cancer Inst. Monograph No. 22.

Lilly, F., Boyse, E. A., and Old, L. J., 1964. Genetic basis of susceptibility to viral leukemogenesis. *Lancet* 2:1207.

Lukes, R. J., Tindle, B. H., and Parker, J. W., 1969. Reed-Sternberg-like cells in infectious mononucleosis. *Lancet* 2:1003.

Mackay, I. R., 1969. Autoimmune disease. *Med. J. Aust.* 1:696.

Mackay, I. R., and Morris, P. J., 1972. Association of autoimmune active chronic hepatitis with HL-A1,8. *Lancet* 2:793.

Marchalonis, J. J., and Cone, R. E., 1973. Biochemical and biological characteristics of lymphocyte surface immunoglobulins. *Transpl. Rev.* 14:3.

Marchalonis, J. J., Cone, R. E., and Atwell, J. L., 1972. Isolation and partial characterization of lymphocyte surface immunoglobulins. *J. Exp. Med.* 135:956.

Marsh, D. G., Bias, W. B., Hsu, S. H., and Goodfriend, L., 1973. Association of the HL-A7 Cross-Reacting Group with a Specific Antibody Response in Allergic Man. *Science* 179:691.

Martin, W. J., Ellman, L., Green, I., and Benaceraff, B., 1970. Histocompatibility type and immune responsiveness in random bred Hartley strain guinea pigs. *J. Exp. Med.* 132:1259.

McDevitt, H. O., and Benaceraff, B., 1969. Genetic control of specific immune responses. *Adv. Immunol.* 11:31.

McDevitt, H. O., Deak, B. D., Shreffler, D. C., Klein, J., Stimpfling, J. H., and Snell, G. D., 1972. Genetic control of the immune response: mapping of the IR-1 locus. *J. Exp. Med.* 135:1259.

Mempel, W., Albert, E., and Burger, A., 1972. Further evidence for a separate MLC locus. *Tissue Antigens* 2:250.

Mickey, M. R., Kreisler, M., Albert, E., Tanaka, N., and Terasaki, P. I., 1971. Analysis of HL-A incompatibility in human renal transplants. *Tissue Antigens* 1:57.

Mickey, M. R., Kreisler, M., and Terasaki, P. I., 1970. Leukocyte antigens and disease. 2.

Alterations in frequencies of haplotypes associated with chronic glomerulonephritis. In P. I. Terasaki (ed.), *Histocompatibility Testing 1970*, Munksgaard, Copenhagen, pp. 237–241.

Mitchell, G. F., Grumet, F. C., and McDevitt, H. O., 1972. Genetic control of the immune response. The effect of thymectomy on the primary and secondary antibody response of mice to poly-L (Tyr,Glu)-poly-D, L-Ala-Poly-L-lys. *J. Exp. Med.* **135**:126.

Morris, P. J., and Dumble, L., 1972. A possible association between anti-HL-A2 production and the presence of HL-A3 and/or HL-A11 in the serum donor. *Transplantation* **13**:546.

Morris, P. J., and Forbes, J. F., 1971a. HL-A and Hodgkin's disease. *Transpl. Proc.* **3**:1275.

Morris, P. J., and Forbes, J. F., 1971b. HL-A in follicular lymphoma, reticulum cell sarcoma, lymphosarcoma, and infectious mononucleosis. *Transpl. Proc.* **3**:1315.

Morris, P. J., and Mackay, I. R. HL-A and autoimmune disease. In preparation.

Morris, P. J., Bashir, H., McGregor, S. A., Batchelor, J. R., Case, J., Kirk, R., Ting, A., Hornabrook, R., Boyle, A., Dumble, L., Law, W., Lightfoot, A., Johnston, J., Guinan, J., and Brotherton, J., 1973a. Genetic studies of HL-A in New Guinea. In J. Dausset and W. Bodmer (eds.), *Histocompatibility Testing 1972*, Munksgaard, Copenhagen. pp. 267-274.

Morris, P. J., Lawler, S., and Oliver, R. T., 1973b. HL-A and Hodgkin's disease. In J. Dausset and W. Bodmer (eds.), *Histocompatibility Testing 1972*, Munksgaard, Copenhagen. pp. 669-677.

Morris, P. J., Ting, A., Alpers, M. P., and Simons, M., 1971. Leukocyte antigens in a New Guinea population. *Tissue Antigens* **1**:49.

Naito, S., Namerow, N., Mickey, M. R., and Terasaki, P. I., 1972. Multiple sclerosis: association with HL-A3. *Tissue Antigens* **2**:1.

Ordal, J., and Grumet, F. C., 1972. The effect of graft versus host reaction on the antibody response to (T,G)-A–L in nonresponder mice. *Fed. Proc.* **31**:777.

Piazza, A., Belvedere, M. C., Bernoco, D., Conighi, C., Conti, L., Curtoni, E. S., Mattiuz, P. L., Mayr, W., Richiardi, P., Scudeller, G., and Ceppellini, R., 1973. HL-A variation in four Sardinian villages under differential selective pressure by malaria. In J. Dausset and W. Bodmer (eds.), *Histocompatibility Testing 1972*, Munksgaard, Copenhagen. pp. 73-84.

Pietsch, M., and Morris, P. J., 1973a. HL-A in lung cancer. In preparation.

Pietsch, M., and Morris, P. J., 1973b. An Association of HL-A3 and HL-A7 with Paralytic Poliomyelitis. *Tissue Antigens* (in press).

Roege, V., Patel, R., and Briggs, W., 1972. Leucocyte antigens and disease. II. Association of HL-A5 and lymphomas. *Am. J. Clin. Pathol.* **58**:14.

Rogentine, G. N., Yankee, R. A., Gart, J. J., Nam, J., and Trapani, R. J., 1972. HL-A antigens and disease. Acute lymphocytic leukemia. *J. Clin. Invest.* **51**:2420.

Rosenthal, I., Scholz, S., Klimmek, R., Albert, E., and Bluha, H., 1973. HL-A antigens and haplotypes in patients with tuberculosis. *Z. Immun.-Forsch.* (in press).

Russell, T. J., Schultes, L. M., and Kuban, D. J., 1972. Histocompatibility (HL-A) antigens associated with psoriasis. *New Engl. J. Med.* **287**:738.

Sanderson, A. R., Mahour, G., Jaffe, N., Das, G., 1973. Incidence of HL-A Antigens in Acute Lymphocytic Leukemia. *Transplantation* (in press).

Sasportes, M., Lebrun, A., Rapaport, F. T., and Dausset, J., 1972. Studies of skin allograft survival and mixed lymphocyte culture reaction in HL-A genotyped families. *Transpl. Proc.* **4**:209.

Schlosstein, L., Terasaki, P. I., Bluestone, R., Pearson, C. M., High Association of an HL-A antigen, W27, with Ankylosing Spondylitis. *New Eng. J. Med.* **288**:704.

Shreffler, D. C., 1973. IN M. Landy and H. McDevitt (eds.), *Genetic Control of Immune Responsiveness*, Academic Press, New York. pp. 79–88.

Simons, M. J., Wee, G. B., Day, N. E., Morris, P. J., Shanmugaratnam, K., and de Thé, G. B. 1973. Immunogenetic Aspects of Nasopharyngeal Carcinoma. 1. Differences in HL-A Antigen Profiles between Patients and Comparison Groups. *Int. J. Cancer* (in press).

Singal, D. P., Naipaul, N., Berry, R., Pai, M. K., and Zipursky, A., 1971. HL-A genotype of patients with acute lymphoblastic leukemia. *Humangenetik* **13**:234.

Snell, G. D., 1968. The H-2 locus of the mouse: observations and speculations concerning its comparative genetics and its polymorphism. *Folia Biol.* **14**:335.

Stokes, P. L., Asquith, P., Holmes, G. K. T., Mackintosh, P., and Cooke, W. T., 1972. Histocompatibility antigens associated with adult coeliac disease. *Lancet* **2**:162.

Svejgaard, A., Svejgaard, E., and Jersild, C., 1973. HL-A and psoriasis. *Scand. J. Immunol.* (in press).

Svejgaard, A., Bratlie, A., Hedin, P. J., Högman, C., Jersild, C., Kissmeyer-Nielsen, F., Lindblohm, B., Lindblohm, A., Low, B., Messetor, L., Moller, E., Sandberg, L., Staub-Nielsen, L., and Thorsby E., 1971. The recombination fraction of the HL-A system. *Tissue Antigens* **1**:81.

Takasugi, M., Terasaki, P. I., Henderson, B., Mickey, M. R., Menck, H., and Thompson, R. W., 1973. HL-A antigens in solid tumors. *Cancer Res.* **33**:648.

Tennant, J. R., 1968. Additional evidence for implication of histocompatibility factors in resistance to viral leukemogenesis in the mouse. In J. Dausset, G. Mathe, and J. Hamburger (eds.), *Advance in Transplantation,* Munksgaard, Copenhagen, pp. 507–514.

Thorsby, E., and Lie, S. O., 1971. Relationship between the HL-A system and susceptibility to diseases. *Transpl. Proc.* **3**:1305.

Thorsby, E., Engeset, A., and Lie, S. O., 1971. HL-A antigens and susceptibility to diseases: a study of patients with acute lymphoblastic leukemia, Hodgkin's disease and childhood asthma. *Tissue Antigens* **3**:147.

Ting, A., Mackay, I. R., and Morris, P. J., 1973. HL-A in autoimmune diseases and infectious mononucleosis. In *Symposia Series in Immunobiological Standardisation,* Kayer, Basel, New York. **18**:276.

van Rood, J. J., and van Leeuwen, A., 1971. HL-A and the Group Five System in Hodgkin's disease. *Transpl. Proc.* **3**:1283.

Vermylen, C., Goethals, Th., and van de Putte, I., 1972. Healthy carrier state and Australia antigen liver disease. *Lancet* **1**:1119.

Walford, R. D., Waters, H., Smith, G. S., and Sturgeon, P., 1973. Anomalous reactivity of certain HL-A typing sera with leukemic lymphocytes, *Tissue Antigens* **3**:222.

Walford, R. L., Zeller, E., Combs, L., and Konrad, P., 1971. HL-A specificities in acute and chronic lymphatic leukemia. *Transpl. Proc.* **3**:1297.

Walford, R. L., Finkelstein, S., Neerhout, R., Konrad, P., and Shanbrom, E., 1970. Acute childhood leukemia in relation to the HL-A human transplantation genes. *Nature* **225**:461.

Waters, H., Konrad, P., and Walford, R. L., 1971. The distribution of HL-A histocompatibility factors and genes in patients with systemic lupus erythematosus. *Tissue Antigens* **1**:68.

Waters, H., Colebatch, J., and Morris, P. J., 1973. HL-A in acute lymphatic leukemia, unpublished.

Wells, J. V., Fudenberg, H. H., and Mackay, I. R., 1971. Relation of the human antibody response to flagellin to GM genotype. *J. Immunol.* **107**:1505.

Whisnant, J. K., Mann, D. L., Rogentine, G. N., and Robbins, J. B., 1971. Human cell-surface structures related to haemophilus influenzae type B disease. *Lancet* **11**:895.

White, A. G., Barnetson, R. St. C., Da Costa, J. A., and McClelland, D. B., 1973. HL-A and disordered immunity. *Lancet* **1**:108.

White, S. H., Newcomer, V. D., Mickey, M. R., and Terasaki, P. I., 1972. Disturbance of HL-A antigen frequency in psoriasis. *New Engl. J. Med.* **287**:740.

Whittingham, S., Morris, P. J., and Mackay, I. R., 1973. Genetic markers in thyrogastric autoimmune disorders, in preparation.

Wilson, D., and Nossal, G. J. V., 1971. Identification of human T and B lymphocytes in normal peripheral blood and in chronic lymphatic leukemia. *Lancet* **2**:788.

Yunis, E., 1971. HL-A and lymphoma. *Transpl. Rev.* **7**:95.

Yunis, E. J., Plate, J. M., Ward, F. E., Seigler, J. F., and Amos, D. B., 1971. Anomalous MLR responsiveness among siblings. *Transpl. Proc.* **3**:118.

Zervas, J. D., Delamore, I. W., and Israels, M. C., 1970. Leucocyte phenotype in Hodgkin's disease. *Lancet* **2**:634.

Chapter 7

Antigen-Binding Receptors on Lymphocytes

Joseph M. Davie

Departments of Pathology and Microbiology
Washington University School of Medicine
St. Louis, Missouri

and

William E. Paul

Laboratory of Immunology
National Institute of Allergy and Infectious Diseases
National Institutes of Health
Bethesda, Maryland

INTRODUCTION

The concept that activation of immunocompetent cells by antigen depends upon the presence of specific antigen-binding receptors on the cell surface has been central to immunologic theory since it was originally proposed by Paul Ehrlich (1900). Direct evidence for the existence of such receptors has been amassed in recent years. In particular, it has been demonstrated that in nonimmunized animals, rare lymphocytes will bind a given substance to their surface and that the frequency of such cells increases upon immunization (Naor and Sulitzeanu, 1967; Byrt and Ada, 1969; Davie and Paul, 1971; Humphrey and Keller, 1970; Davie *et al.*, 1971a).

Although the demonstration of individual antigen-binding cells (ABC) has been accomplished in many laboratories and by a variety of techniques, controversy on several crucial issues exists. This may be due, in part, to the use of different antigens, different species of animals and different methods of measuring ABC. It is the purpose of this paper to summarize experiments from our laboratory concerning ABC of the guinea pig and to compare them to studies of others on ABC of the mouse. Particular attention will be given to controversial points and no attempt at completeness will be made.

171

METHODS FOR MEASURING ABC

The interaction of antigenic determinants and antigen-specific receptors on lymphocyte surfaces can be detected directly by the use of antigens bearing markers which allow their visualization. In general, the antigen can be linked to markers which can be detected by properties such as enzymatic activity (Miller et al., 1971), radioactivity (Ada et al., 1964; Naor and Sulitzeanu, 1967) or fluorescence (Julius et al., 1972) in which a simple relation exists between the amount of marker and the amount of antigen bound to the cell. Alternatively, markers such as erythrocytes (Zaalberg et al., 1968) or bacteria (Mäkelä and Nossal, 1961) which can be detected by virtue of their size may be used. These latter markers do not lend themselves as easily to quantitation of the amount of antigen bound. Although no studies which directly compare the sensitivities of the various techniques have appeared, comparison of results from different laboratories suggests that techniques based on antigen-coated erythrocytes (rosette techniques) are of greater sensitivity than the more quantitative methods, with the possible exception of procedures involving some enzymatic markers. As an example, consider the question about which considerable dispute exists: whether thymocytes or thymus-derived (T) lymphocytes can be demonstrated to bind antigen to their surface. In general, those who use rosette techniques are able to show antigen binding by T cells (Hogg and Greaves, 1972; Wilson, 1971; Bach and Dardenne, 1972; Möller and Mäkelä, 1973), although this is not always the case (Schlesinger, 1970; Takahashi et al., 1971; Crone et al., 1972). On the other hand, those who use conventional radioautography are usually unable to demonstrate antigen binding by T cells (Byrt and Ada, 1969; Davie and Paul, 1971; Lamelin et al., 1972). This suggests that T lymphocytes have fewer antigen-binding receptors than thymus-independent (B) lymphocytes, as the binding of antigen to the latter cells can be detected by either technique. If the differences in results achieved by using radioautography and rosette formation are indeed based on the relative sensitivity of the methods, then extended time of exposure of radioautographs or increased specific activity of the antigen which would increase the sensitivity of this technique should allow the demonstration of antigen binding by T cells. Indeed, it has recently been reported (Dwyer et al., 1972) that antigen binding T cells may be detected if long-term radioautography is used. In addition, Roelants (1972) found θ-bearing ABC in mouse spleen by using highly labeled antigens. Further support for the inference that T cells have fewer receptors than B cells may be drawn from studies of surface immunoglobulin on these cells. The B cell appears to have of the order of 10^5 surface immunoglobulin molecules while the T cell has been reported to bear fewer than 10^3 immunoglobulin molecules (Rabellino et al., 1971). Indeed, in one study, T lymphocytes did not appear to have more surface immunoglobulins than erythrocytes (Nossal et al., 1972).

The sensitivities of the methods used to measure antigen binding to cells are important since the number and type of cells which are detected depend on the methods chosen. Thus, those experiments involving rosette-forming cells possibly consider antigen binding by both T and B lymphocytes, while short-term radioautography measures, to a large extent, only B lymphocytes.

Our experiments have utilized short-term radioautography exclusively. We have considered lymphocytes in guinea pigs which have the capacity to bind ^{125}I-dinitrophenyl-guinea pig albumin (^{125}I-DNP-GPA) to their surface. Briefly, the method involves the incubation of 10 to 50 × 10^6 lymphoid cells with low concentrations (200 ng/ml) of relatively high specific activity (15-30 μCi/μg) ^{125}I-DNP-GPA for 30 minutes at 4C. Unbound antigen is removed by washing the cells repeatedly and individual ABC are enumerated in radioautographs which have been exposed for 1 to 7 days. Much of the remainder of this paper deals with the number of cells, from nonimmune and immune guinea pigs, which bind DNP-GPA, the nature and specificity of their surface receptors, the changes in receptors during ontogeny and during immune responses and the likelihood that these ABC are largely precursors of antibody-secreting cells.

ABC IN NONIMMUNE ANIMALS

Various lymphoid organs from normal guinea pigs contain rare lymphocytes which bind ^{125}I-DNP-GPA (Davie and Paul, 1971). As shown in Table I, these cells are present in lymph nodes, peripheral blood, and spleen and bone marrow,

Table I. Organ Distribution of ABC

Organ	Frequency of DNP-specific ABC (per 10^5 lymphocytes)	
	Newborn	Adult
Thymus	<1	<1
Lymph nodes	N.D.[a]	38.6
Spleen	46.0	33.5
Peripheral blood	18.2	24.4
Bone marrow	6.6	38.5

[a] N.D.—not done.

but absent from the thymus, in both normal adult and newborn guinea pigs. The binding of antigen to the surface of these cells appears to be specific since prior treatment of the cells with unlabeled antigen inhibits the binding of the radio-labeled DNP-GPA. In addition, the specificity of the receptor appears to be largely directed toward the haptenic group. DNP coupled to a variety of protein carriers inhibits the binding of ^{125}I-DNP-GPA to cells. In quantitative terms, these DNP conjugates inhibit binding as well as does DNP-GPA. Indeed, higher molecular weight carriers with many DNP groups inhibit more efficiently than DNP-GPA. Furthermore, DNP-lysine at a high concentration will inhibit the majority of cells from binding ^{125}I-DNP-GPA. The specificity of the receptors for the DNP group has also been demonstrated by a series of experiments using solid immunoadsorbents. Lymphoid cells from nonimmune guinea pigs were mixed with agarose beads to which various DNP-protein conjugates had been covalently linked. After agitating the mixture to ensure contact between cells and beads, the beads and the cells which had adsorbed to them were removed from the cell suspension by filtration. The number of lymphocytes in the depleted population which could bind ^{125}I-DNP-GPA was compared to the number of such lymphocytes in the initial population or in a cell population which had been adsorbed with agarose beads to which an unrelated protein had been linked. Many fewer (<20%) DNP-GPA binding cells were found in the cell suspension which had been adsorbed with DNP-protein agarose beads than in either control population, and the degree of diminution was not related to the nature of the protein carrier. Thus, ^{125}I-DNP-GPA binding lymphocytes will adsorb to beads to which DNP moieties have been coupled regardless of the protein carrier. Furthermore, populations depleted of DNP-specific ABC were depleted of their capacity to transfer primary anti-DNP antibody responses to irradiated syngeneic guinea pigs.

The hapten specificity of the receptors of ABC by itself suggests that ABC are precursors of antibody-secreting cells since cells involved in cellular immune responses rarely exhibit a high degree of specificity for the haptenic group alone, while serum antibody and precursors of antibody-forming cells are often highly hapten specific (Paul, 1970).

A more compelling reason to consider ABC as members of the B lympho-cyte pool comes from experiments where cells were simultaneously examined for surface immunoglobulin and for the capacity to bind ^{125}I-DNP-GPA. It has been clearly demonstrated in the mouse that B lymphocytes have sufficient immunoglobulin on their surfaces to be detected by the binding of fluorescein- or ^{125}I-labeled anti-immunoglobulin, while T lymphocytes do not bind suffi-cient anti-immunoglobulin to be detected by these conventional procedures (Raff, 1970) (see above). Similarly, the study of immunoglobulin on guinea pig lymphocytes indicates that large amounts are found only on lymphocytes

(Shevach *et al.*, 1972). THus, identification of immunoglobulin on a lymphocyte by immunofluorescence strongly suggests that that cell is a B lymphocyte.

When lymph node cells from nonimmune guinea pigs are treated sequentially with ^{125}I-DNP-GPA followed by fluoresceinated rabbit antiguinea pig immunoglobulin and then observed by combined immunofluorescence-radioautography (Davie *et al.*, 1971*b*), nearly all ABC possess easily detectable immunoglobulin on their surface and are thus likely to be of the B lymphocyte line (Davie and Paul, 1971). A typical ABC and its surface immunoglobulin is shown in Fig. 1. The further finding that preincubation of lymphocytes with excess anti-immunoglobulin antibody prior to the addition of ^{125}I-DNP-GPA blocks binding of the radioactive ligand indicates that not only does the ABC possess surface Ig but that Ig is probably responsible for the binding of the antigen.

Similar results have been found by other investigators studying ABC of the mouse (Warner *et al.*, 1970). However, a significant difference exists between these two species when one considers the class of immunoglobulin which functions as the receptor of the B lymphocyte. Investigators who have measured ABC in the mouse have concluded that the receptors for antigen on most lymphocytes have μ determinants. This finding has been confirmed recently in our laboratory. On the other hand, we have found that the majority of ABC from adult guinea pigs have γ_2 determinants on their surface (Table II), and that anti-γ_2 antibody inhibits antigen binding. The latter results are of particular interest in view of recently obtained evidence concerning normal B cell maturation.

Studies of the ontogeny of immunoglobulin-bearing and immunoglobulin-secreting cells in the chicken strongly suggest that cells which secrete IgG antibody have a precursor which bears surface IgM and that a switch from IgM to IgG production occurs during differentiation, very likely as an event independent of antigenic stimulation (Cooper, M. D., *et al.*, 1972). Thus, IgM-containing cells may be found in the bursa of Fabricius of 13-day chick embryos. The peripheral lymphoid tissue of these embryos lacks IgM-containing cells, and IgG-containing cells are not detectable either in the bursa or the peripheral lymphoid tissue (Kincade and Cooper, 1971). Treatment of such embryos with anti-μ antibody followed by bursectomy on the day of hatching results in suppression of the subsequent synthesis of both IgM and IgG (Kincade *et al.*, 1970). This strongly suggests that IgG production depends on an IgM-bearing precursor cell.

However, if treatment with anti-μ antibody is delayed until the day of hatching, at which time precursors of both IgM and IgG immunoglobulin-secreting cells have already migrated from the bursa to the peripheral lymphoid tissue, only IgM synthesis is suppressed. Chickens treated in this way produce normal amounts of IgG (Kincade *et al.*, 1970). Thus, it would appear the *peripheral* precursors of IgG- and IgM-secreting cells are independent, and that, outside the

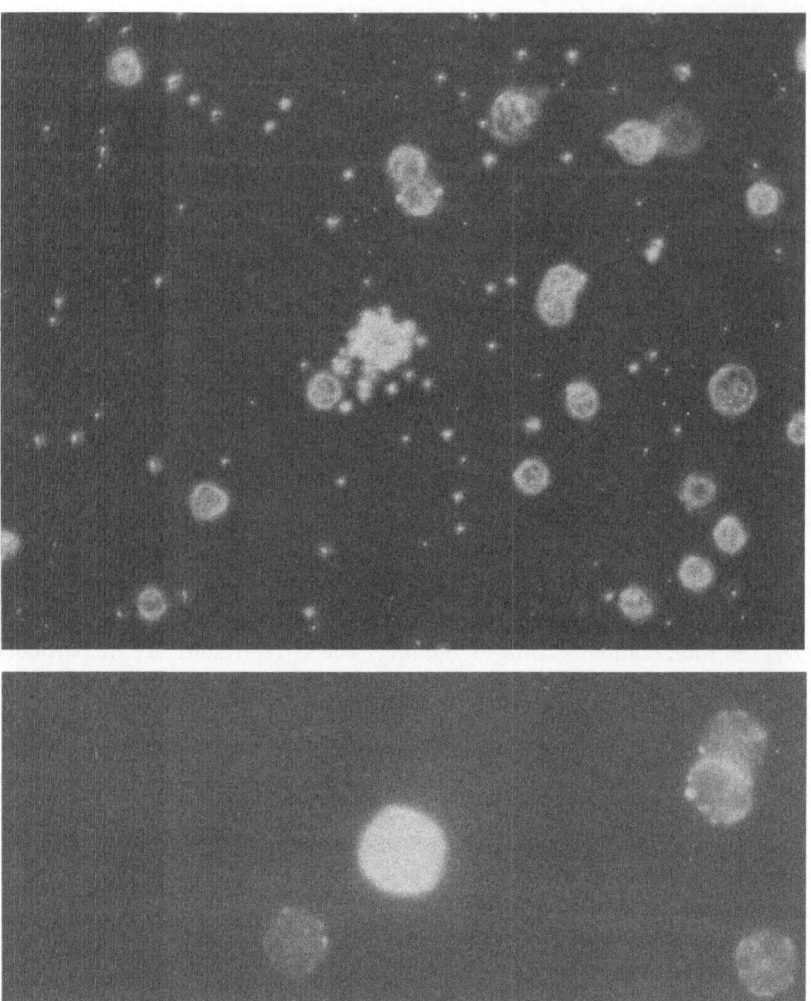

Figure 1. Simultaneous localization of antigen and membrane-associated immunoglobulin. A lymph node cell suspension from a nonimmune guinea pig was incubated with ^{125}I-DNP-GPA for 30 minutes at 4C in medium containing azide. After washing away unbound antigen the cell suspension was incubated with rabbit F1-anti-guinea pig γ_2-immunoglobulin for 30 minutes at 25C in azide. The washed cells were processed for radioautography and examined sequentially with a tungsten and ultraviolet light source. The upper frame shows a DNP-specific ABC as shown by the white-appearing silver grains. The lower frame shows the same ABC when viewed with ultraviolet light at higher magnification. The ABC shown here bears γ_2 immunoglobulin.

Table II. Ig Class of Receptors on ABC in Nonimmune Guinea Pigs and Mice

Heavy chain class	Guinea pig lymph node			Mouse spleen		
	% of total lymphocytes[a]	% of Ig-bearing cells	% of DNP-GPA binding cells[b]	% of total lymphocytes[a]	% of Ig-bearing cells	% of ferritin binding cells[b]
μ	13	28	25	31	69	91
γ_1	14	30	18	0.1	0.2	9
γ_2	16	35	63	7	16	2
α	3	7	N.D.[c]	8	18	9
total Ig	46			45		

[a] Determined by binding of fluorescein-labeled anti-immunoglobulins.
[b] Determined by binding of ^{125}I-DNP-GPA or ^{125}I-ferritin and fluorescein-labeled anti-immunoglobulins.
[c] N.D.—not done.
[d] Determined by pcoling fluorescein-labeled anti-μ, anti-γ_1, anti-γ_2, and anti-α.

bursa, the precursor of the IgG-producing cell either lacks surface IgM or can no longer be suppressed by anti-μ.

In addition, consideration of the effects of bursectomy at various times suggests that *peripheral* IgM-bearing cells do not differentiate into IgG-secreting cells. Embryos bursectomized at 18 or 19 days of age develop into chickens with normal or somewhat elevated serum IgM concentrations but without detectable serum IgG. This is consistent with the emigration of precursors of IgM-secreting cells from the bursa prior to the emigration of precursors of IgG-secreting cells and the inability of the former cells to give rise to appreciable numbers of IgG producers (Cooper, M. D., *et al.*, 1972).

This line of evidence would suggest that in mature animals peripheral precursors of cells which secrete anti-DNP of the IgG class of immunoglobulin should bear surface immunoglobulin which is not IgM and which, very likely, would be of the IgG class.

Recent studies of development of immunoglobulin-synthesizing cells in the mouse suggest a somewhat different ontogeny. Administration of anti-μ antibody to neonatal mice suppresses the subsequent appearance of IgM- and IgG-bearing cells and of IgM and IgG synthesis in these animals (Lawton *et al.*, 1972; Manning and Jutilla, 1972). This is consistent with the IgG-producing cells being descended from an IgM-bearing precursor in the mouse as in the chicken. Study of *in vitro* antibody responses to sheep erythrocytes of mouse spleen suggests a major difference in the pattern of B cell differentiation from that observed in the chicken. Pierce *et al.* (1972a) have reported that *in vitro* primary antisheep erythrocyte antibody responses of both the IgM and IgG class are suppressed by anti-μ antibody, but that anti-γ antibody suppresses antisheep erythrocyte antibody responses of the IgG but not the IgM class. Similar findings were reported by Herrod and Warner (1972) using an adoptive primary response to sheep erythrocytes. This observation is consistent with precursors of antibody-secreting cells bearing IgM immunoglobulin receptors. Upon antigenic stimulation, some of these cells would express surface IgG and differentiate into secretors of IgG. In *in vitro* secondary response, at certain times after priming, anti-μ antibody fails to suppress the IgG antibody response, whereas the anti-γ antibody suppresses quite effectively (Pierce *et al.*, 1972b).

The evidence from the study of mouse responses suggests that in the peripheral lymphoid tissue an IgM-bearing cell is the precursor of the IgG-secreting cell and that a "switch" in immunoglobulin class occurs as a result of antigenic stimulation. After initial immunization, IgG-bearing precursors may predominate, at least for a brief period of time. On the basis of this hypothesis, one would anticipate that in an unimmunized adult mouse the great majority of the ABC would possess receptors of the IgM class. Indeed, as alluded to above, this appears to be the case for mouse ABC. Furthermore, the majority of mouse immunoglobulin-bearing cells have surface IgM (Table II).

The apparent distinction in B cell differentiation pattern between the chicken and mouse is perhaps not surprising, as the chicken has a central lymphoid organ for B cell differentiation whereas no such organ has yet been identified in mammals. It is possible that the commitment of a pluripotent precursor (in regard to Ig class) occurs as a normal ontogenetic event in the bursa, but in animals lacking such an organ this step in differentiation depends upon antigenic stimulation.

Our observations on the ABC of the unimmunized guinea pig complicate this simple interpretation. We observe in the guinea pig a very substantial frequency of ABC and immunoglobulin-bearing cells with surface IgG (γ_2). Thus, γ_2 immunoglobulin is found on 35% of all immunoglobulin-bearing cells and 63% of all DNP-binding cells. Twenty-eight percent of all immunoglobulin-bearing cells in the lymph nodes of adult guinea pigs bear surface IgM, and only 25% of lymphocytes which bind ^{125}I-DNP-GPA have surface IgM. In the mouse spleen, on the other hand, we find that 69% of all immunoglobulin-bearing cells have surface IgM and 91% of ferritin-binding cells have surface IgM (Table II).

Not only do γ_2-bearing cells predominate among those guinea pig cells capable of binding DNP-GPA to their surface, but they appear to be the major precursors of anti-DNP antibody-secreting cells in the guinea pig. Experiments demonstrating this involve the treatment of lymph node and spleen cells from nonimmune guinea pigs with either normal rabbit serum, rabbit anti-γ_2 antiserum or rabbit anti-μ antiserum. The cells were then treated with complement (C), washed and transferred to irradiated, syngeneic guinea pigs. The recipients were immunized with DNP-hemocyanin and their anti-DNP antibody responses measured. Animals which received cells treated with anti-γ_2 antiserum had a marked diminution in their anti-DNP antibody response, whereas animals which received cells treated with anti-μ had little or no change in their anti-DNP responses. Thus, the bulk of the precursors of anti-DNP secreting cells appear sensitive to anti-γ_2 and C but not to anti-μ and C (Davie and Paul, 1971).

The difference between the ABC of mice and guinea pigs might be explained in two general ways. First, it is possible that the guinea pig has had prior contact with antigens bearing the DNP group or cross reactive with it, and that such environmental immunization has provided the antigenic drive for a transition from an IgM-bearing ABC to an IgG-bearing ABC. This possibility is difficult to rule out. Nonetheless, the finding that immune responses of guinea pigs to DNP-proteins resemble primary responses in general is somewhat against it. Moreover, γ_2 immunoglobulin is present on guinea pig lymphocytes which bind human γ-globulin as well as those which bind DNP-proteins (Davie and Paul, 1971). The other major possibility is that mammals retain an antigen-independent differentiation mechanism by which precursor cells become differentiated in regard to class of immunoglobulin which their descendants produce, and that different mammalian species utilize the antigen-independent and antigen-dependent differentiation mechanisms to different extents.

In order to test this latter hypothesis, suppression experiments utilizing anti-μ antibody on fetal guinea pigs at various degrees of gestation would be most helpful. Such experiments have not yet been carried out. However, we have begun to analyze the immunoglobulin-bearing cells in the spleen of fetal guinea pigs for the class of heavy chain present, and we have measured the frequency of DNP-binding cells and determined the class of Ig which such cells bear (Davie *et al.*, 1972*a*).

The gestational period in the guinea pig is approximately 68 days. Two weeks prior to term, significant numbers of IgM-bearing cells are found in the spleen, but few if any γ_1- or γ_2-bearing cells are detected. The γ_1- and γ_2-bearing cells increase in frequency rapidly so that by term the relative frequency of immunoglobulin-bearing cells of each class is similar to that of the adult. What must be established, of course, is whether the IgM-bearing cell of the 54-day guinea pig fetus resembles the chicken bursal cell and the mouse spleen cell in the ability to generate IgG-secreting cells, or, alternatively, is similar to the IgM-bearing cell in the peripheral lymphoid organs of the chicken with its specialization as a precursor of IgM producers.

Lymphocytes which bind ^{125}I-DNP-GPA to their surface are found in the 54-day fetus. They have a frequency approximately half that of adult animals ($\sim$23 per 100,000) and rise to the adult level by birth. Using combined radioautography and immunofluorescence, it was found that 2 weeks prior to birth virtually all ABC have surface IgM and that at the time of birth only 20% of DNP-GPA binding cells have surface γ_2 immunoglobulin (Table III). This is considerably lower than the adult percentage of γ_2-bearing DNP-binding cells ($>$ 60%). As noted above, whether the appearance of γ_2-bearing ABC of the guinea pig is an antigen-independent maturational event or is a response to unrecognized immunization is not yet resolved.

Table III. Ig Class of Receptors on DNP-Specific ABC in Guinea Pigs at Various Ages

| Gestational age, days | Class of immunoglobulin on DNP-GPA binding cells | | | |
| | μ | | γ_2 | |
	ABC/10^5	% of total ABC	ABC/10^5	% of total ABC
54–60 (spleen)	20	83	1	4
61–term (spleen)	16	75	4	20
adult (lymph node)	13	24	32	60

ABC IN IMMUNE ANIMALS

We have considered so far the characteristics of DNP-specific ABC under conditions where purposeful stimulation of these cells by antigen was not a factor. The administration of antigen sets in play a series of events leading to the differentiation of B cells into antibody-secreting cells. The process sometimes requires the collaboration of several cell types including macrophages and thymus-derived lymphocytes; but, above all, the process is initiated and depends upon interaction of antigen and cellbound receptor molecules on B lymphocytes. This section will summarize experiments concerning DNP-specific ABC in immune guinea pigs.

When guinea pigs are immunized to DNP coupled to the homologous protein GPA, they produce significant amounts of antibody capable of binding ^{125}I-DNP-GPA. The appearance of serum antibody in these immunized animals is preceded by a marked increase in the number of lymphocytes with surface receptors specific for DNP-GPA (Davie et al., 1971a). Figure 2 illustrates this increase in frequency of ABC in draining lymph nodes of strain 13 guinea pigs which have received 50 μg DNP-GPA in complete Freund's adjuvant (CFA) in

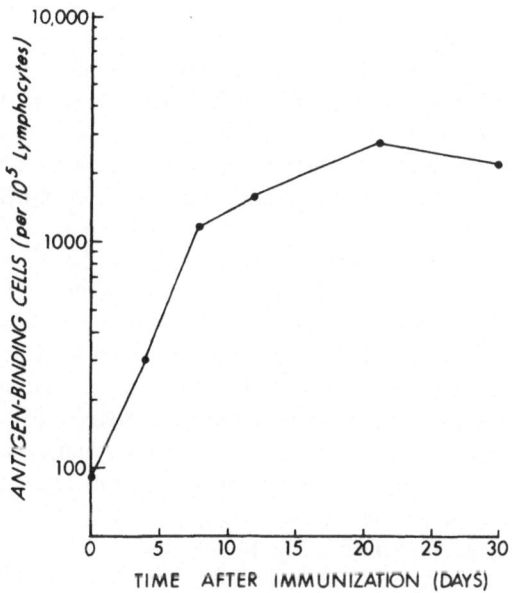

Figure 2. Increased frequency of DNP-specific ABC after immunization. Guinea pigs were immunized by injection, in the footpads, of 50 μg DNP-GPA in CFA. At various times after immunization, the frequency of ABC in the draining lymph nodes was determined (modified from Davie et al., 1971a).

the footpads. The increase in number of specific antigen-binding lymphocytes in immune animals seems not to be due to adsorption of serum antibody to lymphocyte surfaces, as attempts to increase the frequency of ABC by passive administration of anti-DNP antibody to nonimmune animals have not been successful.

The ABC of the immunized animal again appear to be largely members of the B cell pool. Guinea pig B lymphocytes and plasma cells adsorb to glass bead columns and may thus be separated from T cells. When a population of lymph node cells from an immunized guinea pig is passed over a glass bead column, there is a marked depletion of ABC, immunoglobulin-bearing cells, and anti-body-secreting cells (Rosenthal *et al.*, 1972). On the other hand, antigen-sensitive T lymphocytes appear to be enriched, as the emerging population displays increased production of macrophage inhibitory factor and of DNA in response to antigen. Thus, binding of radioactive antigen mainly detects specific B lymphocytes in populations from immune guinea pigs.

The receptor class of DNP-specific ABC in immune guinea pigs is dependent somewhat on the manner of immunization (Davie *et al.*, 1972*a*). For example, when guinea pigs are immunized with 100-μg DNP-BGG emulsified in CFA, the serum anti-DNP antibody elicited is primarily of the γ_2 class. Substantial numbers of DNP-specific ABC have surface Ig of μ, γ_1, and γ_2 classes, respectively, although γ_2-bearing cells are more numerous than cells bearing either of the other classes. However, when guinea pigs are immunized with the same amount of antigen incorporated in incomplete Freund's adjuvant (IFA), there is little proliferation of γ_2-bearing cells while γ_1- and μ-bearing cells increase in numbers to the same degree as they do in animals immunized with antigen in CFA. Furthermore, in response to immunization with DNP-BGG in IFA little anti-DNP antibody of the γ_2 class is produced. Although the mechanisms by which adjuvants cause these selective effects is obscure, the relationship between the class of immunoglobulin on ABC and in the serum antibody is striking.

The specificity of receptors of DNP-GPA-binding cells in immune animals, like that of the serum antibody, is primarily directed toward the hapten (Davie *et al.*, 1971*a*). This may be shown both by inhibition of binding of ^{125}I-DNP-GPA by DNP coupled to heterologous protein carriers and by the univalent ligand ϵ-DNP-L-lysine. Furthermore, ABC bind to solid immunoadsorbents bearing hapten coupled to various protein carriers. In this respect, the receptors resemble serum antibody which is also highly hapten-specific in animals which have been immunized with DNP-GPA. Studies by Claflin *et al.* (1974) which show similarity of class, specificity, and idiotype between receptors and secreted antibody provide support for the thesis that receptor on a precursor cell is identical to the immunoglobulin secreted by the descendants of that cell. This is one of the central postulates of clonal selection theories (Burnet, 1959). It must be stressed, however, that the problem of μ-bearing cells as antecedents of γ-secreting cells which was discussed earlier is still not entirely resolved.

The immune response to most antigens which have been studied has been shown to be a remarkably dynamic process. In the course of many responses a dramatic increase in the affinity for antigen of antibody present in the serum occurs (Eisen and Siskind, 1964). This "maturation" process is believed to result from competition among a population of precursor cells heterogeneous with regard to the affinity of their receptors for available antigen (Siskind and Benacerraf, 1969). Our ability to directly enumerate the precursor population allowed a direct study of immune maturation at the cellular level.

It was necessary in the course of these studies to develop means of determining the relative avidity of cell-bound receptors. Two procedures were used. The first is based upon the relative capacity of the monovalent ligand ϵ-DNP-L-lysine to inhibit ^{125}I-DNP-GPA from subsequently binding to ABC. Receptors which bind hapten with high affinity may be saturated with low concentrations of free ligand and thus inhibited from subsequently binding polyvalent ^{125}I-DNP-GPA. Receptors which bind hapten with low affinity require high free ligand concentrations for saturation. Thus, populations of ABC with receptors of low affinity are only inhibited by high concentrations of ϵ-DNP-L-lysine while populations of ABC with receptors of high affinity are inhibited by both low or high hapten concentrations. The results achieved by hapten inhibition show striking changes in the relative affinity of ABC at different times after immunization (Table IV). The concentrations of hapten

Table IV. Change in Avidity for Hapten of DNP- Specific ABC after Immunization

Time after immunization, days	Frequency of ABC (per 10^3 lymphocytes)	I_{50}[1] $(\log_{10})$
0	0.6	−2.8
8	13.8	−3.4
12	27.5	−5.4
21	31.4	−6.6
29	25.1	−8.6
171	2.0	−9.0

[1] Concentration of ϵ-DNP-L-lysine which blocks 50% of ABC from binding ^{125}I-DNP-GPA.

needed to inhibit half the ABC in nonimmune animals from being detected, the I_{50} value, is about $10^{-3}M$. Within 30 days following injection of 50 μg of DNP-GPA in CFA, the I_{50} value decreases to approximately $10^{-9}M$ and remains at this value for at least 6 months (Davie and Paul, 1972a). This establishes that a "maturation" equal to or, indeed, of a more striking degree than that of antibody occurs in the precursor populations.

A similar approach was used by Möller and Mäkelä (1973) who studied hapten-specific ABC in the mouse by a rosette technique. They also found that the effective inhibitory concentration of hapten needed to block B cell rosette formation decreased strikingly during a 3-month period.

The second approach to measuring the relative avidity of binding of ^{125}I-DNP-GPA to receptors is by calculation of the rates of association and dissociation of antigen-receptor complexes and by determining the concentration of ^{125}I-DNP-GPA at which half saturation of cell receptors occurs (Davie and Paul, 1972b). Both of these more direct methods supported the conclusion that affinity of the antigen-binding receptors is higher late in the immune response than early in the response. However, the absolute values for equilibrium constants calculated from the two direct approaches differ, suggesting that additional factors are involved in the binding of antigen to cell surfaces which are not at present appreciated. A more detailed discussion of these experiments appears elsewhere (Davie and Paul, 1972b).

Since there is now pursuasive evidence that individual clones of cells produce antibody of a single specificity and affinity (Klinman, 1971), the large changes in apparent affinity of ABC must involve preferential expansion of the subpopulations of ABC with high affinity receptors. The "high affinity" ABC may either exist prior to immunization or may arise as mutants during the antigen-driven proliferation of lower affinity ABC. Direct measurement of small subpopulations among the already sparse pool of DNP-specific ABC in the nonimmune animal would be technically difficult, so an attempt to answer this question by indirect means was made. Since antibody-secreting cells are considered the direct descendants of ABC, change in the affinity of antibody produced by individual antibody-secreting cells, by inference, will reflect changes in the ABC population. The relative affinity of antibody secreted by individual cells can be measured by a hapten inhibition technique using hapten-coated erythrocytes in a modified Jerne plaque method (Pasanen and Mäkelä, 1969). Using the same line of reasoning as for ABC, cells secreting low affinity anti-DNP antibody are inhibited from forming plaques by high concentrations of ligand, whereas cells secreting high affinity antibody can be inhibited by low concentrations of hapten.

Furthermore, the data obtained from hapten inhibition experiments can be analyzed to give information as to the distribution of PFC into groups secreting antibody of a given avidity range (Davie and Paul, 1972a). PFC which can be inhibited by 10^{-8}M ϵ-DNP-L-lysine are considered the highest avidity group. Those which are not inhibited by 10^{-8}M but are inhibited by 10^{-7}M fall into the next highest avidity group and so forth. One can, by this approach, estimate the number of PFC in each of several different avidity groups. By determining the number of PFC in each avidity group at various times in the course of the immune response, a considerable clarification of the cellular dynamics leading to the increase in antibody affinity has been achieved. It was found that the earliest indirect PFC which appeared in draining lymph nodes were highly heterogeneous and contained cells in each avidity group. Moreover, even the highest affinity PFC were relatively plentiful in the earliest animals tested. This strongly suggests that antigen-driven mutational events are not responsible for the appearance of high affinity precursor cells. With increasing time after immunization, PFC of all avidity groups increase in frequency until about 8–12 days when the lowest avidity groups begin to decrease in frequency. From then on, the maturation of

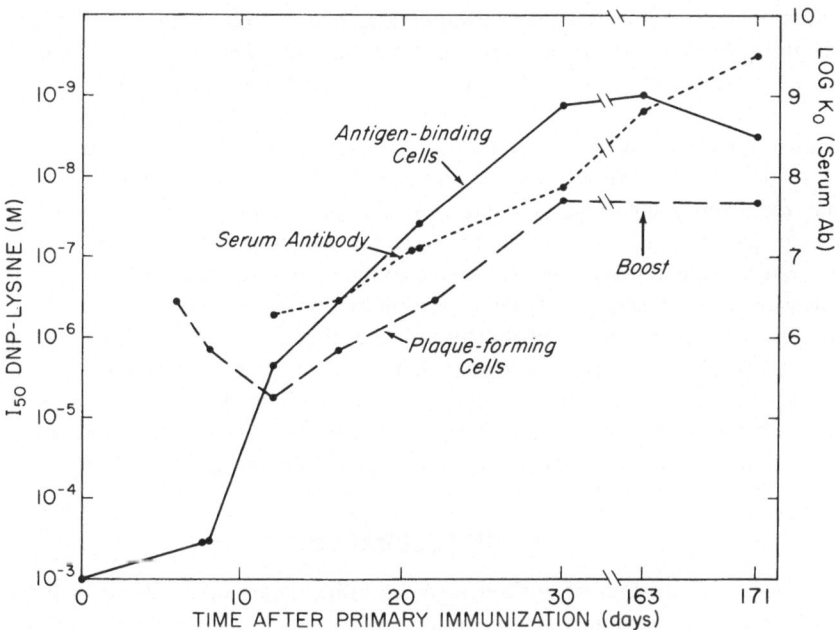

Figure 3. "Maturation" of avidity for hapten of ABC, PFC, and serum anti-DNP antibody after immunization. Guinea pigs were immunized by injection, in the footpads, of 50 μg DNP-GPA in CFA. At various times after immunization, the relative avidities for hapten (the I_{50} values) of DNP-specific ABC and of anti-DNP PFC were measured by the hapten inhibition technique (see text). In addition, the K_0 of the serum anti-DNP antibody was measured by a modified Farr technique. Animals were boosted at 163 days with 50 μg DNP-GPA in IFA in the footpads (from Davie and Paul, 1972a).

the immune response is characterized by the sequential loss of low avidity populations and a striking preservation of the high avidity PFC, rather than a sequential appearance of new populations. Recent studies in the mouse support the changes in PFC avidity which are seen here (Claflin *et al.*, 1973).

When the relative avidities of ABC are compared to those of PFC and serum anti-DNP antibody at various times after immunization, it is seen that the rates of change in these three immunologic compartments are similar (Fig. 3), supporting the contention that ABC indeed represent precursors of PFC.

The most straightforward explanation of the avidity changes and, in fact, the explanation proposed initially to explain immune maturation, addresses itself to differential proliferation rates among precursor cells. We have recently obtained direct evidence to support this concept (Davie and Paul, 1973). The earliest PFC, it will be remembered, are distributed among a wide range of avidities. This heterogeneity of avidities persists for a few days as if no selective proliferation of precursors were occurring. However, later in the immune response selective retention of high avidity PFC occurs. The precursors with lower avidity receptors appear to stop proliferating before those with higher avidity receptors. We injected ^{3}H-thymidine into immunized guinea pigs 2 days before sacrifice and analysis of PFC. The PFC assay was performed as usual in a manner to allow avidity determinations. In addition, the agar slides were processed for radioautography. PFC were identified after radioautography, and it was determined whether the central cell in a plaque was labeled or not. When PFC were analyzed from guinea pigs immunized 8 days previously, a similar fraction of PFC in low and high avidity groups were labeled. However, when PFC from 15–16-day animals were studied, it was found that low avidity PFC were not labeled while high avidity PFC were, even though the frequencies of total PFC in the different groups were similar. This indicates that precursors of cells secreting low avidity antibody have ceased to proliferate while precursors of cells producing high avidity antibody are still actively dividing. Thus, the increase in affinity of serum antibody during immune maturation is the result of the preferential proliferation of the precursor cells bearing high affinity receptors.

ABC IN TOLERANCE

The administration of antigen in doses either larger or smaller than those which result in immunity often results in a state of specific tolerance to subsequent administration of immunogenic doses of antigens. The cellular defect in tolerance has been shown to reside in the T and/or B cell pools, depending on the dose of antigen used and the time after tolerance induction (Chiller and Weigle, 1972). Considerable interest has arisen as to whether B cell tolerance involves an absence of precursor cells or whether the tolerant precursors are present but unable to respond to subsequent antigen contact.

Several groups of investigators have measured the frequency of ABC in tolerant animals. Ada and coworkers have failed to find differences in frequency of specific ABC in either flagellin-tolerant (Ada *et al.*, 1970) or hemocyanin-tolerant rats (Cooper, M. G. *et al.*, 1972). Sjöberg and Möller (1970), similarly, failed to observe decreased numbers of ABC in lipopolysaccharide-tolerant mice. On the other hand, others have reported a diminution of specific ABC in tolerant mice. Humphrey and Keller (1970) observed fewer highly labeled hemocyanin-binding cells in hemocyanin-tolerant mice, and Naor and Sulitzeanu (1969) reported fewer BSA-binding ABC in mice which had been rendered tolerant by a high dose regime. Part of the controversy concerning numbers of ABC in tolerant animals may stem from differences in the degree of tolerance achieved in the B cell pool by various tolerance-inducing methods. Since it is known that B cell tolerance is more difficult to achieve and of shorter duration than T cell tolerance, it is possible that animals which fail to make antibody upon immunization, and are therefore operationally tolerant, may not have a tolerant pool of B cells. Indeed, Möller *et al.* (1971), who enumerated both B and T cell ABC by the rosette technique, found that mice rendered tolerant to dinitrophenylacetyl-BSA had fewer ABC of the T class but, in fact, had equal numbers of ABC of the B class compared to those of control animals.

We have evaluated the number of cells capable of binding ^{125}I-DNP-GPA in tolerant guinea pigs. In order to diminish the confusion inherent in the analysis of B cell ABC in a situation in which tolerance may be, at least in part, a function of the T cell pool, we have chosen a tolerance induction regime in which B cell tolerance is the prime or sole outcome. The DNP conjugate of the random copolymer *D*-glutamic acid and *D*-lysine (DNP-*D*-GL) causes little or no anti-DNP antibody response and is a potent tolerogen. Guinea pigs or mice treated with DNP-*D*-GL fail to produce anti-DNP antibody upon subsequent immunization with DNP-proteins provided a sufficient dose of DNP-*D*-GL is used. This tolerance is largely in the B cell pool on the basis of the following evidence:

1. It can be induced in thymus deprived mice (adult thymectomy, lethal irradiation, bone marrow reconstitution). Spleen cells from such animals, when mixed with normal thymus cells, prepare a lethally irradiated recipient for a markedly diminished primary anti-DNP response to DNP-proteins (Breitner, 1973).

2. Guinea pigs tolerized with DNP-*D*-GL have absent (or markedly depressed) anti-DNP antibody responses upon subsequent immunization with DNP-GPA but normal cellular immune (T cell) responses to this antigen (Cohen *et al.*, 1973).

Guinea pigs which have received 3 mg of DNP-*D*-GL have a striking depression in the number of cells capable of binding DNP-GPA (Katz *et al.*, 1971).

Thus, animals tolerized in this way have 2.2 ± 1.9 ABC per 10^5 lymphocytes as compared to 21.3 ± 4.3 ABC per 10^5 lymphocytes in control animals. This depression in the frequency of ABC occurs within 1 day of the administration of DNP-D-GL and persists for at least 2 weeks.

The degree of tolerance induced by DNP-D-GL depends upon the dose of tolerogen used and the interval between tolerance induction and immunization. When a state of partial tolerance has been induced, immunization with DNP-GPA leads to a modest degree of anti-DNP antibody synthesis. The number of ABC in such animals is markedly lower than the number in control immunized guinea pigs. The anti-DNP antibody which is produced is of lower affinity than that made by control animals (Davie et al., 1972b). This is consistent with partial tolerance preferentially affecting the precursor cells with high affinity antigen-binding receptors. Moreover, it is conceivable that the failure of others to note marked depression in ABC of the B cell pool may have been due to a preservation of low affinity ABC in functionally tolerant mice.

Thus, specific B cell tolerance, at least in this model system, seems to be characterized by an absence of, or a marked reduction in, the number of detectable specific ABC. The reason for the failure to detect ABC could be due to (1) absence of specific B cells, (2) failure of specific B cells to display receptors on their surface, or (3) blockage of specific receptors by tolerogen. The chronicity of the tolerant state and the rapid turnover rate of surface receptors make the latter explanation unlikely, although our understanding of the membrane events following antigen-receptor interaction is sufficiently incomplete so that it cannot be excluded. Distinguishing between the two former and more likely alternatives will require further study.

SUMMARY

We have considered the characteristics of guinea pig lymphocytes which have the ability to bind ^{125}I-DNP-GPA to their surface. These cells appear to be predominantly, if not exclusively, members of the bone marrow-derived pool of lymphocytes. In the nonimmune animal, the cells are rare, and the receptors responsible for binding of antigen are, on most cells, γ_2 immunoglobulins which have specificity for the haptenic portion of the antigen. These cells appear to be precursors of antibody-secreting cells and are crucial to immune function. Selective physical removal of the cells from cell suspensions by hapten immuno-adsorbents or by inactivation using anti-γ_2 antibody and complement results in depressed ability of the cell populations to transfer primary immune responsiveness to irradiated recipients. The class of receptor of DNP-specific ABC changes with the age of the animal. In fetal life, the predominant immunoglobulin determinant on DNP-specific ABC is μ, and only just before birth do γ_2-bearing ABC appear. Throughout adult life γ_2-bearing ABC predominate.

Immunization of guinea pigs with DNP-GPA results in a striking increase in the frequency of cells which bind [125] I-DNP-GPA. The receptors of ABC in immune animals are similar to those in nonimmune animals with regard to specificity and immunoglobulin class. A striking difference, however, is apparent when the avidity of the receptors for antigen is measured. The receptors on ABC from nonimmune animals require high free hapten concentration in order to achieve saturation of the binding sites, indicating that such receptors have low affinity for hapten. However, with increasing time after immunization the free hapten concentration needed for saturation falls, so that by 30 days after immunization saturation is reached at a hapten concentration 6 logs lower than before immunization. The changes in affinity of the cell receptors are reflected by similar affinity changes in secreted antibody. A detailed study of the process showed that "maturation" is the result of preferential proliferation by high affinity precursor cells. The data support the concept that maturation is the result of competition by precursor cells (ABC) for available antigen. As the free antigen concentration falls, only cells with receptors of sufficiently high avidity for the antigen can capture antigen and continue to proliferate and mature to antibody-secreting cells.

By using a method of tolerance induction which affects only B cells it was conclusively shown that one type of B cell tolerance is characterized by decreased numbers of ABC.

A large body of information on surface immunoglobulin and antigen-binding characteristics of B lymphocytes has been collected. Although as may be clear from this brief review, controversy still exists on many issues, the approach has led to a considerable simplification in our understanding of immune phenomena. However, we have an incomplete picture of the mechanism by which antigen-receptor interaction leads either to immunity or tolerance. Similarly, the nature of the integration of receptor into the membrane and the important changes in receptor attendant upon antigen binding are only beginning to be explored. It is on these exciting and crucial issues that considerable attention will be focused.

REFERENCES

Ada, G. L., Byrt, P., Mandel, T., and Warner, N., 1970. A specific reaction between antigen labelled with radioactive iodine and lymphocyte-like cells from normal, tolerant and immunized mice or rats. In J. Sterzl and I. Riha (eds.), *Developmental Aspects of Antibody Formation and Structure,* Vol. II, Academic Press, New York, p. 503.

Ada, G. L., Nossal, G. J. V., and Pye, J., 1964. Antigens in immunity. III. Distribution of iodinated antigens following injection into rats via the hind footpads. *Aust. J. Exp. Biol. Med. Sci.* 42:295.

Bach, J. F., and Dardenne, M., 1972. Antigen recognition by T lymphocytes. I. Thymus and marrow dependence of spontaneous rosette-forming cells in the mouse. *Cell. Immunol.* 3:1.

Breitner, J. C. S., 1973. Induction of hapten-specific tolerance in mouse B cells. *Fed. Proc.* 32:1002 (abstr.).

Burnet, F. M., 1959. *The Clonal Selection Theory of Acquired Immunity.* Cambridge University Press, Cambridge.

Byrt, P., and Ada, G. L., 1969. An *in vitro* reaction between labelled flagellin or haemocyanin and lymphocyte-like cells from normal animals. *Immunology* 17:503.

Chiller, J. M., and Weigle, W. O., 1972. Cellular basis of immunological unresponsiveness. *Contemp. Topics Immunobiol.* 1:119.

Claflin, J. L., Lieberman, R., and Davie, J. M., 1974. Clonal nature of the immune response to phosphorylcholine. I. Specificity, class, and idiotype of phosphorylcholine binding receptors on lymphoid cells. *J. Exp. Med.* in press.

Claflin, L., Merchant, B., and Inman, J., 1973. Antibody binding characteristics at the cellular level. I. Comparative maturation of hapten-specific IgM and IgG plaque-forming cell populations. *J. Immunol.* 110:241.

Cohen, B. E., Davie, J. M., and Paul, W. E., 1973. Hapten-specific tolerance: Depressed humoral and normal cellular immune responses. *J. Immunol.* 110:213.

Cooper, M. G., Ada, G. L., and Langman, R. E., 1972. The incidence of hemocyanin-binding cells in hemocyanin-tolerant rats. *Cell. Immunol.* 4:289.

Cooper, M. D., Lawton, A. R., and Kincade, P., 1972. A developmental approach to the biological basis for antibody diversity. *Contemp. Topics Immunobiol.* 1:33.

Crone, M., Koch, C., and Simonsen, M., 1972. The elusive T cell receptor. *Transpl. Rev.* 10:36.

Davie, J. M., and Paul, W. E., 1973. Immunological maturation: Preferential proliferation of high affinity precursor cells. *J. Exp. Med.* 137:201.

Davie, J. M., and Paul, W. E., 1972a. Receptors on immunocompetent cells. V. Cellular correlates of the "maturation" of the immune response. *J. Exp. Med.* 135:660.

Davie, J. M., and Paul, W. E., 1972b. Receptors on immunocompetent cells. IV. Direct measurement of avidity of cell receptors and cooperative binding of multivalent ligands. *J. Exp. Med.* 135:643.

Davie, J. M., and Paul, W. E., 1971. Receptors on immunocompetent cells. II. Specificity and nature of receptors on dinitrophenylated guinea pig albumin- ^{125}I-binding lymphocytes of normal guinea pigs. *J. Exp. Med.* 134:495.

Davie, J. M., Paul, W. E., and Asofsky, R., 1972a. Immunoglobulin class of receptors on DNP-specific antigen binding cells of guinea pigs. *Fed. Proc.* 31:735 (abstr.).

Davie, J. M., Paul, W. E., Katz, D. H., and Benacerraf, B., 1972b. Hapten-specific tolerance: Preferential depression of the high-affinity antibody response. *J. Exp. Med.* 136:436.

Davie, J. M., Rosenthal, A. S., and Paul, W. E., 1971a. Receptors on immunocompetent cells. III. Specificity and nature of receptors on dinitrophenylated guinea pig albumin- ^{125}I-binding lymphocytes of immunized guinea pigs. *J. Exp. Med.* 134:517.

Davie, J. M., Paul, W. E., Mage, R., and Goldman, M. B., 1971b. Membrane-associated immunoglobulin of rabbit peripheral blood lymphocytes: Allelic exclusion at the *b* locus. *Proc. Nat. Acad. Sci.* 68:430.

Dwyer, J. M., Warner, N. L., and Mackay, I. R., 1972. Specificity and nature of the antigen-combining sites on fetal and mature thymus lymphocytes. *J. Immunol.* 108:1439.

Ehrlich, P., 1900. On immunity with special reference to cell life. *Proc. Roy. Soc.* 66:424.

Eisen, H. N., and Siskind, G. W., 1964. Variations in affinities of antibodies during the immune response. *Biochemistry* 3:996.

Herrod, H. G., and Warner, N. L., 1972. Inhibition by anti-μ chain sera of the cellular transfer of antibody and immunoglobulin synthesis in mice. *J. Immunol.* 108:1712.

Hogg, N. M., and Greaves, M. F., 1972. Antigen-binding thymus-derived lymphocytes. II. Nature of the immunoglobulin determinants. *Immunology* 22:967.

Humphrey, J. H., and Keller, H. U., 1970. Some evidence for specific interaction between immunologically competent cells and antigens. In J. Sterzl, and I. Riha (eds.), *Developmental Aspects of Antibody Formation and Structure*, Vol. II, Academic Press, New York, p. 485.

Julius, M. H., Masuda, T., and Herzenberg, L. A., 1972. Demonstration that antigen-binding cells are precursors of antibody-producing cells after purification with a fluorescence-activated cell sorter. *Proc. Nat. Acad. Sci.* 69:1934.

Katz, D. H., Davie, J. M., Paul, W. E., and Benacerraf, B., 1971. Carrier function in anti-hapten antibody responses. IV. Experimental conditions for the induction of hapten-specific tolerance or for the stimulation of anti-hapten anamnestic responses by "non-immunogenic" hapten-polypeptide conjugates. *J. Exp. Med.* 134:201.

Kincade, P. W., and Cooper, M. D., 1971. Development and distribution of immunoglobulin-containing cells in the chicken. An immunofluorescent analysis using purified antibodies to μ, γ and light chains. *J. Immunol.* 106:371.

Kincade, P. W., Lawton, A. R., Bockman, D. E., and Cooper, M. D., 1970. Suppression of immunoglobulin G synthesis as a result of antibody-mediated suppression of immunoglobulin M synthesis in chickens. *Proc. Nat. Acad. Sci.* 67:1918.

Klinman, N. R., 1971. Purification and analysis of "monofocal" antibody. *J. Immunol.* 106:1345.

Lamelin, J. P., Lisowska-Bernstein, B., Matter, A., Ryser, J. E., and Vasalli, P., 1972. Mouse thymus-independent and thymus-derived lymphoid cells. I. Immunofluorescent and functional studies. *J. Exp. Med* 136:984.

Lawton, A. R., Asofsky, R., Hylton, M. B., and Cooper, M. D., 1972. Suppression of immunoglobulin class synthesis in mice. I. Effects of treatment with antibody to μ-chain. *J. Exp. Med.* 135:277.

Mäkelä, O., and Nossal, G. J. V., 1961. Bacterial adherence: A method for detecting antibody production by single cells. *J. Immunol.* 87:447.

Manning, D. D., and Jutilla, J. W., 1972. Immunosuppression of mice injected with heterologous anti-immunoglobulin heavy chain antisera. *J. Exp. Med.* 135:1316.

Miller, A., DeLuca, D., Decker, J., Ezzell, R., and Sercarz, E. E., 1971. Specific binding of antigen to lymphocytes. Evidence for lack of unispecificity in antigen-binding cells. *Am. J. Pathol.* 65:451.

Möller, E., Sjöberg, O., and Mäkelä, O., 1971. Immunological unresponsiveness against the 4-hydroxy-3,5-dinitro-phenacetyl (NNP) hapten in different lymphoid cell populations. *Eur. J. Immunol.* 1:218.

Naor, D., and Sulitzeanu, D., 1969. Binding of ^{125}I-BSA to lymphoid cells of tolerant mice. *Intern. Arch. Allergy Appl. Immunol.* 36:112.

Naor, D., and Sulitzeanu, D., 1967. Binding of radioiodinated bovine serum albumin to mouse spleen cells. *Nature* 214:687.

Nossal, G. J. V., Warner, N. L., Lewis, H., and Sprent, J., 1972. Quantitative features of a sandwich radioimmuno-labeling technique for lymphocyte surface receptors. *J. Exp. Med.* 135:405.

Pasanen, V. J., and Mäkelä, O., 1969. Effect of the number of haptens coupled to each erythrocyte on hemolytic plaque formation. *Immunology* 16:399.

Paul, W. E., 1970. Functional specificity of antigen-binding receptors of lymphocytes. *Transpl. Rev.* 5:130.

Pierce, C. W., Solliday, S. M., and Asofsky, R., 1972a. Immune responses in vitro. IV. Suppression of primary γM, γG, and γA plaque-forming cell responses in mouse spleen cell cultures by class-specific antibody to mouse immunoglobulin. *J. Exp. Med.* 135:675.

Pierce, C. W., Solliday, S. M., and Asofsky, R., 1972b. Immune responses in vitro. V. Suppression of γM, γG, and γA plaque-forming cell responses in cultures of primed mouse spleen cells by class-specific antibody to mouse immunoglobulins. *J. Exp. Med.* 135:698.

Rabellino, E., Colon, S., Grey, H. M., and Unanue, E. R., 1971. Immunoglobulins on the surface of lymphocytes. I. Distribution and quantitation. *J. Exp. Med.* 133:156.

Raff, M. C., 1970. Two distinct populations of peripheral lymphocytes in mice distinguishable by immunofluorescence. *Immunology* 19:637.

Roelants, G. E., 1972. Quantitation of antigen specific T and B lymphocytes in mouse spleens. *Nature New Biol.* 236:252.

Rosenthal, A. S., Davie, J. M., Rosenstreich, D. L., and Blake, J. T., 1972. Depletion of antibody-forming cells and their precursors from complex lymphoid populations. *J. Immunol.* **108**:279.

Schlesinger, M., 1970. Anti-θ antibodies for detecting thymus-dependent lymphocytes in the immune response of mice to SRBC. *Nature* **226**:1254.

Shevach, E., Green, I., Ellman, L., and Maillard, J., 1972. Heterologous antiserum to thymus-derived cells in the guinea pig. *Nature New Biol.* **235**:19.

Siskind, G. W., and Benacerraf, B., 1969. Cell selection by antigen in the immune response. *Adv. Immunol.* **10**:1.

Sjöberg, O., and Möller, E., 1970. The presence of antigen-binding cells in tolerant animals. *Nature* **228**:780.

Takahashi, T., Old, L. J., McIntire, K. R., and Boyse, E. A., 1971. Immunoglobulin and other surface antigens of cells of the immune system. *J. Exp. Med.* **134**:815.

Warner, N. L., Byrt, P., and Ada, G. L., 1970. Blocking of the lymphocyte antigen receptor site with anti-immunoglobulin sera *in vitro. Nature* **226**:942.

Wilson, J. D., 1971. Immunoglobulin determinants on rosette-forming cells. Their changing nature during an immune response. *Aust. J. Exp. Biol. Med. Sci.* **49**:415.

Zaalberg, O. B., van der Meul, V. A., and van Twisk, M. J., 1968. Antibody production by isolated spleen cells. A study of cluster and plaque techniques. *J. Immunol.* **100**:451.

Chapter 8

Modification of B Lymphocyte Differentiation by Anti-Immunoglobulins

Alexander R. Lawton, III and Max D. Cooper

Spain Immunology Research Laboratories
Departments of Pediatrics and Microbiology
University of Alabama in Birmingham
Birmingham, Alabama

INTRODUCTION

The discovery that in birds and mammals lymphoid cells mediating delayed sensitivity are developmentally and, in part, functionally independent from those involved in antibody production has greatly stimulated research on the cellular aspects of immunity. Recognition that B and T cells are separate populations has led to the definition of morphologic and functional markers for these cell lines. These markers have made it feasible to study the early events of lymphoid differentiation.

Among the markers described for B cells are receptors for antigen-antibody complexes (Basten *et al.*, 1972), aggregated IgG (Dickler and Kunkel, 1972), and activated C3 (Bianco *et al.*, 1970), as well as membrane antigens such as MBLA (Raff *et al.*, 1971; Lamelin *et al.*, 1972) and PC-1 (Takahashi *et al.*, 1970). Functionally, a more important B lymphocyte marker is the immunoglobulin present in high density on the cell surface (Coombs *et al.*, 1969; Pernis *et al.*, 1970; Raff, 1970). The available evidence indicates that the membrane-bound immunoglobulin on B lymphocytes serves as the receptor for antigen and is a critical component of the triggering mechanism which initiates proliferation to form memory cells and terminal differentiation to antibody-secreting plasma cells (reviewed in Davie and Paul, 1973; Wigzell, 1973).

Supported by USPHS-NIH Grants CA 13148, RR 055349, and the American Cancer Society.

Following the leads provided by experiments demonstrating suppression of synthesis of immunoglobulins bearing specific allotypic markers by antiallotype antibodies in rabbits and mice, several groups of investigators have used heterologous antibodies directed toward various classes of immunoglobulins to study expression of immunoglobulin in the surface of B lymphocytes as it relates to differentiation of this cell line. In this chapter we will attempt to bring together information obtained from this approach in several species and using different experimental designs. Allotype suppression has been reviewed elsewhere and will be mentioned only briefly (Mage, 1967; Herzenberg and Herzenberg, 1973).

We will begin by outlining the conceptual framework on which our interpretations will be based. B lymphocyte differentiation is a discontinuous process, divisible into two major stages. The first stage involves the initial expression of genes coding for antibodies and incorporation of receptor antibody into the cell membrane. The clonal selection hypothesis and its forerunners predicted that this process precedes recognition of exogenous antigens, and a considerable amount of direct evidence supports this view. The second stage is initiated by contact with antigen and includes all of the events comprising a humoral immune response. This oversimplified restatement of the clonal selection hypothesis is important to this review, since experiments using antibodies to various classes of immunoglobulins to manipulate the development of B cells have been directed primarily at either first or second stage events, and the results can be viewed more clearly in this context.

SUPPRESSION OF FIRST STAGE B LYMPHOCYTE DIFFERENTIATION: *IN VIVO* MODELS

In a study of the ontogeny of immunoglobulin-producing cells in the chicken using immunofluorescent techniques, Kincade and Cooper (1971) made observations supporting the idea that IgG producing cells were the progeny of cells which previously had synthesized IgM. First, as had been previously shown by Thorbecke *et al.* (1968), IgM synthesis preceded IgG synthesis in the developing bursa by a period of several days. Second, it was found that the first cells synthesizing IgG always appeared in the medullary areas of follicles which already contained many IgM producers, although other follicles in the same section might contain only IgM. Third, a substantial number of individual bursal cells which contained stainable cytoplasmic IgG also contained IgM, while a very small proportion of IgG-producing spleen cells were apparent "double producers."

The idea that antibody-producing cells might switch from IgM to IgG synthesis has been the subject of many investigations since it was determined that IgM antibodies could be detected earlier than IgG antibodies during a primary immune response. In all instances, the question had been posed within the context of what we have termed second-stage B cell differentiation; that is, whether such a switch occurs within a population of cells engaged in response to an antigen. Although in several studies simultaneous production of IgM and IgG antibodies by single cells was demonstrated, the frequency of such cells was low (Nossal *et al.*, 1964; Nordin *et al.*, 1970; Ivanyi and Dresser, 1970; Nossal *et al.*, 1972). Together with evidence that most immunoglobulin-producing cells were restricted to synthesis of a single type of heavy and light chain (Pernis *et al.*, 1965; Cebra *et al.*, 1966), these results argued that cells committed to IgG and IgM synthesis were largely independent populations.

Knowledge of the effects of embryonic bursectomy on the development of IgM and IgG serum concentrations in chickens placed the idea of a switch in a different perspective. Chickens bursectomized sufficiently early in embryonic life were found to be agammaglobulinemic, whereas chicks bursectomized 2 or 3 days prior to hatching frequently attained IgM levels many times normal, but had very low or undetectable IgG in serum (Cooper *et al.*, 1969). By the time of hatching bursectomy usually does not prevent development of IgM or IgG synthesis. These observations suggested that expression of both immunoglobulin classes, and their relative rates of production, was in some way controlled by the bursa. It has since been possible to relate these findings to the numbers and commitment with regard to immunoglobulin class of precursor B lymphocytes emigrating from the bursa prior to its removal. The first cells to differentiate in this site synthesize IgM, and on leaving the bursa they and their progeny are apparently permanently committed to synthesis of IgM. These cells, or the clones they comprise, have a long functional life-span and must be capable of replication, since chickens subjected to early bursectomy continue to produce large amounts of IgM, have stable (although lower than normal) percentages of circulating B lymphocytes, and make antibodies to complex antigens if repeatedly stimulated. Despite antigen-driven replication, they do not switch from IgM to IgG production, as evidenced by the persistent deficiency of circulating IgG (Kincade *et al.*, 1973). Together with the previously cited studies indicating the rarity of cells simultaneously producing IgM and IgG during an immune response, or among immunoglobulin producers populating peripheral lymphoid tissues, these results argue against the frequent occurrence of a switch from IgM to IgG among post-bursal lymphocytes. The dichotomy between these results and the frequency of apparent "double producers" within the developing bursa strengthened our suspicion of a switch from IgM to IgG synthesis during the primary stage of B lymphocyte differentiation.

It was to investigate this possibility that experiments involving administration of antibodies to μ chains to chick embryos were initiated. Briefly, Kincade *et al.* found that a sufficient dose of purified anti-μ antibodies given *in ovo* just before IgM synthesis begins in the bursa resulted in a profound depression in synthesis of both IgM and IgG. If this treatment were combined with bursectomy at hatching, permanent agammaglobulinemia was the result; birds given anti-μ but not bursectomized recovered the capacity to synthesize both immunoglobulin classes within a period of a few weeks (Cooper et al., 1971; Kincade et al., 1970). Birds made agammaglobulinemic by anti-μ treatment and bursectomy were shown to (1) lack lymphocytes in peripheral blood or spleen with membrane-bound immunoglobulin (Kincade et al., 1971); (2) lack cells capable of forming rosettes with sheep erythrocytes or binding ^{125}I labeled antigens (Kincade et al., unpublished observations; Webb and Cooper, 1973); and (3) lack germinal centers and cells with stainable cytoplasmic immunoglobulin of any class. These agammaglobulinemic birds rejected wattle grafts as rapidly as normal controls and have since been shown to develop delayed sensitivity to tuberculin, DNP-guinea pig albumin, and ferritin.

Kincade and Cooper (1973) have analyzed the development of the recently described chicken IgA as regards the effects of bursectomy. In normal chickens, IgA is not detectable in serum before about 19 days after hatching, and thus lags considerably behind IgM. The effects of embryonic bursectomy on development of IgA indicate that cells committed to synthesis of this class develop in and immigrate from the bursa later than IgG precursors. Bursectomy before 18 days of incubation resulted in absence of detectable IgA at 5 months of age. IgA was not detectable in the serum of any bird which was markedly deficient in IgG, and was also absent in some birds with substantial amounts of serum IgG. Birds deficient in circulating IgA also lacked IgA-containing cells in lymphoid tissue, including the lamina propria of the intestine. Finally, it was determined that chickens made agammaglobulinemic by treatment with anti-μ and bursectomy at hatching lacked IgA as well as IgM and IgG.

We have interpreted the suppression of IgG and IgA synthesis which follows treatment with anti-μ antibodies and bursectomy as indicating that the precursor B lymphocytes for the latter classes are derived from cells which have synthesized and expressed IgM on their surface. From the evidence mentioned previously which attests to the infrequency of a switch from IgM to IgG synthesis during the antigen-driven stage of B lymphocyte differentiation, we further concluded that this switch in chickens occurs in and under the control of the bursa of Fabricius. One of the most convincing pieces of evidence supporting this statement, and also the best control for the specificity of the effects of anti-μ, was obtained by analyzing the effects of anti-μ treatment on chicks which had been allowed to hatch, were bursectomized, and then treated with anti-μ antibodies. This treatment brought about significant reductions in serum IgM concentrations, but did not suppress IgG synthesis (Kincade et al., 1971).

Primarily on the basis of these results in chickens we have formulated a model for B cell differentiation which has been discussed in detail elsewhere (Cooper et al., 1972a,b). Since the ideas expressed in this model have provided the stimulus for our research as well as the conceptual framework, or bias, of our interpretations it will be briefly recapitulated. The model divides B lymphocyte differentiation into two stages. The first stage involves the conversion of stem cells to antigen-sensitive B lymphocytes and takes place within and under the direct influence of a specific inductive microenvironment. A major event in development of immunocompetence is the expression of genes for the synthesis of antibody and the incorporation of this antibody into the cell membrane. The developing stem cell first synthesizes and expresses IgM on its surface. In subsequent generations some of the progeny of this cell repress the gene for the constant region of the μ chain ($C\mu$) and switch to expression of $C\gamma$ without any necessary alteration in the expression of genes coding for other components of the receptor antibody (C_L, V_L, V_H). A similar switch among progeny of IgG-committed B cells would lead to expression of $C\alpha$. This switch in genetic commitment of B cells may not be immediately reflected in the class of membrane-bound immunoglobulin, since it has been demonstrated that cells committed to IgG synthesis may have IgM surface immunoglobulin (Pernis *et al.,* 1971). Since the turnover rate of cell surface immunoglobulin is high (Vitetta and Uhr, 1972), it seems necessary to postulate that this surface immunoglobulin, if made by the cell bearing it, may be coded by a long-lived messenger RNA.

B lymphocytes randomly exit from this microenvironment in the order of their development; IgM committed cells appear first in peripheral lymphoid tissues, then IgG cells, and finally IgA cells. The place of IgD and IgE in this sequence has not been established. The second stage of differentiation begins when a clone of cells having the same specificity for antigen but with members committed to synthesis of each immunoglobulin class makes contact with its antigen. All of the differentiative events initiated by direct antigen contact comprise this stage; our model simply proposes that a switch in synthesis of heavy chain class occurs rarely during antigen-driven terminal differentiation.

Suppression of Immunoglobulin Synthesis in Mice

Our studies on suppression of immunoglobulin synthesis in mice by anti-immunoglobulins have been designed to obtain evidence supporting or contradicting this model. The primary goals were to determine (1) whether the switch from IgM to IgG synthesis during initial B lymphocyte differentiation which had been demonstrated in the chicken was also a fundamental aspect of differentiation of this cell line in mammals, and (2) whether the postulated developmental sequence, IgM→IgG→IgA, could be verified experimentally. The germfree mouse was chosen as the experimental subject with consideration of these goals. IgM synthesis and secretion in germfree mice cannot be detected until a few days following birth, and synthesis of IgG_1 begins still later. The failure of anti-μ antibodies given after hatching to depress IgG synthesis in chickens emphasized the importance of introducing the antibodies during the earliest period of B lymphocyte development. Adult germfree mice have low serum concentrations of IgG_1 and often lack detectable IgG_2. The levels of maternally derived IgG immunoglobulins in the young are correspondingly low. The probability of delivering antibodies specific for IgG to the appropriate target cells without interference from circulating IgG would thus be enhanced in germfree offspring, making it feasible to determine the effects of IgG suppression on IgA synthesis. Our experience with the chicken model also suggested the necessity for continued administration of antiglobulins, since recovery from suppression was very rapid if the bursa was left *in situ* (Kincade *et al.*, 1970). Each of these considerations proved to be important, although not absolutely critical, as Manning and Jutila (1972c,d) have demonstrated the feasibility of suppressing immunoglobulin synthesis in conventional mice with antibodies to μ chain.

The same basic protocol has been used for experiments involving treatment of mice with antibodies to various classes of immunoglobulins and for analysis of the results (Lawton *et al.*, 1972d). Purified goat antibodies have been used in all experiments. The mouse myeloma proteins MOPC 104E (IgMλ), RPC-23 (IgG$_1$, κ), RPC-24 (IgG$_{2a}$, κ), and MOPC 315 (IgA λ) coupled to Sepharose 2B, served as immunoadsorbents. In each case the antiserums were cross absorbed to remove unwanted specificities before elution of antibody from the homologous column. Germfree BALB/c mice were injected intraperitoneally with 0.5 mg of antibody on the day of birth, an additional 1.5 mg to 2 mg at intervals during the first week, and then 1.0 mg each week until the termination of the experiments. Control animals received injections of normal goat γ globulin or no injections. When the mice were 8–10 weeks old, half of each group was immunized 3 times with soluble ferritin or once with ferritin in complete Freund's adjuvant. Three to four w eks later the animals were sacrificed. Serum was obtained for measurement of immunoglobulin concentrations and determination of hemagglutination titers to ferritin, goat IgG, a crude preparation of goat serum globulins, and sheep erythrocytes. Spleens, mesenteric lymph nodes, and a large segment of small intestine were removed for histologic and immunofluorescent study. The percentage of B lymphocytes bearing immunoglobulins M, G_1, G_2, and A in spleen was determined by direct immunofluorescence. Immunoglobulin biosynthesis by cultured spleen fragments was estimated by immunoelectrophoresis and autoradiography. Other assays of B and T lymphocyte function have been done in selected experiments and will be discussed in following sections (these experiments result from collaborative efforts with Dr. Richard Asofsky, Ms. Martha Hylton, Dr. Joseph Davie, and Dr. Robert Tigelaar).

Suppression of Immunoglobulin Synthesis by Anti-μ Antibodies

To date more than 40 mice treated with anti-μ antibodies according to the protocol outlined above have been studied. Excepting one animal, which provided an important clue to the biologic activity of anti-μ, the results have been remarkably consistent. Two gross alterations of lymphoid tissue occurred in anti-μ treated mice. Spleens from such animals, except those given complete Freund's adjuvant, were very small, having a mean weight of less than 40 mg as compared to 74 mg for uninjected controls and 86 mg for animals given normal goat γ-globulin. This difference was correlated histologically with extreme rarity or absence of germinal centers in spleens of suppressed mice. The second striking morphologic difference between anti-μ treated and other groups of mice was the absence of visible Peyer's patches in the former. Although small aggregates of lymphocytes could be found microscopically in sections of the intestines, corticomedullary differentiation was lacking. Runting, as recently described by Murgita *et al.* (1973) in conventional Swiss mice given anti-μ, has never occurred in our experiments.

Immunoglobulin production in anti-μ treated mice has been measured using three different assays: determination of serum immunoglobulin concentrations, of biosynthesis of immunoglobulin by cultured spleen fragments, and a semi-quantitative analysis of numbers of immunoglobulin-producing cells in spleen, mesenteric lymph node, and gut. The results have been quite complementary. The immunofluorescence assay has been particularly valuable in determining the effects of treatment with anti-globulin on IgA production.

In Table I the geometric mean immunoglobulin concentrations and frequency of detectable levels in serum from anti-μ treated mice is compared to those of two control groups. One group of controls received normal goat γ-globulin (NGG) according to the same dosage schedule as was used for anti-μ antibody. Other controls were uninjected. Anti-μ treated mice, excluding the one animal which will be discussed subsequently, lacked detectable IgM. IgG_1 concentrations were higher than in uninjected controls, but lower than in NGG treated mice. Mean levels of IgG_2 and IgA were similar in uninjected controls and anti-μ treated mice, both being considerably lower than in NGG controls. Differences between the groups were magnified by analysis of the frequency of detectable immunoglobulins. One anti-μ treated animal was agammaglobulinemic, and nearly half (18/42) lacked immunoglobulins other than IgG_1. Comparisons of frequency of detectable IgM, IgG_2, and IgA in anti-μ treated mice *vs.* either control group showed highly significant differences with the exception of IgG_2 in anti-μ *vs.* uninjected controls. Although mean levels of IgG_1 were not significantly different in anti-μ treated animals and NGG controls, the distribution of concentrations was quite different, the former having a higher proportion of low levels (<1 mg/ml) and a lower proportion of very high levels (>10 mg/ml), as shown in Table II. Similar results emerge from comparisons of the frequency of detectable immunoglobulin biosynthesis by cultured spleen fragments (Table III). This technique reveals that more than half of anti-μ treated animals are not completely suppressed, in that they do synthesize small amounts of IgM. Compared to uninjected germfree controls, anti-μ treated mice have a significantly decreased frequency of IgM, IgG_2, and IgA synthesis.

Table I. Serum Immunoglobulins in Mice Treated with Anti-μ, Uninjected Controls, and Controls Given Normal Goat IgG[1]

Treatment	IgM		IgG$_1$		IgG$_2$		IgA	
	Mean[2]	Frequency[3]	Mean	Frequency	Mean	Frequency	Mean	Frequency
Normal goat IgG	1.56	26/26	9.04	26/26	0.13	26/26	0.18	26/26
p[4]		<0.001		NS		<0.001		<0.001
Anti-μ[5]	<0.02	0/42	5.11	41/42	<0.02	13/42	<0.03	8/42
p		<0.001		NS		<0.1		<0.001
None	0.23	49/49	0.18	49/49	<0.02	24/49	<0.04	38/49

[1] Pooled results from 4 separate experiments
[2] Geometric mean, mg/ml
[3] Proportion with Ig concentrations > 0.02 mg/ml
[4] Chi square test for significance of difference in frequency of detectable immunoglobulin
[5] Data on one animal in this group were not included, as explained in the text

Table II. Distribution of Serum IgG_1 Concentrations[a]

	Number of animals with		
Group	< 1 mg/ml	1–10 mg/ml	> 10 mg/ml
Anti-μ	8	18	16
Normal goat IgG	0	10	16

[a] $\chi^2 = 6.9; p < 0.05$

Table III. Frequency of Detectable Immunoglobulin Biosynthesis by Cultured Spleen Fragments from Anti-μ Treated and Control Mice

Treatment	IgM	IgG_1	IgG_2	IgG_{2b}	IgA
Goat IgG	25/25	25/25	24/25	9/10	21/25
p	<0.001	NS	<0.1	<0.001	<0.05
Anti-μ	20/32	32/32	25/32	4/18	18/32
p	<0.001	NS	<0.005	<0.001	<0.001
None	41/41	41/41	41/41	37/41	41/41

The major additional information obtained from immunofluorescent examination of tissues relates to the distribution of IgA positive cells in gut. Such cells were either very rare or absent in the lamina propria of anti-μ treated animals; in controls IgA cells were present in all suitably sectioned villi, in numbers usually exceeding 10 per longitudinal section (Lawton et al., 1972d). Surprisingly, this high frequency of IgA positive cells was found in all uninjected germfree mice as well as controls given goat IgG. The frequency of IgA positive cells in gut has proven to be a much better index of suppression of IgA synthesis than their frequency in spleen or mesenteric node where they are rare in all germfree animals. The latter tissues from anti-μ treated mice sometimes contained as many IgA cells as did those from controls.

The incomplete suppression of immunoglobulin synthesis was more than balanced by the profound depression of antibody responsiveness in mice treated with anti-μ. With the exception to be discussed later, none of the 19 mice immunized with ferritin have produced detectable antibodies (Table IV). This number includes 4 animals which received ferritin in complete Freund's adjuvant (see Table VII). All immunized control animals responded. In order to determine the effects of chronic antigenic stimulation by the goat antibodies, titers to two fractions of goat serum were measured. One fraction was goat IgG, eluted from DEAE under conditions of low ionic strength. The second was a heterogeneous fraction of goat globulins, including immunoglobulins. We expected that many control animals would respond to minor contaminants but might exhibit neo-natal tolerance to goat IgG, which is the major component in the antibody preparation. In fact, most of the controls given normal goat IgG had antibodies to pure IgG, although the titers to goat globulins were much higher. No antibody to goat IgG was found in anti-μ treated mice. Three-fourths had antibodies to goat globulins, but the titers were lower than in goat IgG treated controls.

The primary target for the suppressive effect of anti-μ antibodies on immu-noglobulin synthesis and specific antibody production is the B lymphocyte. This conclusion is supported by both morphologic and functional observations. (1) Lymphoid tissues from anti-μ treated mice lacked or were very deficient in germinal centers and primary follicles in the lymph node cortex, which are the major homing sites for B lymphocytes (Lawton et al., 1972d). (2) Fewer than 2% of spleen cells from these mice had membrane-bound immunoglobulin, as detected by direct immunofluorescence (see Table VI). In our own studies, as

Table IV. Frequency of Detectable Antibody Responses in Anti-μ Treated and Control Mice[a]

Treatment	Ferritin	Antigens goat IgG[b]	Goat globulins[c]
Goat IgG	10/10	17/25	20/20
p	<0.001	<0.001	<0.05
Anti-μ	0/19	0/42	29/36
p	<0.001		
None	28/28	–	–

[a] Antibodies were detected by passive hemagglutination, using antigens coated to sheep erythrocytes. Equivocal (±) agglutination is scored as negative.

[b] Fraction of goat serum eluted from DEAE with 0.01 M phosphate, pH 8.0.

[c] Fraction of goat serum eluted from DEAE with 0.2 M NaCl in 0.01 M phosphate, pH 8.0.

well as those of other groups, about 45% of spleen cells from normal (including germfree) mice carry this B lymphocyte marker (Lamelin *et al.*, 1972; Raff, 1970; Rabellino *et al.*, 1971; Jones *et al.*, 1971). (3) The reduction in spleen size and cell yield in anti-μ treated mice (about 40% less than controls) correlated closely with the deficiency of B lymphocytes. The complement of T lymphocytes in these spleens was not measured directly, but a functional assessment indicated that the proportion of T cells was increased by a factor of 2. In a quantitative graft-*vs.*-host assay, the spleen enlargement produced by injection of 2.5×10^6 spleen cells from anti-μ treated mice into BALB/c $\times$ C57 B1 recipients was greater than that produced by 5×10^6 cells from control spleens (Asofsky *et al.*, submitted for publication). These data suggest that the absolute numbers of T cells per spleen are normal, and that the reduction in spleen size is attributable to B cell deficiency. (4) The frequency of spleen cells binding ^{125}I ferritin in anti-μ treated mice was less than $1/10^5$, and was not increased following immunization. (5) The deficiency of ferritin-binding lymphocytes in spleens from anti-μ treated mice was correlated with the failure of their spleen cells to adoptively transfer a secondary response to ferritin when given to irradiated recipients (Lawton *et al.*, 1972a; Asofsky *et al.*, submitted for publication).

The suppressive effects of anti-μ were found to be highly dependent upon the timing and duration of anti-μ treatment (Lawton *et al.*, 1973). The initial clues to the importance of these factors came from the exceptional mouse, which has been omitted from the preceding data. This animal, recognized at autopsy because of the presence of a large spleen and Peyer's patches, was analyzed separately. It had high immunoglobulin levels, normal proportions of B lymphocytes in spleen, large numbers of cells binding ^{125}I ferritin ($140/10^5$), and produced antibodies in response to ferritin (Asofsky *et al.*, submitted for publication). Since this mouse was housed with several other fully suppressed animals and must have received anti-μ injections, we guessed that one or more injections given during the first week of life might have leaked from its peritoneal cavity. To investigate this possibility, groups of mice were begun on treatment with anti-μ (1 mg/week) at 1 or 2 weeks of age, and injections were continued until 1 week before sacrifice. Other mice were treated with 2.5 mg anti-μ during the first week of life and received no subsequent injection.

The major differences observed in groups of mice treated with anti-μ by the 3 different protocols is given in Tables V–VII. Neither the LAG (delayed treatment) nor the SHORT (early treatment) mice showed any evidence for suppression of immunoglobulin synthesis or antibody responses. SHORT animals had immunoglobulin levels which were comparable to uninjected controls, while LAG animals had high levels, similar to mice given normal goat globulin. IgM concentrations of LAG mice were even higher than those of NGG controls.

Two observations in the LAG animals were particularly striking. First, their

Table V. B-Cell Development in Mice Treated with Anti-μ According to Different Schedules[a]

	Full	Short	Lag
Peyer's patches	0	N[c]	N
Spleen weight	↓	N	↑
Germinal centers	↓↓	N	↑
B lymphocytes	↓↓	N	↑(IgG$_1$)
Antibody response	0	N	N (↑)[b]
IgA cells in gut	↓↓	N	N

[a] FULL: 2 mg anti-μ during first week of life, 1 mg each week thereafter.
SHORT: 2 mg anti-μ during first week, none thereafter.
LAG: 1 mg anti-μ each week, beginning at 1 or 2 weeks of age.

[b] 12/13 unimmunized LAG animals had measurable levels of antibodies to ferritin (mean $\log_2$ titer, 3.4 ± 1.4). 1/12 immunized animals did not respond. 17/25 LAG mice had natural agglutinins to SRBC (3.2 ± 2.5), as compared to 4/30 mice given NGG (0.4 ± 1.1).

[c] N, normal as compared to uninjected controls.

spleens contained a variable but high proportion of cells which stained for membrane-bound IgG$_1$ (Table VI). In combined immunofluorescence-autoradiography studies, 30-45% of spleen cells binding ^{125}I ferritin stained for IgG$_1$, and 40-60% for IgM. No γ2-bearing antigen binding cells (ABC) were found in either unimmunized or immunized groups. These results are quite different from those obtained in control mice (discussed more fully below), where nearly all ABC in unimmunized animals stain for IgM, while following immunization approximately 60% stain for IgM and 30% for IgG$_2$ (Asofsky *et al.*, submitted for publication). With the fluorescein conjugated antibodies we have used, no other group of animals has had more than 2% IgG$_1$ positive cells. The high proportion of γ1-B lymphocytes in LAG mice might be an artifact. For example, it could be due to the presence of a complex of goat anti-μ and mouse anti-goat γ-globulin of the IgG$_1$ class coated on IgM bearing B lymphocytes *in vivo;* such cells would stain for the mouse IgG$_1$. However, the fact that these cells have not been seen in mice treated with anti-γ1, anti-γ2, anti-a, or normal

Table VI. Percentage of B Lymphocytes in Spleen[a]

Group	Number of pools[b]	IgM	IgG$_1$	IgG$_2$	IgA
Anti-μ, FULL[c]	10	<0.5 ± 0.2	<0.3 ± 0.1	<0.4 ± 0.3	<0.8 ± 0.8
Anti-μ, LAG[c]	6	31.5 ± 7.3	15.5 ± 12.8	4.2 ± 3.4	<0.5 ± 0.4
Anti-μ, SHORT[c]	4	28.7 ± 2.5	<0.3 ± 0.1	5.5 ± 3.4	2.6 ± 1.1
Normal goat γ-globulin	6	27.8 ± 10.5	1.2 ± 0.8	13.8 ± 9.2	<0.8 ± 0.8
Control	12	32.8 ± 7.0	<0.2 ± 7.0	10.1 ± 8.4	3.0 ± 2.3

[a] Mean ± S.D.
[b] 2–6 spleens/pool.
[c] See footnote, Table V, for treatment schedule.

Table VII. Antibody Responses in Mice Immunized with Ferritin

	Type of immunization				
	75 μg in saline X4		100 μg in complete Freund's adjuvant		
Group	No.	Log$_2$ HA titer	Group	No.	Log$_2$ HA titer
Anti-μ[b] complete	15	0	Anti-μ complete	4	0
Anti-μ LAG[b]	6[a]	10.0 ± 5.2	Anti-μ LAG	6	10.7 ± 1.2
Anti-μ SHORT[b]	9	8.4 ± 2.9	Anti-γ2	6	13.2 ± 2.0
Anti-γ1	8	5.9 ± 2.6	Anti-γ1 + γ2	6	10.0 ± 2.7
Normal goat γ-globulin	5	7.0 ± 1.6	Normal goat γ-globulin	9	14.2 ± 1.6
Control	21	7.4 ± 1.8	Control	7	14.7 ± 1.4

[a] 1 animal did not respond.
[b] See footnote, Table V, for treatment schedule.

goat IgG, all of which were making antibodies to goat γ-globulin, raises the possibility that anti-μ has modulated in some way the expression of immunoglobulin by B lymphocytes. The second observation may be consistent with this possibility. Unimmunized LAG mice, with one exception, had low but significant antibody titers to ferritin (Table V). In addition, most had antibodies to sheep erythrocytes, which are almost always lacking in germfree mice. This effect may be similar to that sought in a recent study by Katz and Unanue (1972). These investigators asked whether treatment of primed mouse spleen cells with doses of anti-immunoglobulin sufficient to cause capping and endocytosis of surface immunoglobulin would cause the cells to be nonspecifically triggered when injected into irradiated recipients. They failed to find evidence for differentiation to antibody production induced by antiglobulin alone, but they did show that this treatment in conjunction with secondary immunization resulted in an enhanced response in the adoptive host. A similar adjuvant effect was observed in LAG animals immunized with ferritin in saline (Table VII). Excluding one animal which did not respond, titers to ferritin were significantly higher in LAG animals than any other group. This difference was not seen when ferritin was given in complete Freund's adjuvant to LAG and appropriate control animals.

A possible explanation for the different effects of anti-μ given by different schedules has come from studies of the ontogeny of B lymphocytes in mouse spleen (Möller, 1961; Nossal and Pike, 1973; Gelfand et al., 1973; Spear et al., 1973). B lymphocytes are first detectable about 4 days before birth. At the time of birth the proportion of B lymphocytes detected by anti-μ or anti-κ is <4%. Between 24 and 72 hours of life there is a dramatic rise in both percentage and total numbers of B cells, followed by a more gradual increase to adult levels by 3–4 weeks. As seems true in the chicken model, the suppressive effects of anti-μ may be demonstrable only when the antibody contacts the cells at a critical stage of their differentiation.

The same general conclusions on the suppressive effects of anti-μ antibodies given in vivo have been reached by Manning and Jutila (1972c,d). These investigators have used conventional, rather than germfree, BALB/c mice and have examined the effects of anti-μ treatment on immunoglobulin concentrations and plaque-forming responses to sheep erythrocytes. Antiserum to IgM, given chronically from birth, suppressed synthesis of all immunoglobulin classes and eliminated direct and indirect PFC responses. This suppressive effect was shown not to depend upon T cells, since suppression could be achieved in thymusless (nude) animals. Rejection of allogeneic skin grafts by suppressed animals was normal (Manning and Jutila 1972a). Finally, it was shown that complete suppression of PFC responses was dependent upon initiation of anti-μ treatment early in life, and that recovery from suppression had occurred by 1 month following the last injection of anti-μ.

In summary, effective suppression with anti-μ seems to depend upon contact between the antibody and the μ-bearing B lymphocyte at an early stage of its differentiation. The majority of these cells are either killed or prevented from proliferating, resulting in an absolute deficiency of B lymphocytes. Recovery, probably due to differentiation of new waves of stem cells, occurs rapidly when anti-μ treatment is stopped. Some clones, probably those stimulated by antigenic contact to differentiation involving loss of μ receptors, escape from suppression and are stimulated by antigens to synthesize large amounts of IgG_1 antibody. It is known from experiments in chickens that a few B lymphocytes may give rise to many plasma cells and normal or even supernormal serum immunoglobulin concentrations, so that immunoglobulin levels are a relatively insensitive index of the degree of suppression (Kincade et al., 1973). Finally, the evidence is consistent with the concept that μ-bearing B lymphocytes are the precursors of cells committed to synthesis of the other immunoglobulin classes.

Treatment of Mice with Antibodies to $\gamma 1$, $\gamma 2$, and a Determinants

The effects of treatment with antibodies specific for any of these classes have been distinctly different from those produced by anti-μ. All of the animals have had prominent Peyer's patches and normal or large spleens at autopsy. Their spleens have contained normal proportions of B lymphocytes, many germinal centers, and large numbers of plasma cells. Antibody responses to ferritin were comparable to those of controls (Table VII). These negative results strongly reinforce the hypothesis that primary development of immunocompetent B lymphocytes is uniquely related to expression of IgM.

Suppression of IgG_1

Of 17 mice treated with purified anti-$\gamma 1$, only 1 had detectable IgG_1 in serum. This result was in part due to rapid elimination of IgG_1 from circulation, since IgG_1 containing plasma cells were present in spleen and lymph nodes, and biosynthesis of IgG_1 occurred in spleen cultures (Asofsky et al., submitted for publication). By both of these assays, animals treated with anti-$\gamma 1$ synthesized as much or slightly more IgG_1 than uninjected germfree controls, although much less than mice given equivalent amounts of normal goat IgG in other experiments.

The effects of anti-$\gamma 1$ treatment on synthesis of IgG_2 and IgA immunoglobulins were difficult to interpret. IgG_2 concentrations were significantly higher ($p < 0.05$) than in any other group of mice in this series which did not receive complete Freund's adjuvant. Mean levels of IgA were higher than those of uninjected controls studied in the same experiment. However, 6 of the 17 animals lacked detectable IgA in serum, a situation which was never found in controls given normal goat IgG. Guts of these animals contained, on the average, fewer IgA containing plasma cells than the uninjected controls, but many more than were present in anti-μ treated mice. Finally, B lymphocytes bearing IgG_2 and IgA determinants were present in normal to increased numbers in spleen. This experiment provided no firm evidence for the hypothetical differentiation sequence, $M{\rightarrow}G{\rightarrow}A$.

As in the LAG experiments with anti-μ, suggestive evidence for modulation of the immune response was obtained in the anti-γ_1 group. The incidence of spleen cells binding ^{125}I ferritin in unimmunized control mice was ~$10/10^5$; in a combined immunofluorescence-autoradiography assay more than 90% of antigen-binding cells scored had stained for surface IgM. Spleens of ferritin immunized controls contained an average of 44 $ABC/10^5$, of which approximately 70% were μ positive and 30% stained for $\gamma2$. Smaller percentages of cells were stained for $\gamma1$ (7%) and a (15%) as well. This shift in distribution of the classes of immunoglobulin on ABC consequent to immunization of controls was observed in *unimmunized* anti-$\gamma1$ treated mice. This group had approximately the same frequency of ABC ($8/10^5$), but only 63% were μ-bearing, while 20% stained for $\gamma2$. On immunization there was a 20-fold increase in frequency of ABC, as compared to a 4-fold increase in controls. This difference was correlated with an increase of antibody titers in recipients of adoptively transferred spleen cells from this group as compared to controls. The proportion of μ-bearing ABC in immunized anti-$\gamma1$ treated mice was 60%, while 7% stained for $\gamma1$, 36% for $\gamma2$, and 24% for a. In both control and anti-$\gamma1$ treated groups immunized with ferritin, the cumulative percentage of ABC stained for each immunoglobulin class was greater than 100, indicating that some cells either expressed or had passively absorbed more than one immunoglobulin class (Asofsky *et al.*, submitted for publication).

It is not entirely clear that the specificity of the anti-$\gamma1$ was involved in either the adjuvant effect or the change in class distribution of antigen-binding B lymphocytes, since a control group treated with normal goat IgG was not included in this particular experiment. It is perhaps significant that a different sort of shift in the class of immunoglobulin on ABC was observed in animals treated with anti-μ by the LAG protocol. In the latter group, a major proportion of ABC in both immunized and unimmunized animals stained for $\gamma1$ determinants, and no $\gamma2$ ABC were found. Unfortunately, attempts to correlate these shifts with changes in the class of ferritin antibody produced have failed for technical reasons.

Manning and Jutila (1972*b*) have reported somewhat different results in animals treated with anti-$\gamma1$. The doses of antiserum given were not sufficient to eliminate IgG_1 from serum, although the levels were transiently depressed. Nevertheless, they observed partial suppression of the direct PFC response and nearly complete suppression of indirect plaques. The latter observation apparently involved both $\gamma 1$ and $\gamma 2$ PFC. They suggested that the observed suppression of μ and $\gamma 2$ plaques might have been due to contaminants in their antiserum. Since the class of antibody to ferritin was not determined in our experiments, the results cannot be easily compared. However, antibody responses in our anti-$\gamma 1$ animals were slightly higher than in controls. Since IgG_1 was lacking from serum and IgG_2 levels were high, it is likely that the antibody was of IgM and/or IgG_2 classes. Normal germfree mice, similarly immunized with ferritin in saline, have been shown to synthesize antibodies predominantly of the IgG_1 class (Barth et al., 1965; Asofsky et al., 1968).

Suppression with Anti-IgG$_2$ and Anti-IgA

Results of attempts to suppress synthesis of IgG_2 and IgA by administration of their respective antibodies may be summarized very briefly. In neither case was the concentration of circulating immunoglobulin lowered significantly. Responses to ferritin of animals given anti-$\gamma 2$ were substantial, and similar to LAG animals, low titers to ferritin occurred in unimmunized mice. No effect on IgA synthesis was demonstrated in anti-$\gamma 2$ treated mice. Three of five mice treated with anti-a had diminished numbers of IgA containing cells in gut, but this deficiency was not reflected in serum IgA levels, which were quite high (Lawton et al., 1973). Manning has reported transient suppression of IgA synthesis, as manifested by decreased amounts of IgA in serum and feces, in mice treated with anti-a. In his study, recovery of the capacity to synthesize IgA occurred during the course of treatment with anti-a; IgA levels in control and anti-a treated animals were identical by about 50 days of age (Manning, 1972). The animals in our experiments were not studied until 90 days of age. Murgita et al. (1973) have recently reported strikingly different results in anti-a treated mice. They found suppression of serum IgA levels and reduction of IgA producers in spleen, while IgA cells in gut were present in normal numbers. The reasons for this difference are not known.

Evidence That IgA Committed Cells
Are Derived from IgG Bearing Precursors

To this point neither treatment with anti-$\gamma 1$ nor with anti-$\gamma 2$ had produced convincing evidence for suppression of IgA synthesis. Treating mice with antisera reactive with both $\gamma 1$ and $\gamma 2$, Manning and Jutila (1972b) also failed to affect IgA synthesis. In each case, however, suppression of the IgG classes was incomplete. Observations that anti-μ suppression was effective only if begun very early in life, together with the supposition that maternally transferred immunoglobulins might interfere with the effects of antibodies to IgG during this early period of B cell differentiation suggested a modification in experimental design. Thus we attempted to delay differentiation of B lymphocytes for a period of time by treatment with anti-μ, in the hope of permitting catabolism of maternally transferred IgG, before attempting to suppress IgG synthesis. It had already been established that recovery from the effects of anti-μ given during the first week of life was complete by 12 weeks of age.

A group of 12 mice were given 0.5 mg anti-μ on days 1, 2, 3, and 4, and 1 mg on day 7. On days 5, 6, and 8 they received 1 mg of purified antibody specific for shared determinants of $\gamma1$ and $\gamma2$. (The latter antibodies had been prepared by passage of antiserum to IgG_1 over an IgG_2 immunoadsorbent column, and passage of antiserum to IgG_2 over an IgG_1 column. The pooled eluates, after absorption on IgM and IgA columns, reacted strongly with IgG_1 and IgG_2, but failed to react with IgM and IgA myeloma proteins of either κ or λ type.) After the first week of life these animals received no further injections of anti-μ but continued to receive 1 mg anti-$\gamma1 + \gamma2$ weekly. At 8 weeks, half of the mice were immunized with 100 μg ferritin in complete Freund's adjuvant. They were sacrificed at 11 weeks, 1 week following the last injection of anti-$\gamma1$ + $\gamma2$.

The mean level of IgM in serum of these mice was high (2.36 mg/ml), and all immunized animals responded to ferritin. In 6/12 animals (5/6 in the unimmunized group), IgM was the only immunoglobulin detectable in serum. Eight of the twelve animals had no detectable serum IgA. There was a definite correlation between absence of detectable IgG immunoglobulins and of IgA. None of the 6 animals lacking IgG_1 and IgG_2 had detectable IgA, while IgA was present in 4/6 animals having detectable IgG_1. Three of the four mice which had detectable

Table VIII. Frequency of IgA Deficiency

Treatment	No. with IgA <0.02 mg/ml/total	%	Significance[a]
Anti-μ, FULL	34/42	81	
Anti-μ, SHORT	14/21[b]	67	
Anti-$\gamma1 + \gamma2$	8/12	67	
Anti-$\gamma1$	6/17	35	
None	11/49	22	
Anti-a	0/5	0	
Anti-$\gamma2$	0/11	0	
Anti-μ, LAG	0/25	0	
Normal goat IgG	0/26	0	

[a] Chi square test between individual groups. Groups not connected by vertical lines differ at the significance level $p < 0.05$.

[b] The frequency of absent IgA in this group did not differ from that of uninjected controls in the same experiment (7/13, $\chi^2 = 0.6$, $p > 0.3$).

IgA had the highest levels of IgG_1 observed in this group (2.9, 7.3, and 9.5 mg/ml), and 2 of these 3 were the only ones having detectable IgG_2.

In Table VIII the frequency of less than threshold concentrations of IgA in serum is given for all suppression experiments. The first 3 groups, anti-μ FULL, anti-μ SHORT, and anti-γ1 + γ2, differed significantly from both uninjected controls and controls given normal goat IgG. Anti-γ1 treated mice had a significantly higher frequency of IgA deficiency than did controls given equivalent amounts of goat γ-globulin, although they did not differ significantly in this respect from uninjected controls.

The critical question is whether suppression of IgA synthesis in the γ1 + γ2 group was produced by early treatment with anti-μ or by IgG suppression. SHORT animals, who received anti-μ in the same way as the γ1 + γ2 group, had a similar frequency of IgA deficiency in serum. However, the former group had not been given repeated injections of goat IgG, a factor which has a major effect on IgA levels (Table I). A convincing answer to this question was provided by analysis of IgA containing cells in gut. The consistent abundance of IgA containing cells in this location (more than 10 cells per longitudinally sectioned villus) in all controls, including unmanipulated germfree animals, contrasted with their rarity in mice treated with a full suppressive course of anti-μ (less than one cell per 20–30 villi) has given us considerable confidence in this assay.

In Fig. 1 the frequency of IgA positive cells in intestine in animals treated with anti-γ1 + γ2 is compared to that in mice given anti-μ during the first week of life (SHORT group) and no other treatment. Only 2/12 mice in the anti-γ1 + γ2 group were scored as having normal numbers of IgA producing cells, while in 5/12 these cells were very rare. All of the 21 animals in the SHORT group had a high frequency of IgA cells in gut. This difference was highly significant (χ^2 = 20.1, $p < 0.001$). In the anti-γ1 + γ2 group, the frequency of detectable

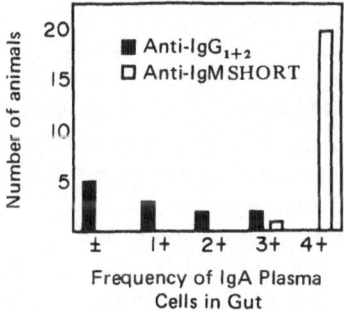

Figure 1. IgA containing cells in gut were scored by direct immunofluorescence. The scoring system ranges from ±, indicating fewer than one cell per 5–10 villi, to 4+, indicating more than 10 cells per villus. The two groups of mice are discussed in the text.

IgA in serum was correlated with numbers of IgA plasma cells in gut; 7 of the 8 mice having low numbers of cells in gut lacked detectable serum IgA, while gut scores were 2–3+ in 3 of 4 animals having serum IgA.

These positive results suggest that the proposed switch from γ to α synthesis during primary B lymphocyte differentiation may be correct. We are hopeful that the early treatment with anti-μ may provide a means whereby any immunoglobulin class may be fully suppressed, thus allowing more precise analysis of differentiation relationships among the two major IgG classes and IgA.

SUPPRESSION OF SECOND STAGE DIFFERENTIATION BY ANTI-IMMUNOGLOBULINS: *IN VITRO* MODELS

Our purpose in this section is not to exhaustively review the results that have been obtained using anti-immunoglobulins to modify B cell responses *in vitro*, but rather to emphasize the fundamental differences between these approaches and the *in vivo* suppression experiments just described. In essence, the *in vitro* models have been used to probe the nature of receptors expressed on B lymphocytes already committed to synthesize antibody of a given specificity. We believe the major effects of *in vivo* treatment with anti-immune globulins are exerted at an earlier stage of differentiation, and provide information on primary development of immunocompetent cells. This distinction will be irrelevant if either of two circumstances holds: (1) the entire process of B cell differentiation is driven by specific antigen contact, or (2) B lymphocytes are differentiated independently of specific antigen contact, but all virgin B lymphocytes have IgM receptors.

That exogenous antigens are not required for primary B lymphocyte differentiation is a basic tenet of the clonal selection hypothesis (Burnet, 1959) and its ancestor (Ehrlich, 1900). Since antigenic influence cannot be entirely excluded in any living organism, this concept is not amenable to formal proof. The closest approach in mammals has come from studies of the ontogeny of B lymphocytes. In the human fetus, IgM and IgG B lymphocytes are present in liver by 8–9 weeks of gestation, and IgA positive cells by 11–12 weeks. By 14 weeks, the proportion of B lymphocytes in blood and spleen are the same as in adults. At these early ages, mature antibody producing cells (taken as evidence of antigen stimulation) are either absent or extremely rare (Lawton et al., 1972b). Proportions of B lymphocytes in spleens of germfree mice are the same as in conventional animals of the same strain, and have the same developmental pattern during ontogeny (Lawton and Asofsky, unpublished data). Specific antigen-binding cells are present before birth in guinea pig (Davie et al., 1972) and mouse (Spear et al., 1973). In the latter species, antigen-binding cells of different specificities were found prior to birth (Spear et al., 1973). Antigen-binding cells, presumably B lymphocytes, are also present in the germfree colostrum-deprived piglet (Decker *et al.*, 1973). The clear implication of these observations is that environmental antigens are not required for generation of B lymphocytes.

The possibility that functional antigen receptors of unprimed B lymphocytes consist exclusively of IgM antibodies has been most convincingly put forth by the studies of Pierce *et al.* (1972*a,b;* 1973). This group has studied the effects of specific antiheavy chain reagents on *in vitro* primary or secondary responses of mouse spleen cells to sheep erythrocytes. Anti-μ was found to inhibit the primary PFC response of all immunoglobulin classes: IgM, IgG$_1$, IgG$_2$, and IgA. Antibodies to $\gamma 1$ suppressed IgG$_1$ PFC, and to a variable extent, IgG$_2$ PFC; anti-$\gamma 2$ behaved in a reciprocal manner. Only IgA PFC were suppressed by anti-a. *In vivo* priming produced definite changes in susceptibility of PFC classes to suppression which were both time and dose dependent. Following immunization with 10^9 SRBC there was a gradual loss of suppression of $\gamma 1$ and $\gamma 2$ PFC by anti-μ which was maximal at 10–14 days. By 21 days, responses in both classes were again fully suppressed by anti-μ. This apparent shift from μ to γ receptors among precursors of IgG-PFC was amplified in both magnitude and duration by increasing the dose of antigen used in priming (Pierce *et al.*, 1973). No such shift occurred in IgA-PFC, which were always inhibited by anti-μ.

The simplest interpretation of these data is that all virgin precursor cells have μ receptors, and that γ receptors are developed (or become functional) only after differentiation events provoked by antigen (Pierce *et al.*, 1973). This is consistent with observations that most (80–90%) antigen-binding cells in unimmunized mice have μ receptors, and that a major proportion of cells with γ receptors can be found after immunization (Davie and Paul, 1973; Wigzell, 1973; Asofsky *et al.*, submitted for publication; Warner *et al.*, 1970; Greaves and Hogg, 1971; Warner, 1972).

Herrod and Warner have used an adoptive transfer system to study the nature of cell receptors. Incubation of unprimed mouse spleen cells with anti-μ at low temperatures or incubation with heavily labeled ^{125}I anti-μ produced reduction of IgM responses to sheep erythrocytes (direct PFC) and to brucella in irradiated recipients of the cells (Herrod and Warner, 1972). However, little or no inhibition of indirect PFC response occurred as a consequence of anti μ treatment, the responses averaging 77-87% of the control (Warner, 1972). In another type of experiment, spleen cells from donor mice having 1 set of IgG$_1$ and IgG$_2$ allotypes were treated with anti-μ and then transferred to congenic recipients with different IgG allotypes. Depression of synthesis of donor allotype in immunized recipients was observed. From the latter data the authors conclude that unprimed B lymphocytes destined for IgG, as well as IgM synthesis had μ receptors. The failure to inhibit IgG antibody responses with anti-μ was felt to be inconclusive, as the absolute magnitude of the indirect response was small in both control and experimental groups.

Warner (1972) and Pierce *et al.* (1973) have proposed similar models for antigen-driven differentiation of B lymphocytes. Both begin with a virgin B cell expressing only μ receptors. Under the influence of antigen, these cells proliferate, and some differentiate to the point of expressing multiple classes of receptor antibodies. Restriction, as regards expression of a single class of receptor antibody, is then a property of memory cells. This concept is supported by the observations of Greaves on changes in the receptor class of rosette forming cells (RFC) during the course of an immune response to sheep erythrocytes. Using inhibition of RFC by antibodies to various immunoglobulin classes as an assay, Greaves observed that early in the immune response the sum of RFC inhibited by anti-μ and anti-$\gamma 1$ or anti-$\gamma 1$ and anti-$\gamma 2$, used independently, was consistently greater than when the two antiglobulins were used together. After about 15 days this additive phenomenon was no longer observed. These results suggested that B-cells early in the response simultaneously expressed more than one immunoglobulin class (Greaves and Hogg, 1971).

These models and ours are in agreement as regards the existence of a switch in expression of CH genes ($\mu \rightarrow \gamma$) during differentiation of a single clone of B lymphocytes. This concept has received additional strong support from demonstration that immunoglobulins of different classes may share identical V regions and light chains (Wang *et al.*, 1970, 1969). The models differ on the role of antigen in this switch: Our model proposes that switching occurs during the primary, antigen-independent, stage of B lymphocyte differentiation.

Evidence for the existence of a major population of virgin B lymphocytes committed to IgG (or IgA) and having homologous receptors is largely circumstantial, but in our view, compelling. (1) IgG-bearing B lymphocytes develop in the avian bursa at a specific time in embryogenesis, apparently not influenced by antigen (Kincade and Cooper, 1971). Extrabursal IgM-bearing lymphocytes are unable to convert to IgG and IgA producing cells (Cooper *et al.*, 1969; Kincade *et al.*, 1973). Neither IgM- nor IgG-producers switch to IgA production outside of the bursa (Kincade and Cooper, 1973). (2) IgG- and IgA-bearing B lymphocytes appear in adult proportions within hemopoietic and lymphoid tissues of the human fetus very early in ontogeny, and probably independently of antigen (Lawton *et al.*, 1972*b*). B lymphocytes with μ or γ receptors have been demonstrated in the fetal pig, shielded from antigen by an impermeable 6-layered placenta (Binns *et al.*, 1972). (3) In the unimmunized adult guinea pig, the majority of lymphocytes binding the antigen dinitrophenyl-guinea pig albumin have IgG_2 receptors; a few IgG_2 antigen-binding cells are present before birth (Davie and Paul, 1973, 1972). Treatment of unprimed spleen or lymph node cells with anti-$\gamma 2$ and complement diminish their capacity to transfer an antibody response to DNP, while anti-μ and complement does not (Davie and Paul, 1971). (4) The numbers and class distribution of B lymphocytes in mouse spleen are identical in germfree and conventional animals of the same strain (Lawton and Asofsky, unpublished data). The thrust of these data is that B lymphocytes bearing γ and α determinants appear under conditions of minimal antigenic influence; presumably they express variable as well as constant region determinants and are potentially capable of binding antigens and being triggered to terminal differentiation.

Anderson's experiments on suppression of IgG allotype responses in mice have provided evidence for existence of a functional population of virgin cells with γ receptors (Anderson, 1972). When F1 (Ig^a/Ig^b) spleen cells were given to irradiated Ig^a recipients together with antiserum to Ig1-b (allotype of IgG_{2a}) and sheep erythrocytes, suppression of specific Ig1-b plaques was obtained, but only after a lag period of 4–5 days. In addition, IgG_1 and Ig-1-a plaques were suppressed, while IgM was unaffected. These results suggested that IgM and IgG precursors were separate populations, but the latter were not restricted with regard to IgG class or allotype. The lag period before onset of suppression implies a population of IgG committed cells with μ receptors, and could clearly be interpreted in terms of an antigen driven switch from μ to γ receptors. However, in other experiments in which anti-Ig1-b was given to irradiated recipients prior to stimulation with sheep erythrocytes, the specific Ig1-b PFC response was suppressed for as long as 46 days following antiserum treatment. Ig1-b protein was detected in serum much earlier, making it unlikely that residual anti-Ig1-b persisted this long. This observation suggests that precursor cells with Ig1-b receptors must have existed prior to antigen contact. Since the B lymphocyte appears to be the target cell for neonatal allotype suppression (Harrison *et al.*, 1973), these and other experiments involving suppression of IgG constant region allotypes would seem to require a population of virgin B lymphocytes with γ receptors (Mage, 1967; Herzenberg and Herzenberg, 1973).

If a population of virgin IgG committed cells with γ receptors exists, why has it been so difficult to demonstrate in functional assays? A useful approach to this question might be to consider some characteristics of IgM and IgG responses in terms of the "receptor equals product" hypothesis. Two aspects will be compared: maturation in affinity and the role of T lymphocytes.

That a major increase in affinity of IgG antibodies occurs with time after immunization has long been recognized (reviewed in Siskind and Benacerraf, 1969). In contrast, affinity of IgM antibodies appears to change very little (Mäkelä *et al.*, 1970; Sarvas and Mäkelä, 1970). Several recent studies have extended these observations to the level of single antibody-forming cells (Andersson, 1970; Davie and Paul, 1972; Claflin *et al.*, 1973; Claflin and Merchant, 1973; Huchet and Feldmann, 1973; Möller *et al.*, 1973). It has been shown that (1) early in the primary response a broad spectrum of affinities exists; (2) maturation involves selection of high affinity cells at the expense of low affinity cells; and (3) the increase in affinity of IgG producers is several orders of magnitude greater than that of IgM producers; in some studies almost no maturation of the latter population was found (Huchet and Feldmann, 1973; Möller *et al.*, 1973). The selection process is viewed as a consequence of cells with receptors of high affinity competing more successfully for diminishing concentrations of antigen. If receptor equals product, the greater selective pressure exerted on IgG precursors than on IgM precursors would suggest that at a given level of receptor affinity, cells with μ receptors are more easily triggered than cells having γ receptors. Mäkelä *et al.* (1970) have previously suggested this possibility and have proposed that the increased efficiency of IgM as a receptor could be based on multivalent binding. The likelihood of the latter idea has been somewhat lessened by indications that cell bound IgM is monomeric rather than pentameric (Vitetta and Uhr, 1972). However, the molecular size of dissociated membrane IgM cannot be taken as firm evidence for its spatial orientation *in situ.*

The concept that μ receptors are more efficient than γ receptors in transmitting the antigen mediated signal for proliferation could explain the class-related differences in requirement for T-cell collaboration (Taylor and Wortis, 1968). Current evidence reviewed by Mitchell (1973) and Gershon (1973) in this volume indicates that IgG responses are much more thymic-dependent than IgM responses. Studies on thymectomized animals have suggested that IgA committed precursors may have a still greater requirement for T-cell help (reviewed in Lawton, *et al.*, 1972c). Athymic mice have a profound deficiency in IgA synthesis, although large numbers of IgA bearing B lymphocytes are present in their circulation (Crewther and Warner, 1972; Bankhurst and Warner, 1972). The deficiency in IgA synthesis can be repaired by transplantation of embryonic thymus epithelium (Wortis, personal communication). A T-cell defect may also be involved in isolated IgA deficiency in humans. Most patients with this abnormality have normal numbers of IgA bearing B lymphocytes (Lawton *et al.*, 1972c), and these cells can be triggered *in vitro* to synthesize and secrete IgA when stimulated by pokeweed mitogen (Wu *et al.*, 1973), suggesting that the *in vivo* differentiation defect may involve another cell line.

The role of T cells in triggering B-cell responses of different antibody classes can be viewed in two ways. The T cell could promote an antigen-driven "switch" in commitment from μ to γ (a). This does not seem to be a prerequisite for the expression of the various immunoglobulin classes on the surface of B lymphocytes, since the development of B lymphocytes bearing each of the immunoglobulin classes is unimpaired in athymic mice (Bankhurst and Warner, 1972) and humans (Cooper and Lawton, 1972). Alternatively, the T cell could facilitate triggering of a population of B cells *already* committed to synthesize IgG or IgA, but incapable of responding with plasma cell differentiation in the absence of T-cell help. Implicit in the second hypothesis is the notion that γ or a receptors may be less efficient than μ receptors in antigen binding or in generating the signal for initiation of terminal differentiation.

The presence of carrier primed T cells greatly enhances the production of hapten-specific antibody (Mitchison, 1969; Katz et al., 1970). Although both IgM and IgG responses may be enhanced (Scherrmacher and Rajewsky, 1970), in some systems the effect seems to be based on selective recruitment of IgG precursors (Claflin and Merchant, 1973; Cheers and Miller, 1973). Cheers and Miller showed that carrier priming of mice dramatically enhanced development of primary hapten-specific IgG plaque-forming cells, but had no effect on the IgM response. The same result was obtained using carrier educated thymus cells in a double adoptive transfer system (Cheers and Miller, 1973). Claflin and Merchant (1973) obtained a similar selective enhancement of primary IgG PFC by carrier priming. Their experiments were designed to study the affinity of early primary IgG plaque-forming cells. The data suggest that in animals immunized with an optimal dose of hapten-carrier conjugate, carrier priming results in a higher proportion of very low affinity IgG PFC. At an equivalent response level in terms of numbers of IgG PFC/10^6 cells, the average affinity of hapten-specific PFC is clearly lower in carrier primed mice than in mice responding to a secondary immunization with hapten-carrier conjugate. While these observations could be interpreted in terms of an antigen-driven switch, it is difficult to understand why a switch mechanism should favor low affinity PFC.

Based on these considerations the following alternative interpretations of the *in vitro* suppression experiments which do not require an antigen-driven switch can be proposed. For this discussion we assume that (1) virgin B lymphocytes with γ or α receptors exist, and (2) the differential requirement for T-cell helper function among different antibody classes is related to receptor class on the precursor cell.

In the first alternative, IgG committed cells are present in two populations, one having μ receptors, and the other γ receptors. Some evidence for the existence of the former population has come from the work of Pernis et al. (1971) and of Anderson (1972). The ease of B-lymphocyte triggering is based on the class of receptor, so that IgG cells with μ receptors respond similarly to IgM precursors: both responses may be enhanced by T-cell function, but some members may be triggered with minimal help. In contrast, the population of IgG committed cells with γ receptors has a more stringent requirement for T-cell help. The less than optimal conditions offered by *in vitro* culture systems could permit function of only the most easily triggered IgG cells, those with μ receptors, in the primary response. Thus nearly all of the IgG response would be suppressed by anti-μ antibodies (Pierce et al., 1972a). A better environment, such as provided by an irradiated host, could account for the failure of Warner and Herrod to suppress IgG antibody responses with anti-μ (Warner, 1972). The inhibition of synthesis of donor IgG_1 and IgG_2 immunoglobulins in recipients of anti-μ treated cells observed by Herrod and Warner (1972) might be related to the fact that no antigenic stimulation was given, as this is another way of selecting for the most easily triggered cells.

Two effects of antigen priming might account for the escape of IgG responses from the suppressive effects of anti-μ. First, educated T-cells are provided. Second, the population of IgG committed cells is selected for those clones having high affinity γ receptors and therefore favored for stimulation by antigen.

A conceptual difficulty with models proposing μ receptors for γ-committed B cells should be mentioned. Since the turnover rate of surface immunoglobulin is high (Vitetta and Uhr, 1972), it is necessary to postulate either the presence of a long-lived messenger RNA or simultaneous expression of two C_H genes to account for IgG cells with μ receptors. This problem applies to any model in which receptor does not strictly equal product.

A second alternative arises from observations suggesting that specific IgM antibody may facilitate immune responses. Such antibody might be a product of either T cells (Feldmann, 1972) or B cells (Henry and Jerne, 1968). Particularly intriguing is the possibility that T-cell helper function is mediated by a diffusible product with μ determinants, IgT. Feldmann has presented evidence that activated T cells produce an antigen-specific product which binds, together with antigen, to macrophages, and that these macrophages can then stimulate a "thymic-dependent" response of B cells. This antigen-specific factor can be inhibited by antibodies to mouse immunoglobulins or to μ chains (Feldmann, 1972). Inactivation of such a factor could conceivably account for the suppressive effects of anti-μ in the primary *in vitro* response.

Pierce *et al.* (1972*a*) showed that anti-μ did not interfere with the capacity of either macrophages or lymph node cells (as a source of T cells), treated independently, to restore the ability of anti-θ treated nonadherent spleen cells to respond to sheep erythrocytes. Conversely, anti-μ did inhibit the response of B cells in cultures reconstituted with normal macrophages and T cells. While this result indicates that the B cell is an important target for anti-μ, it may not exclude a role for a specific IgT. First, the effect of anti-μ on T cells might be reversible when the antibody is removed. Second, the inhibitory activity of anti-μ on responses of intact spleen cultures was reversible by addition of soluble IgM protein for up to 48 hr in culture, indicating that the antibody was still present on cells and could be displaced. This result leaves open the possibility that anti-μ carried on the surface of B cells might still be capable of inactivating a T-cell product.[1] The escape of IgG responses from anti-μ suppression in the secondary response might again be attributed to maturation in affinity of cell receptors.

---

[1] It is unlikely that the suppressive effects of anti-μ treatment of mice could be primarily due to inactivation of a T-cell antibody, since an absolute reduction in numbers of B cells has been demonstrated, and there is no defect in rejection of skin allografts or in the capacity of spleen cells to induce graft *vs.* host reactions. Experiments to determine whether T-cell helper function is altered in anti-μ treated animals are underway.

This argument emphasizes some of the difficulties in relating results of culture experiments to *in vivo* phenomena. Feldmann's experiments utilized primed T cells and B cells. Although IgG response was not determined, one would predict that none would be found in the absence of activated T cells or their products. This prediction, if true, would be difficult to reconcile with Pierce's observation that secondary IgG responses could be obtained in the continuous presence of anti-μ antibody. Resolution of this apparent conflict will require more direct comparisons of the effects of anti-μ on the two systems.

Table IX outlines evidence from several species bearing on the question of an antigen-driven switch in diversification of classes of B cells. The balance of data favors the view that this process, like generation of diversity of specificities, is not dependent on contact with exogenous antigens. It is for this reason that a critical evaluation of the evidence in mice suggesting an antigen-driven switch seems particularly important.

The relationship between receptor class and commitment for primed B lymphocytes, at least in mice, appears to be more straightforward. Walters and Wigzell used anti-IgG_1 or anti-IgG_{2a} to block the binding of primed precursors to antigen columns. They observed that in the presence of anti-IgG_1, precursors of IgG_1 antibody passed through the column, while precursors of IgG_{2a} antibody were specifically retained (Wigzell, 1973; Walters and Wigzell, 1970). The reverse was true if the same cell population was treated with anti-IgG_{2a}. Pierce and coworkers have studied the effects of anti-heavy chain reagents on the *in vitro* secondary response to sheep erythrocytes. Following a sufficient priming dose, IgM, IgG_1, and IgG_2 responses were inhibited only by the corresponding class of antiglobulin. Two exceptions to this rule were demonstrated. First, if the priming dose were relatively low, IgG responses only transiently escaped the suppressive effects of anti-μ. Second, IgA responses were always suppressed by both anti-μ and anti-a (Pierce *et al.*, 1972*b*, 1973).

Kishimoto and Ishizaka have studied the effects of anti-μ and anti-γ on the *in vitro* secondary response of rabbit spleen cells to hapten-carrier conjugates (Kishimoto and Ishizaka, 1971; Ishizaka and Kishimoto, 1972; Kishimoto and Ishizaka, 1972). They found that anti-γ consistently suppressed IgM, as well as IgG, responses while anti-μ suppressed IgG responses to a variable degree. IgG responses of hyperimmunized animals were more consistently suppressed by anti-μ than were those of animals given a single priming immunization.

The results of suppression experiments were confirmed by use of antibody immunoabsorbent columns to fractionate the cells. Passage of the cells over either anti-γ or anti-μ columns reduced both the IgG and IgM responses of the passed cells. Cells retained on the anti-γ column, when reconstituted with a source of T cells, were able to make both IgM and IgG responses (Kishimoto and Ishizaka, 1972). A critical control for these experiments was provided by assaying for IgE antibody production. Neither anti-γ nor anti-μ treatment, in

Table IX. Evidence Supporting Antigen-Dependent or Antigen-Independent Generation of Class Diversity for B-Lymphocytes

Species	Antigen-independent	Antigen-dependent
Man	μ, γ, and α B lymphocytes are present in adult proportions by 14 wks gestation when few or no plasma cells are present (Lawton et al., 1972b).	
Pig	μ and γ B lymphocytes are present in adult proportions 2 wks before term, whereas few plasma cells are found and serum immunoglobulins are < 1/1000 adult level (Binns et al., 1972).	
Mouse	Proportion of μ, γ, and α B lymphocytes is similar in germfree and conventional animals (Lawton and Asofsky, unpublished data).	80–90% of antigen binding cells (ABC) in unprimed mice have μ receptors (Davie and Paul, 1973). γ and α ABC's are proportionately increased by immunization.
	Pretreatment of unprimed spleen cells with anti-μ suppressed IgM, but not IgG response in irradiated recipients of the transferred cells (Warner, 1972).	Anti-μ suppressed primary IgM, IgG$_1$, IgG$_2$, and IgA responses in vitro. IgG$_1$ and IgG$_2$ responses were not suppressed following antigen priming in vivo (Pierce et al., 1972a,b, 1973).

Unprimed spleen cells treated with antiallotype serum (to determinants of IgG_{2a}) failed to generate an IgG_{2a} response when the recipient was given antigen more than 30 days later (Anderson, 1972).

Pretreatment of unprimed spleen cells with anti-μ suppressed expression of IgG allotype synthesis in congenic recipients (Herrod and Warner, 1972).

Guinea pig

Most antigen binding cells (ABC) in unprimed adults have $\gamma 2$ receptors. ABC with $\gamma 2$ receptors are present in fetal life, but cells with μ receptors predominate. Anti-$\gamma 2$ plus complement treatment prevented transfer of an adoptive response to irradiated recipients, while anti-μ complement did not (Davie and Paul, 1973).

Chicken

Development of IgG precursors is bursa-dependent, and not influenced by antigen (Kincade and Cooper, 1971). Extrabursal IgG precursors cannot be suppressed by anti-μ (Kincade et al., 1970). Extrabursal IgM or IgG committed cells cannot be induced to "switch" to synthesis of the other classes by intensive antigen stimulation (Kincade et al., 1973; Kincade and Cooper, 1973).

soluble form or bound to the immunoabsorbent, suppressed IgE production (Kishimoto and Ishizaka, 1972).

These results suggest that a significant proportion of hapten-specific memory cells committed to IgM synthesis have both μ and γ receptors. Most IgG precursors would appear to have only γ receptors, although cells having both μ and γ appear following sufficient antigen stimulation. IgE precursors presumably express neither μ nor γ receptors.

The reasons for the discrepancy between these data and that obtained on primed cells from mice is unclear. If preconceived bias is ignored, the rabbit experiments might be viewed more comfortably as suggesting a switch from γ to μ than μ to γ. An additional problem brought out by these studies is the apparent lack of correspondence between the class of receptor on B lymphocytes determined by functional assays and by direct techniques. Pernis *et al.* (1970) failed to find γ-bearing B lymphocytes in the rabbit using antibodies to Fc determinants, although a small proportion was detected with antibodies to hinge region allotypic determinants of IgG. However, 90% of the total B lymphocytes had IgM receptors.

CONCLUSION

The use of antibodies to heavy chains as probes for studying B-lymphocyte differentiation has provided a considerable amount of information and has raised a variety of questions. The *in vivo* suppression experiments with anti-μ in chickens and mice would seem to establish the expression of IgM synthesis as the primary event in B-lymphocyte differentiation. Evidence in man that myeloma proteins of different heavy chain classes may have identical light chains and heavy chain V regions suggests that a switch in commitment from IgM to IgG or IgA may occur without any change in antibody specificity. Evidence suggesting that primary differentiation of IgA precursors occurs through an intermediate cell which expresses IgG has been given. In trying to relate the results of *in vivo* suppression experiments to studies in which anti-immunoglobulins have been used to modify specific antibody responses *in vitro*, what we believe to be a fundamental difference between the experimental systems has been emphasized. The primary ontogenetic development of B lymphocytes constitutes a separate stage of differentiation, apparently dependent upon inductive influences of a specific microenvironment rather than exogenous antigens. Neonatal anti-immunoglobulin suppression seems to be directed primarily at this stage of development, and we propose that a switch from IgM→IgG→IgA occurs during this stage. The *in vitro* and combined *in vitro* and *in vivo* experiments have been, in contrast, clearly directed toward an antigen-driven differentiation process which begins with clones of B lymphocytes, either virgin or memory cells, and ends with production of a specific antibody. Results of these experiments have suggested the possibility of an antigen-driven switch from μ to γ receptors within the population of B lymphocytes committed to IgG synthesis. Basically similar models for this differentiation process have been presented by Warner (1972), Pierce *et al.* (1973), and Kishimoto and Ishizaka (1972). We have presented alternate interpretations of these data based on (1) evidence that the switch from IgM to IgG in the chicken occurs predominantly, if not exclusively, within the bursa, (2) evidence that development of IgG and IgA B lymphocytes is not antigen dependent in several species, (3) some functional evidence for the existence of virgin B lymphocytes with γ receptors, and (4) analysis of the role of T lymphocytes in primary IgG responses. Determination as to which of these is the correct interpretation will require direct analysis of the class or classes of immunoglobulin expressed on the surface of individual B lymphocytes at various stages of the immune response, and more precise understanding of the mechanisms by which T cells control the response of different immunoglobulin classes.

ACKNOWLEDGMENTS

Ms. Karen Prude and Ms. Jo Nell Reynolds provided capable technical assistance. We are greatly indebted to our collaborators, Drs. Richard Asofsky, Joseph Davie, and Robert Tigelaar, and Ms. Martha Hylton, for their willingness to share observations while permitting us to differ on some interpretations.

REFERENCES

Anderson, H. R., 1972. *Eur. J. Immunol.* **2**:11.
Andersson, B., 1970. *J. Exp. Med.* **132**:77.
Asofsky, R., Cooper, M. D., Davie, J. M., Hylton, M. B., Lawton, A. R., and Tigelaar, R., submitted for publication.
Asofsky, R., Ikari, N. S., and Hylton, M. B., 1968. In M. Miyakawa and T. D. Luckey (eds.), *Advances in Germfree Research and Gnotobiology*, Chemical Rubber Co., Cleveland, p. 219.
Bankhurst, A. D., and Warner, N. L., 1972. *Aust. J. Exp. Biol. Med. Sci.* **50**:661.
Barth, W. F., McLaughlin, C. L., and Fahey, J. L., 1965. *J. Immunol.* **95**:781.
Basten, A., Miller, J. F. A. P., Sprent, J., and Pye, J., 1972. *J. Exp. Med.* **135**:610.
Bianco, C., Patrick, R., and Nussenweig, V., 1970. *J. Exp. Med.* **132**:702.
Binns, R. M., Feinstein, A., Gurnes, B. W., and Coombs, R. R. A., 1972. *Nature New Biol.* **239**:114.
Burnet, F. M., 1959. *The Clonal Selection Theory of Acquired Immunity*, Vanderbilt University Press, Nashville.
Cebra, J. J., Colberg, J. E., and Dray, S., 1966. *J. Exp. Med.* **123**:547.
Cheers, C., and Miller, J. F. A. P., 1973. *J. Exp. Med.* **137**:254.
Claflin, L., and Merchant, B., 1973. *J. Immunol.* **110**:252.
Claflin, L., Merchant, B., and Inman, I., 1973. *J. Immunol.* **110**:241.
Coombs, R. R. A., Feinstein, A., and Wilson, A. B., 1969. *Lancet* **2**:1157.
Cooper, M. D., and Lawton, A. R., 1972. *Am. J. Pathol.* **69**:513.
Cooper, M. D., Lawton, A. R., and Kincade, P. W., 1972*a. Clin. Exp. Immunol.* **11**:143.
Cooper, M. D., Lawton, A. R., and Kincade, P. W., 1972*b*. In M. G. Hanna (ed.), *Contemporary Topics in Immunobiology*, Vol. 1, Plenum Press, New York, p. 33.

Cooper, M. D., Kincade, P. W., Bockman, D. E., and Lawton, A. R., 1971. In K. Lindahl-Kiessling, G. Alm, and M. G. Hanna, Jr. (eds.), *Advances in Experimental Medicine and Biology*, Vol. 12, Plenum Press, New York, p. 17.

Cooper, M. D., Cain, W. A., Van Alten, P. J., and Good, R. A., 1969. *Intern. Arch. Allergy* 35:242.

Crewther, P., and Warner, N. L., 1972. *Aust. J. Exp. Biol. Med. Sci.* 50:625.

Davie, J. M., and Paul, W. E., 1973. In M. D. Cooper and N. L. Warner (eds.), *Contemporary Topics in Immunobiology*, Vol. 3, Plenum Press, New York.

Davie, J. M., and Paul, W. E., 1972. *J. Exp. Med.* 135:660.

Davie, J. M., and Paul, W. E., 1971. *J. Exp. Med.* 134:495.

Davie, J. M., Paul, W. E., and Asofsky, R., 1972. *Fed. Proc.* 31:735.

Decker, J., Clarke, J., MacPherson, L., Weinstein, R., and Sercarz, E. E., 1973. In B. D. Janković and K. Isaković (eds.), *Microenvironmental Aspects of Immunity*, Vol. 29, Plenum Press, New York, p. 269.

Dickler, H. B., and Kunkel, H. G., 1972. *J. Exp. Med.* 136:191.

Ehrlich, P., 1900. *Proc. Roy. Soc.* 66:424.

Feldmann, M., 1972. *J. Exp. Med.* 136:737.

Gelfand, M. C., Asofsky, R., and Lawton, A. R., 1973. *Fed. Proc.* 32:1011.

Gershon, R. K., 1973. In M. D. Cooper and N. L. Warner (eds.), *Contemporary Topics in Immunobiology*, Vol. 3, Plenum Press, New York.

Greaves, M. F., and Hogg, N. M., 1971. In B. Amos (ed.), *Progress in Immunology*, Academic Press, New York, p. 111.

Harrison, M. R., Mage, R. G., and Davie, J. M., 1973. *J. Exp. Med.* 137:254.

Henry, C., and Jerne, N. K., 1968. *J. Exp. Med.* 128:133.

Herrod, H. G., and Warner, N. L., 1972. *J. Immunol.* 108:1712.

Herzenberg, L. A., and Herzenberg, L. A., 1973. In M. D. Cooper and N. L. Warner (eds.), *Contemporary Topics in Immunobiology*, Vol. 3, Plenum Press, New York.

Huchet, R., and Feldmann, M., 1973. *Eur. J. Immunol.* 3:49.

Ishizaka, K., and Kishimoto, T., 1972. *J. Immunol.* 109:65.

Ivanyi, J., and Dresser, D. W., 1970. *Clin. Exp. Immunol.* 6:493.

Jones, G., Torrigiani, G., and Roitt, I. M., 1971. *J. Immunol.* 106:1425.

Katz, D. H., and Unanue, E. R., 1972. *J. Immunol.* 109:1022.

Katz, D. H., Paul, W. E., Gordl, E. A., and Benacerraf, B., 1970. *J. Exp. Med.* 132:261.

Kincade, P. W., and Cooper, M. D., 1973. *Science* 179:398.

Kincade, P. W., and Cooper, M. D., 1971. *J. Immunol.* 106:371.

Kincade, P. W., Self, K. S., and Cooper, M. D., 1973. *Cell. Immunol.* 8:93.

Kincade, P. W., Davie, J. M., Paul, W. E., Lawton, A. R., and Cooper, M. D., unpublished observations.

Kincade, P. W., Lawton, A. R., and Cooper, M. D., 1971. *J. Immunol.* 106:1421.

Kincade, P. W., Lawton, A. R., Bockman, D. E., and Cooper, M. D., 1970. *Proc. Nat. Acad. Sci.* 67:1918.

Kishimoto, T., and Ishizaka, K., 1972. *J. Immunol.* 109:1163.

Kishimoto, T., and Ishizaka, K., 1971. *J. Immunol.* 107:1567.

Lamelin, J.-P., Lesowska-Bernstein, B., Matter, A., Ryser, J. E., and Vassalli, P., 1972. *J. Exp. Med.* 136:984.

Lawton, A. R., and Asofsky, R., unpublished data.

Lawton, A. R., Asofsky, R. M., Davie, J. M., and Hylton, M. B., 1973. *Fed. Proc.* 32:1012.

Lawton, A., Asofsky, R., Tigelaar, R., Hylton, M., and Cooper, M., 1972a. *Fed. Proc.* 31:751.

Lawton, A. R., Self, K. S., Royal, S. A., and Cooper, M. D., 1972b. *Clin. Immunol. Immunopathol.* 1:104.

Lawton, A. R., Royal, S. A., Self, K. S., and Cooper, M. D., 1972c. *J. Lab. Clin. Med.* 80:26.

Lawton, A. R., Asofsky, R., Hylton, M. D., and Cooper, M. D., 1972d. *J. Exp. Med.* 135:277.

Mage, R. G., 1967. *Cold Spring Harbor Symp. Quant. Biol.* 32:203.

Mäkelä, O., Ruoslahti, E., and Seppalo, H. T., 1970. *Immunochemistry* 7:917.
Manning, D. D., 1972. *J. Immunol.* 109:1152.
Manning, D. D., and Jutila, J. W., 1972*a. Nature* 237:58.
Manning, D. D., and Jutila, J. W., 1972*b. J. Exp. Med.* 135:1316.
Manning, D. D., and Jutila, J. W., 1972*c. J. Immunol.* 108:282.
Mitchell, G. F., 1973. In M. D. Cooper and N. L. Warner (eds.), *Contemporary Topics in Immunobiology,* Vol. 3, Plenum Press, New York.
Mitchison, N. A., 1969. In M. Landy and W. Braun (eds.), *Immunological Tolerance,* Academic Press, New York, p. 149.
Möller, G., 1961. *J. Exp. Med.* 114:415.
Möller, E., Bullock, W. W., and Mäkelä, O., 1973. *Eur. J. Immunol.* 3:172.
Murgita, R., Mattioli, C., and Tomasi, T. B., Jr., 1973. *J. Exp. Med.* 138:209.
Nordin, A. A., Cosenza, H., and Sell, S., 1970. *J. Immunol.* 104:495.
Nossal, G. J. V., and Pike, B. L., 1973. In B. D. Janković and K. Isaković (eds.), *Microenvironmental Aspects of Immunity,* Vol. 29, Plenum Press, New York, p. 11.
Nossal, G. J. V., Warner, N. L., Lewis, H., and Sprent, J., 1972. *J. Exp. Med.* 135:405.
Nossal, G. J. V., Szenberg, A., Ada, G. L., and Austin, G. J., 1964. *J. Exp. Med.* 119:485.
Pernis, B., Forni, L., and Amante, L., 1971. *Ann. N.Y. Acad. Sci.* 190:420.
Pernis, B., Forni, L., and Amante, L., 1970. *J. Exp. Med.* 132:1001.
Pernis, B., Chiappino, G., Kelus, A. S., and Gell, P. G. H., 1965. *J. Exp. Med.* 122:853.
Pierce, C. W., Asofsky, R., and Solliday, S. M., 1973. *Fed. Proc.* 32:41.
Pierce, C. W., Solliday, S. M., and Asofsky, R., 1972*a. J. Exp. Med.* 135:675.
Pierce, C. W., Solliday, S. M., and Asofsky, R., 1972*b. J. Exp. Med.* 135:698.
Rabellino, E., Colon, S., Grey, H. M., and Unanue, E. R., 1971. *J. Exp. Med.* 133:156.
Raff, M. C., 1970. *Immunology* 19:637.
Raff, M. C., Nase, S., and Mitchison, N. A., 1971. *Nature* 230:50.
Sarvas, H., and Mäkelä, O., 1970. *Immunochemistry* 7:933.
Scherrmacher, V., and Rajewsky, K., 1970. *J. Exp. Med.* 132:1019.
Siskind, G. W., and Benacerraf, B., 1969. *Adv. Immunol.* 10:1.
Spear, P. G., Rutishauser, U., Millette, C. F., Wang, A. L., and Edelmann, G. M., 1973. *Fed. Proc.* 32:1011.
Takahashi, R., Old, L. J., and Boyse, E. A., 1970. *J. Exp. Med.* 131:1325.
Taylor, R. B., and Wortis, H. H., 1968. *Nature* 220:927.
Thorbecke, G. J., Warner, N. L., Hochwald, G. M., and Ohanian, S. H., 1968. *Immunology* 15:123.
Vitetta, E. S., and Uhr, J. W., 1972. *J. Exp. Med.* 136:676.
Walters, C. S., and Wigzell, H., 1970. *J. Exp. Med.* 132:1233.
Wang, A. C., Wilson, S. K., Hopper, J. E., Fudenberg, H. H., and Nisonoff, A., 1970. *Proc. Nat. Acad. Sci.* 66:337.
Wang, A. C., Wang, I. Y. F., McCormick, J. N., and Fudenberg, H. H., 1969. *Immunochemistry* 6:451.
Warner, N. L., 1972. In M. D. Cooper and M. G. Hanna, Jr. (eds.), *Contemporary Topics in Immunobiology,* Vol. 1, Plenum Press, New York, p. 87.
Warner, N. L., Byrt, P., and Ada, G. I., 1970. *Nature* 226:942.
Webb, S. R., and Cooper, M. D., 1973. *J. Immunol.* 111:275.
Wigzell, H., 1973. In M. D. Cooper and N. L. Warner (eds.), *Contemporary Topics in Immunobiology,* Vol. 3, Plenum Press, New York.
Wortis, H., personal communication.
Wu, L. Y. F., Lawton, A. R., Greaves, M. F., and Cooper, M. D., 1973. In F. Daguillard (ed.), *Proceedings of the Seventh Leucocyte Culture Conference,* Academic Press, New York, p. 485.

Chapter 9

The Roles of T and B Lymphocytes in Self-Tolerance and Autoimmunity

A. C. Allison

Clinical Research Centre
Harrow, Middlesex, England

INTRODUCTION

Ehrlich (1906), with his usual perceptiveness, drew attention to the remarkable fact that although vertebrates can readily be immunized with cells or body fluids from other animals they do not as a rule make antibodies against their own tissue constituents. He termed the phenomenon "horror autotoxus," but was unable to advance any satisfactory explanation for it. While developing the clonal selection theory of immunity, Burnet (1959) postulated that autoantigens ("self" antigens) are either secluded from the immune system or that clones of lymphocytes exposed to autoantigens early in the course of ontogenetic development are eliminated or inactivated. Autoimmunity was thought to follow the proliferation of "forbidden clones" of lymphocytes with specificity for autoantigens.

Burnet's postulates attracted widespread interest, but have recently run into serious difficulties. With the development of sensitive methods for quantitation, notably radioimmunoassay, antigens thought to be secluded have been demonstrated in circulating blood. Thus, thyroglobulin is found in serum from normal human newborns and adults in concentrations of about 10–100 ng/ml. Thyroglobulin will be taken as a model autoantigen in this chapter because of the ease with which autoantibodies against this protein can be elicited, for example, by immunization with autologous thyroglobulin in the presence of Freund's complete adjuvant or immunization with heterologous thyroglobulins. Formation of autoantibodies against thyroglobulin in experimental animals is often accompanied by thyroiditis. Such autoimmune reactions are not confined to thyroglobulin; for example, immunization with isologous testicular or brain extracts leads to autoimmune orchitis or encephalomyelitis. It is difficult to understand how such procedures could rapidly induce the proliferation of "forbidden clones" of lymphocytes able to react with the appropriate autoantigens.

TOLERANCE IN T AND B LYMPHOCYTES

Several findings of the past few years have allowed reconsideration of the problem. The first and most important is the distinction between thymus-dependent (T) and other (B) lymphocytes, with the latter cells and their progeny responsible for antibody synthesis and release while the former participate in cell-mediated immunity and exert helper effects in the formation of antibodies against most antigens (Miller and Mitchell, 1969). The second relevant finding is that in the absence of adjuvants administration of heterologous serum proteins at intermediate dosage results in antibody formation, whereas administration of high doses or repeated low doses of the same antigens results in tolerance (Dresser and Mitchison, 1968). The tolerant animals are unable to synthesize antibody even when antigens are subsequently administered in a highly immunogenic form (usually in adjuvant), although their immune responses to other antigens are normal. Hence there is no general impairment of immune responses, but an induced antigen-specific unresponsiveness. It was then found by Taylor (1969) and by Chiller et al. (1971) that, in mice made tolerant by repeated low doses of bovine serum albumin or human gammaglobulin, T-lymphocyte responses to the antigens are markedly depressed, whereas B-lymphocyte responses are normal or nearly normal. This was demonstrated by the capacity of bone marrow lymphocytes (or splenic B lymphocytes) from low-dose tolerant mice to reconstitute an immune response against the tolerogen when transferred to irradiated syngeneic mice together with normal thymus cells, in contrast to the poor immune response when thymus cells from tolerant animals are used together with bone marrow cells from normal donors in irradiated recipients. After a high dose of antigen bone marrow cells also become unresponsive. Moreover, unresponsiveness is rapidly induced and persistent in T lymphocytes, and is more slowly induced and transient in B lymphocytes. These findings led to the postulate by Weigle (1971) and independently by Allison (1971) that with circulating soluble autoantigens two types of tolerance are present. When antigens circulate in low concentrations, such as thyroglobulin, there will be the equivalent of low-dose tolerance; specific T cells become unresponsive but specific B cells are present in normal numbers and are able to respond to autoantigens suitably presented to them. The B cells can be stimulated by immunization with cross-reacting antigens, in which case autoantibodies are made only against those autoantigenic determinants shared with the cross-reacting antigens. Alternatively, autoantibodies would be formed by immunization with autoantigen in the presence of suitable adjuvants, which provide nonantigen-specific T cell stimulation (see Allison, 1973). Other situations allowing stimulation of autoantigen-reactive B cells are discussed below.

In contrast, by analogy with high-dose tolerance, it can be postulated that in the case of soluble autoantigens circulating in high dose, such as serum albumin, both B and T cells become unresponsive. In that case no manipulation would give rise to autoantibody formation.

T CELL HELPER EFFECTS IN IMMUNE RESPONSES

The requirement for T cell helper effects in immune responses is now well defined. Helper effects are dose-dependent, being most marked when the antigen dose is small, and occur with a wide range of antigens. A minority of naturally occurring and synthetic antigens with repeating antigenic determinants in appropriate configurations do not require T cell helper effects, and are known as thymus-independent antigens. Examples are pneumococcus capsular polysaccharide, lipopolysaccharide (endotoxin) of Gram-negative bacteria, levan, and polyvinylpyrrolidone. However, with most naturally occurring antigens T-cell helper effects are well marked; this is known, for example, in formation of antibody against serum albumin, immunoglobulin, thyroglobulin, and erythrocytes.

The third finding that has relevance to autoimmunity concerns the role of T and B lymphocytes in antibody formation against haptens attached to immunogenic carriers. Owing largely to studies in the laboratories of Mitchison and of Benacerraf it has been shown that antihapten antibody is synthesized and released by B cells, but for this to occur an immune response by helper T lymphocytes against the carrier is normally required. This is shown in Fig. 1 (line 1). A development of this approach has been the demonstration by Iversen (1970) and others that animals can also be sensitized so that T cells react against a hapten and that in such animals administration of a normally nonimmunogenic protein (e.g., a myeloma immunoglobulin in an inbred mouse) coupled to the hapten results in formation of antibody (anti-idiotypic). (This is illustrated in Fig. 1, line 5.)

AUTOANTIGEN-BINDING LYMPHOCYTES IN NORMAL SUBJECTS

If the hypothesis of self-tolerance presented above is correct, it should be possible to identify B cells but not T cells capable of reacting with autoantigens circulating in low concentration, such as thyroglobulin, whereas neither B nor T cells able to react with autoantigens circulating in high concentration, e.g., serum albumin, should be demonstrable. Experiments were therefore undertaken to determine, by sensitive autoradiographic techniques, the binding of homologous thyroglobulin and serum albumin by human lymphocytes (Bankhurst et al., 1973). Peripheral blood lymphocytes from normal human subjects were allowed

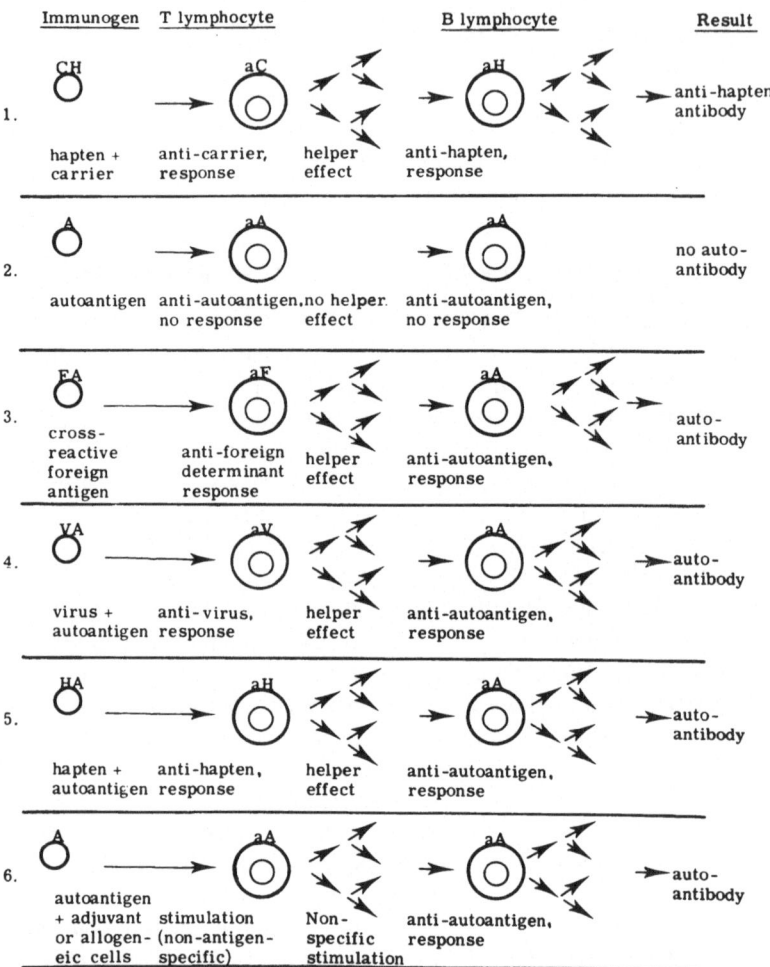

Figure 1. Diagram of the relationships of T and B lymphocytes with different specificities in autoimmune responses.

Antigenic determinants: H—hapten; C—carrier; A—autoantigenic determinant, shared with a foreign antigen; F—foreign antigenic determinant, not shared with autologous antigen; V—virus antigen.

Lymphocyte receptors for antigen: aH—anti-hapten, etc.

Slanted arrows show proliferation and differentiation of cells, accompanied, in the case of B lymphocytes, by antibody production, and in the case of T lymphocytes, by a helper effect. B lymphocytes exposed to antigen (arrow) respond only when there is a helper effect.

to bind high specific-activity ^{125}I human thyroglobulin or human serum albumin. The B lymphocytes were identified by their large amount of surface immunoglobulin, as shown by binding of radioactive anti-immunoglobulin. Selective removal of B cells from the population of lymphocytes was achieved by passing them through columns of beads coated with antibody against human immunoglobulin. The B lymphocytes are retained on such columns, presumably because their large amount of surface immunoglobulin reacts with the antibody on the beads. Studies of the cells that have passed through the columns show marked depletion or absence of B lymphocytes.

Nine out of 11 normal subjects had peripheral blood lymphocytes which bound ^{125}I-thyroglobulin (Table I). In contrast, no lymphocytes which bound human serum albumin were found in 3 normal human subjects. Lymphocytes binding thyroglobulin were absent after passage through the column retaining B cells in three experiments, and were markedly depleted in a fourth experiment. Thus the antigen-binding cells are identified as B lymphocytes.

Antigen-binding lymphocytes have been characterized in the mouse, using radioiodinated antigens, by Ada and by Sulitzeanu and their colleagues (see Ada and Cooper, 1971). Antigen-binding lymphocytes are primarily B lymphocytes; their number is not reduced by treating spleen cells with antitheta serum and complement, and there are normal numbers of antigen-binding lymphocytes in the congenitally athymic mouse. The antigen-binding cells are also the antigen-sensitive lymphocytes; radiation-induced death of lymphocytes which bind a highly radioactive antigen specifically abrogates the immune response to that antigen while leaving other immune responses intact.

Table I. Lymphocytes Binding Homologous ^{125}I-Antigens in Normal People (Bankhurst *et al.*, 1973)

Type of labeled antigen[b]	Number of labeled cells[a]	
	Individual subjects	Average[c]
Human thyroglobulin	175, 455, 150, 0, 100 80, 380, 0, 500, 298, 240	216
Human serum albumin	0, 0, 0	0

[a] Number of labeled lymphocytes per 10^6 lymphocytes.

[b] 5×10^6 lymphocytes were reacted for 30 min with 270–500 ng of labeled antigen in a 0.50 ml volume. Autoradiographs were exposed 8–24 days.

[c] The average was calculated from the 9 positive subjects.

A general criticism of the work carried out on antigen-binding cells is that the cells have been incubated with less than saturating amounts of labeled antigen. However, the concentrations of thyroglobulin used in our experiments were of the same order as found in serum and as are required for radiation-induced death of reactive lymphocytes. The conditions used for studying binding presumably identify the cells on which interest should be focused, namely, antigen-binding immunocompetent cells which are precursors of cells producing reasonably high-affinity antibody. Roberts *et al.* (1973) have also found cells binding homologous thyroglobulin in normal human subjects; the number of binding cells is increased in patients with autoallergic thyroiditis. Moreover, Ada and Cooper (1971) have found lymphocytes binding homologous thyroglobulin in normal rats, and Clagett (1972) has found them in normal mice. Since inbred animals were used, these results confirm that the reactions must be with autologous rather than homologous antigenic determinants.

Several recent findings support the view that the antigen-binding B lymphocytes just described are involved in the production of autoantibody against thyroglobulin, and that T cell helper effects are required to elicit such an immune response. Suicide of CBA mouse spleen cells with highly radioactive isologous thyroglobulin before transfer to irradiated recipients leaves intact antibody formation against heterologous thyroglobulins but abolishes the formation of the thyroglobulin autoantibodies which are seen when no suicide has been performed. If the suicide is carried out with highly radioactive heterologous thyroglobulin, no antibodies against thyroglobulin—heterologous or homologous—can be elicited by immunization with heterologous proteins. In mice which have been thymectomized, irradiated, and reconstituted with syngeneic bone marrow, antibodies against heterologous thyroglobulin and autoantibodies are only seen when recipients have also received a graft of thymus cells. Thus our postulate that tolerance to an autoantigen circulating in low dose thyroglobulin is selective for T lymphocytes is borne out by appropriate experiments.

Playfair and Clarke (1973) have also found that repeated inoculations of mice with rat erythrocytes leads to the production of autoantibodies against erythrocytes. Helper T cells reacting against common antigenic determinants may well be involved, since thymectomy abolished autoantibody formation. The strain which responded best was C57B1, in aging members of which a relatively high incidence of erythrocyte autoantibodies has been reported by Linder *et al.* (1972). Complexes of some erythrocyte antigens and antibodies accumulate in the kidneys, from which it appears that small amounts of the antigens may normally circulate in soluble form, thereby inducing selective T-cell unresponsiveness.

The reason for the absence of lymphocytes binding human serum albumin in normal human subjects is open to speculation. The simplest explanation is that serum albumin is found in very high concentration in extracellular fluids and saturates all the receptor sites for antigen, despite washing of cells. An alternative explanation is that there are very few or no lymphocytes able to bind a soluble autoantigen present in high concentration, and that self-tolerance under these conditions involves a different mechanism, namely, the elimination or inhibition of multiplication of the antigen-sensitive B lymphocyte clones. Observations in experimental animals support the latter interpretation. Unanue (1971) has been unable to find, in the lymph nodes of the mouse, lymphocytes binding autologous albumin, although cells binding autologous growth hormone are observed; the latter would circulate in low dose. Naor and Sulitzeanu (1969) have reported that in mice made tolerant to heterologous albumin the number of antigen-binding lymphocytes falls. Similar findings in mice made tolerant to human gammaglobulin have been reported by Louis et al. (1973). In contrast, mice tolerant to hemocyanin, flagellin, and Escherichia coli lipopolysaccharide have shown normal or increased numbers of antigen-binding cells (Ada and Cooper, 1971). Thus the nature of the antigen and dosage schedule seem to determine whether specific B cells become eliminated or made unresponsive, on the one hand, or remain demonstrable in the recipient.

ALLOGENEIC CELL STIMULATION, ADJUVANTS, AND AUTOANTIBODY FORMATION

The work of Katz (1972) and others has shown that injections of allogeneic immunocompetent cells under conditions that produce mild graft-vs.-host reactions abolish the need for cooperation of carrier T cells in a hapten-carrier system. Evidence has accumulated that T cells are stimulated in a nonantigen-specific fashion. By analogy, inoculations of allogeneic cells should stimulate the formation of autoantibodies. Boyse and his associates (1970) have found that mice injected with allogeneic cells produce autoantibodies against thymocytes. Fialkow et al. (1973) have recently found that repeated injections of F_1 mice with parental cells rapidly induce the formation of antinuclear antibodies; allotype markers were used to establish that these were produced by host and not donor B cells. These results support the view that allogeneic cell stimulation can result in autoantibody formation, and the role of this phenomenon in chronic graft-vs.-host disease deserves further study.

The role of adjuvants in eliciting autoantibody formation in experimental animals is well known. Many adjuvants stimulate proliferation of T cells, and T cells are required for the increase by several adjuvants of antibody formation by B cells (see Allison, 1973). Freund's complete adjuvant may in addition exert a carrier effect if mycobacterial antigens are able to form complexes with host antigens. The human counterpart is the finding of antinuclear and other auto-antibodies in leprosy in which patients carry a heavy mycobacterial load, which may have adjuvant activity—and also in malaria, syphilis, and other infections.

Idiotypic determinants of immunoglobulins were discovered by Oudin and Michel (1963) as a result of immunizing animals with bacteria coated with homologous antibodies. The bacteria may well have been active as carriers (their antigens stimulating T cells, which present the idiotypic determinants of antibacterial antibodies correctly to responsive B cells), and perhaps also as adjuvants: nonantigen-specific stimulators of immunocompetent cells. In the mouse, bacterial lipopolysaccharide (endotoxin) is a powerful direct stimulator of B lymphocytes, and it may well be that one of the consequences of bacterial infection in man will be an adjuvant effect.

VIRUS INFECTIONS

It follows from what has been said that if it were possible to bypass the requirement for T cells responsive against autoantigens autoantibody formation could be elicited. One way by which this might be achieved is by virus infection. Virus-specific antigens are often found on the membranes of infected host cells, and host antigens in the envelopes of lipid-containing viruses. Thus virus antigens and autoantigens could form common immunogenic units which function in a manner analogous to the hapten-carrier system (as shown in Fig. 1, line 4).

An analogous principle has been used by Lindenmann and Klein (1967) to increase immunity against tumor-specific antigens by immunizing mice with influenza virus grown in the tumor cells. Harboe and Haukenes (1966) have found that chickens immunized with influenza virus containing an antigen from the chorioallantoic cells in which it was cultured produce autoantibody against the same antigen present in liver and bile. In the laboratory of Oldstone and Dixon (1969) infection of NZB, NZW, and NZB/NZW hybrid mice with polyoma virus or lymphocytic choriomeningitis virus accelerates the onset of autoimmune manifestations and increases their incidence. As infectious mononucleosis wanes a variety of autoantibodies are often found, and several other human virus infections including influenza, measles, varicella, Coxsackie, and herpes simplex viruses are sometimes followed by autoallergic manifestations, including antibody-mediated thrombocytopenia and positive Coombs tests. The development of cold autoagglutinins, often directed against the I blood group, after *Mycoplasma pneumoniae* infections, may have a similar explanation.

EFFECTS OF HAPTENS AND DRUGS

As mentioned above, another way in which the requirement for specifically reactive T cells can be bypassed is to sensitize an animal against a hapten (such as oxazolone or dinitrophenol) and couple the hapten to host constituents before reinjection into the same or a syngeneic animal. Such procedures have been used to produce autoantibody against thyroglobulin and antibody against the idiotypic determinant of a monoclonal syngeneic immunoglobulin. This may be the way by which in human patients exposure to certain drugs is followed by autoantibody production. Two possible examples are the formation of autoanti-bodies against red cells (often directed against Rh blood groups) in patients treated with a-methyldopa and the presence of antinuclear factors in patients treated with hydrallazine, isoniazid, procaineamide, and other drugs. The postu-late is that patients will have T-cell reactivity against the drugs or their metabo-lites, and that the drugs or metabolites should be associated as haptens with erythrocyte membranes or nucleoproteins, respectively. Both these postulates are testable, especially since the antinuclear factor can be reproduced in experi-mental animals.

CONTROL OF IMMUNE RESPONSES BY T CELLS

If tolerance to autoantigens is due to selective T cell unresponsiveness, it is inevitably precarious, since it can be abrogated by several mechanisms already listed. It is therefore likely that an additional "fail-safe" mechanism for prevent-ing autoimmunity should exist. A second hypothesis put forward by Allison *et al.* (1971) is that T cells can exert specific feedback control on the synthesis of antibodies by B cells and that relaxation of this control—especially in aging humans and experimental animals—may be an important factor in the develop-ment of autoimmunity. A role of T cells in immunological surveillance against malignant cells is supported by observations of an increased incidence of tumors (especially those that are virus-induced) in experimental animals with depressed cell-mediated immunity and the raised probability of developing lymphoreticular neoplasms in humans with immunodeficiency syndromes or immunosuppressed after kidney transplantation. Immunological reactions are known to be subject to feedback control, the most fully studied case being the specific inhibition of antibody formation by administration of antibody. We suggest that a similar inhibition can be exerted by T cells, and that this provides a surveillance mechanism against aberrant immune reactions (Fig. 2).

Evidence in support of this interpretation comes from experiments with NZB mice, which develop a Coombs-positive hemolytic anemia from about the

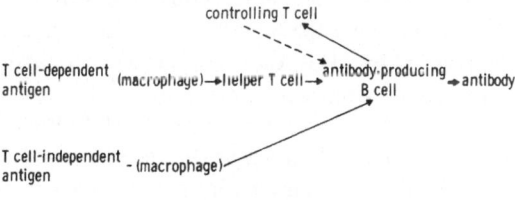

Figure 2

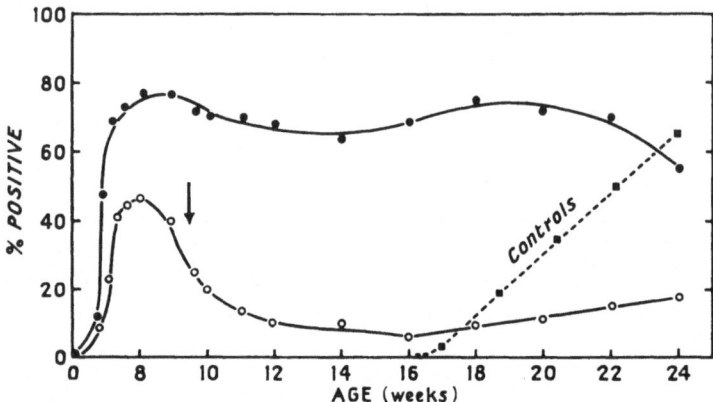

Figure 3. Adoptive transfer of positive antiglobulin (Coombs) reactions to young NZB mice: (1) ●———● Received A.L.G. 2 mg. four times intraperitoneally followed by 200-250 × 10⁶ spleen cells intraperitoneally from old Coombs-positive NZB donors. (2) ○———○ Received normal rabbit IgG (N.R.G.) followed by similar injections of spleen cells. (3) ■····■ Received N.R.G. only.

age of 4 months. Denman and others (1970) have shown that if spleen cells are transferred from old to young NZB mice, about half of the recipients show positive Coombs tests which usually disappear in a few weeks (Fig. 3). If the recipients are given antilymphocytic globulin (ALG), more recipients develop positive Coombs tests and these remain positive usually until the death of the animals. The simplest explanation of these results is that T cells in the young animals exert an inhibitory influence on the B cells from the spleens of old animals that are producing antibody against homologous erythrocytes (as shown by the arrow in Fig. 2) and that T-cell control is abolished by ALG administration. In keeping with this interpretation, Playfair and Allison (1973) have found that transfer of thymus cells from 2-wk old NZB mice monthly to NZB's from the age of one month significantly delayed the onset of positive direct Coombs tests. Further evidence for the positive nature of the control comes from experiments in which spleen cells from NZB mice are transferred into irradiated BALB/c mice; the recipients only develop positive Coombs tests if treated with ALG. Adoptive transfer of renal disease within the NZB/NZW strain is likewise achieved only in ALG-treated recipients. Thus, suppression of autoantibody formation in adoptive transfer experiments dominates over expression, but the suppression can be relieved by ALG. Additional evidence for a role of suppressor T cells in this situation comes from experiments of Playfair and Allison (1973) in which spleen cells from NZB mice were transferred to BALB/c × NZB F₁ hybrids. No positive Coombs tests were observed in the recipients unless the transferred cell population was treated with anti-θ serum and complement, in which case recipients rapidly developed autoantibodies against erythrocytes.

In general, evidence has accumulated that NZB mice and some of their hybrid offspring are especially prone to develop autoimmunity for two reasons. Their T cells are unusually resistant to tolerance induction, as judged by reactions against foreign serum proteins and erythrocytes. Moreover, their T-cell function declines rapidly with age, as judged by capacity to mount graft-*vs.*-host reactions and in other ways. Hence there is a combination of both factors favoring autoimmunity.

Teague and Friou (1969) have found that aging strain A mice frequently develop antibody against deoxyribonucleoprotein (anti-nuclear factor—ANF). Transfers of thymus cells from young to old syngeneic animals that had developed ANF resulted in decreased levels or disappearance of ANF. These workers have also suggested that cells in the thymus and spleen of young mice may participate in homeostatic control of autoantibody formation, and that this control may be less effective in aging animals. The age-dependence of autoantibody formation in humans is well documented.

Two other groups of investigators independently postulated in 1971 the existence of suppressor T cells to explain experimental findings in their laboratories. Since the concept is still relatively novel and of general interest, evidence in support of it will be reviewed briefly. The Herzenbergs (1973) and their colleagues have been concerned with the phenomenon of allotype suppression in mice. Suppression of immunoglobulin allotypes is a remarkable example in higher organisms of the regulation of gene expression by antibodies directed against the products of these genes. In rabbits and mice prenatal and/or early postnatal exposure to antiallotype antibody suppresses the formation of the allotype in animals genetically able to produce it. In many mouse strains the suppression is transient, but in F_1 hybrids of the SJL strain, and in rabbits, long-term suppression lasting the life of the animal often occurs. Sensitive tests show that suppression is not due to antibody against the suppressed allotype, or to the elimination of B cells able to synthesize the allotype. It is due to the presence of T cells which suppress the expression of the allotype. For example, if spleen cells from allotype-suppressed animals are transferred to irradiated recipients, there is a brief burst of synthesis of the suppressed allotype followed by reestablishment of the suppression. If the cells are treated with antitheta serum and complement before transfer, the suppressed allotype emerges permanently in the recipient. Admixture of cells from suppressed animals with those of normal donors before transfer prevents the expression of the allotype in irradiated recipients; as in the NZB example, suppression dominates over expression. Suppression has also been demonstrated *in vitro*. If heterozygous mice are immunized against sheep erythrocytes, approximately equal numbers of cells releasing antibody of each allotype are demonstrated by the Jerne plaque technique. If T cells from suppressed animals are added to the system, the proportion of cells producing the suppressed allotype is significantly reduced.

For several years it has been known that inoculations of large numbers of foreign erythrocytes in rats and mice induce tolerance to this antigen, and McCullagh (1972) has provided evidence that this is due to the presence in tolerant rats of cells suppressing the reaction. If mixtures of lymphoid cells from normal and tolerant animals are transferred to irradiated recipients, tolerance dominates over responsiveness. Gershon and Kondo (1971) have reported similar results in mice and obtained evidence that the suppressor cells are T lymphocytes. Ada and Cooper (1971) have found that tolerance to hemocyanin in mice is due to the presence of suppressor T cells, and Basten has similar results with fowl gammaglobulin in mice. Thus several well-studied examples of T cell suppression of antibody formation have come to light, and the phenomenon may be quite general. Other findings suggest a role for suppressor T cells in graft-*vs.*-host reactions (Gershon *et al.*, 1972) and contact hypersensitivity against a chemical sensitizer in mice (Asherson *et al.*, 1971).

A role for T-cell suppression of autoimmunity in chickens genetically predisposed to thyroiditis (obese chickens) is suggested by the work of Wick and his colleagues (1970). They found that thymectomy accelerated and aggravated thyroiditis, whereas early bursectomy abolished it. Presumably the helper effects were already established at the time of thymectomy. A high incidence of thyroiditis has also been observed in thymectomized and irradiated rats (Penhale *et al.*, 1973).

Two mechanisms by which T cells may exert suppressor effects have been postulated. According to the first, T cells are able to recognize the specific (idiotypic) determinants of immunoglobulin receptors that distinguish one B cell from another; they can then react against the corresponding B cells and suppress immunoglobulin synthesis. Three lines of evidence, none of them yet entirely conclusive, suggest that T cells can recognize idiotypic determinants of syngeneic mice. Experiments on the use of monoclonal immunoglobulins as carriers in the production of antibody against haptens suggest that T cells can react against idiotypes. Experiments of Hannestad *et al.* (1973) show that BALB/c mice given injections of monoclonal immunoglobulins in complete adjuvant become immunized against plasmacytomas producing that immunoglobulin. In the immunized mice, there was strong selection for tumor variants with defective production of immunoglobulin heavy chains. It is likely that T cells in the immunized mice are able to react against idiotypic determinants to which heavy chains make an important contribution. The third argument follows from the postulate of Ramseier and Lindenmann (1969) that F1 animals are able to react against parental strain immunocompetent cells because of the presence of a receptor on the latter for antigens of the other parental strain. The postulate of an immunological reaction against such receptors has wide implications, so that it should be tested rigorously by acceptable methods.

The second mechanism by which T-cell products may suppress B-cell activity arises from the work of Feldmann and his colleagues (Feldmann and Nossal, 1973). They have advanced evidence in support of the view that T cells exposed to antigen release a factor (perhaps an immunoglobulin) which attaches to the surface of a macrophage, where it can stimulate a response by B cells in the vicinity. In the absence of macrophages, or in the presence of excess T-cell product, the product reacts directly with B cells and inhibits their response. On this hypothesis suppressor T cells would give rise to an excessive release of product, with inhibitory consequences. It should be possible to distinguish between these alternatives (for example, on Feldmann's hypothesis transfer of many T cells from suppressed animals to irradiated recipients should result in suppression, whereas smaller numbers should exert a helper effect); but the appropriate experiments have not yet been performed.

CONGENITAL VIRUS INFECTIONS

The work of Traub in the 1930's (Traub 1936) established that in mouse colonies vertical transmission from mothers to offspring of lymphocytic chorio-meningitis (LCM) virus establishes a symptomless lifelong infection in which no antiviral antibody is demonstrable in the circulating blood. Infection of adult mice with LCM leads to an immunopathological disease and antibody formation. The lack of antibody after congenital LCM virus infection was one of the observations which led Burnet and Fenner (1969) to postulate the existence of immunological tolerance. More recently, Oldstone and Dixon (1969) have demonstrated the accumulation in the kidneys of mice congenitally infected with LCM of immune complexes containing viral antigen and antibody. Hence the congenitally infected mice are able to make some antibody against viral antigens. Volkert and Hannover-Larsen (1965) found that if spleen cells from LCM-immune mice (infected as adults) are transferred to syngeneic congenitally infected carrier animals very high levels of antibody are formed, but no immuno-pathological disease results after a short interval.

The simplest interpretation of these findings appears to be that LCM viral antigens produce a tolerance resembling that occurring with autoantigens in low dose, namely, that T cells specific for viral antigens become unresponsive while specific B cells remain able to respond to antigen. In the absence of specific helper cells, only a small amount of antibody is produced, and this combines with antigen liberated into the circulation to form immune complexes which accumulate in the kidney, leading eventually to immunopathological glomerulo-nephritis. However, when virus-specific T cells are supplied by adoptive immunization, a helper effect greatly increases antibody formation in the recipient animals. A helper role for T cells in antibody formation against LCM viral antigens is demonstrated by the recent experiments of Cole et al. (1972). Adoptive immunization of congenitally infected LCM virus carrier mice with

Table II. Antibody Against Lymphocytic Chorio-
meningitis Virus Antigens in BALB/c Mice Neonatally
Infected and Adoptively Immunized
(Cole *et al.*, 1972)

Treatment	C.F. antibody mean (range)	Viremia
None	0 (0)	4.0
10^8 immune spleen cells	3000 (200–12,000)	0.5
10^8 immune spleen cells treated with anti-θ + C^1	0 (0–25)	3.3

spleen cells from syngeneic immune donors resulted in high antibody levels, as already described, but treatment of the spleen cells with antitheta serum before transfer virtually abolished this effect (Table II). Thus, even in the presence of B cells from immune donors, little antibody is formed unless sensitized T cells are also present.

Analogous results have been obtained in other congenital virus infections, for example, accumulation in carrier mice of complexes of antibody and antigens of murine leukemogenic viruses (Hirsch *et al.*, 1969, and Oldstone *et al.*, 1972). Law (1973) has found that injections of solubilized major histocompatibility antigens into newborn mice results in tolerance in respect of capacity to form antibodies against these antigens. It would be of interest to know whether B or T cells or both become unresponsive in experiments of this type. The recipient mice, although unable to make detectable anti-H-2 antibody, reject grafts of tumors from the same donor strain. This supports other evidence suggesting that antigens other than H-2 are involved in graft rejection, and that it is more difficult to induce unresponsiveness to antigens presented in the surface of a cell than those circulating in soluble form.

Indeed the whole problem of tolerance to histocompatibility antigens and other antigens recognized by transplantation tests following neonatal or prenatal exposure to foreign cells or oncogenic viruses is at present being reinvestigated in several laboratories. The evidence in different situations is conflicting, and no definitive general conclusions can yet be drawn.

GENERAL COMMENT

The concept that most autoantigens circulate in low dose and induce unresponsiveness in specific populations of T but not B cells explains many observations that were difficult to reconcile with the clonal deletion of anti-body-forming cells postulated by Burnet (1959). Enough evidence has accumulated to make it likely that the concept of selective unresponsiveness of T cells is correct, at least for those autoantigens so far analyzed in detail. This includes antigens of vertically transmitted viruses as well as autoantigens. The concept is also useful in clinical immunology to explain autoantibody formation after virus and other microbial infections, by certain drug treatments, and in other situations. However, many problems still remain without explanation, e.g., the mechanism by which prolonged exposure to low doses of antigens induces T-cell unresponsiveness, why tolerogenic exposure to some antigens leads to depletion of antigen-binding B cells while exposure to other antigens does not, and why it is easier to induce unresponsiveness to soluble antigens than antigens on the surface of cells recognized by transplantation tests. Enough information has also accumulated to support the validity of the suppressor T-cell hypothesis and its part in the control of autoimmune reactions, but how widespread and important this reaction is remains to be analyzed.

REFERENCES

Ada, G. L., and Cooper, M. G., 1971. *Ann. N.Y. Acad. Sci.* **181**:96.

Allison, A. C., 1973. *Ciba Foundation Symposium on Immunopotentiation,* ASP, Amsterdam.

Allison, A. C., 1971. *Lancet* **2**:1401.

Allison, A. C., Denman, A. M., and Barnes, R. D., 1971. *Lancet* **1**:135.

Asherson, G. L., Zembala, M., and Barnes, R. M. R., 1971. *Clin. Exp. Immunol.* **9**:109.

Bankhurst, A. D., Torrigiani, G., and Allison, A. C., 1973. *Lancet* **1**:226.

Boyse, E. A., Bressler, E., Iritani, C. A., and Lardis, M., 1970. *Transplantation* **9**:339.

Burnet, F. M., 1959. *The Clonal Selection Theory of Acquired Immunity.* Cambridge University Press, Cambridge.

Burnet, F. M. and Fenner, F., 1969. *The production of antibodies.* Macmillan, Melbourne.

Chiller, J., Habicht, G. S., and Weigle, W. O., 1971. *Science* **171**:813.

Clagett, J. A., 1972. *Fed. Proc.* **31**:743.

Cole, G. A., Nathanson, N., and Prendergast, R. A., 1972. *Nature* **238**:335.

Cooper, M. G., and Ada, G. L., 1973. *J. Exp. Med.* (in press).

Denman, A. M., Russell, A. S., and Denman, E. J., 1970. *Series Immunobiol.* **16**:253.

Dresser, D. W., and Mitchison, N. A., 1968. *Adv. Immunol.* **8**:129.

Ehrlich, P., 1906. *Collected Studies on Immunity,* London, Macmillan.

Feldmann, M., and Nossal, G. J. V., 1973. *Transpl. Rev.* **13**:3.

Fialkow, P. J., Gilchrist, C., and Allison, A. C., 1973. *Clin. Exp. Immunol.*

Gershon, R. K., and Kondo, K., 1971. *Immunology* **21**:903.

Gershon, R. K., Cohen, P., Heucin, R., and Liebhaber, S. A., 1972. *J. Immunol.* **108**:586.

Hannestad, I., Kao, M. S., and Eisen, H. N., 1973. *Proc. Nat. Acad. Sci. U.S.A.* **69**:2295.

Harboe, M., and Kaukenes, G., 1966. *Acta Path Microbiol. Scand.* **68**:98.

Herzenberg, L. A., and Herzenberg, L. A., 1973. In M. D. Cooper, and N. L. Warner (eds.), *Contemporary Topics in Immunobiology,* Vol. 3, Plenum Press, New York.

Hirsch, M. S., Allison, A. C., and Harvey, J. J., 1969. *Nature (Lond.)* **223**:739.

Iversen, G. M., 1970. *Nature* (London) **227**:273.

Katz, D. H., 1972. *Transpl. Rev.* **12**:141.

Law, L. W., 1973. Private communication.

Lindenmann, J., and Klein, D. A., 1967. *J. Exp. Med.* **126**:93.

Linder, E., Pasternack, A., and Edgington, T. S., 1972. *Clin. Immunol. Immunopathol.* **1**:104.

Louis, J., Chiller, J., and Weigle, W. O., 1973. *J. Exp. Med.*

McCullagh, P. J., 1972. *Transpl. Rev.* **12**:180.

Miller, J. F. A. P., and Mitchell, G. F., 1969. *Transpl. Rev.* **1**:3.

Mitchison, N. A., 1971. In *Sixth International Immunopathology Symposium,* p. 52. Karger, Basel.

Naor, D., and Sulitzeanu, D., 1969. *Intern. Arch. Allergy* **36**:112.

Oldstone, M. B. A., and Dixon, F. J., 1969. *J. Exp. Med.* **129**:483.

Oldstone, M. B. A., Tishon, A., Tonietti, G., and Dixon, F. J., 1972. *Clin. Immunol. Immunopathol.* **1**:6.

Oudin, J., and Michel, J., 1963. *Compt. Rend. Acad. Sci.* (Paris) **259**:805.

Penhole, W. J., Farmer, A., McKenna, R. P., and Irvine, W. J., 1973. *Clin. Exp. Immunol.* **15**:225.

Playfair, J. H., and Allison, A. C., 1973. Unpublished observations.

Playfair, J. H., and Clarke, M., 1973. *Nature (New Biol.)* **243**:213.

Ramseier, H., and Lindenmann, J., 1969. *Pathol. Microbiol.* **34**:374.

Roberts, I., Whittingham, S., and Mackay, I. R., 1973. *Lancet* **2**:936.

Taylor, R. B., 1969. *Transpl. Rev.* **1**:114.

Teague, P. O., and Friou, G. J., 1969. *Immunology* **17**:665.

Traub, E., 1936. *J. Exp. Med.* **64**:183.

Unanue, E. R., 1971. *J. Immunol.* **107**:1168.

Chapter 10

Immunological Studies of Nude Mice

Henry H. Wortis

Department of Pathology
Tufts University School of Medicine
Boston, Massachusetts

INTRODUCTION

Nude mice pose several interesting biological questions. On the one hand they present a variety of pleiotropic effects, ranging from hairlessness to thymic dysgenesis, which have an unknown common property. On the other hand they may very well be a model for the study of immune reactions in which a single major participant—the thymus—is absent.

Studies of nude mice therefore fall into three categories: (1) their use as an athymic experiment of nature; (2) searches for hitherto unknown defects in nude mice—perhaps defects independent of the thymic dysgenesis; and (3) a search for a thread which connects the varied effects of the mutation. The experiments reviewed here fall into the first category. Of necessity they were carried out under the assumption that effects of the *nude* mutation, other than on the thymus or thymus dependent events, were not likely to be relevant. It seems reasonable to join in this assumption.

GENETICS

Nude is a mutant allele of the nu locus of the VII linkage group (Flanagan, 1966). The only other locus of this group with a known relation to immune responses is df (Ames pituitary dwarf) (Schaible and Gowen, 1961), but the linkage between nu and df is not close. Nude is recessive, and while a relative leukopaenia has been reported in heterozygotes by Pantelouris (1968), I am not aware that this has been confirmed, nor has there been any published report of other phenotypic differences between nu/+ and +/+ mice.

The original mutation arose in noninbred stock. At the moment the *nude* allele is being put onto inbred backgrounds by repeated backcrossing. Among the strains being used for this purpose are CBA, Balb/C, and C57BL/6.

CELLULAR DEFECTS

The Thymus

As first reported by Pantelouris (1968), nudes lack a normal thymus. In the upper anterior mediastinum are two paired structures: one lobulated, with irregularly arranged cells with foamy, slightly basophilic cytoplasm; the other consists of several cysts or vacuoles lined with ciliated columnar epithelium (Pantelouris and Hair, 1970; Wortis *et al.,* 1971). In a mature nude these cysts can be several millimeters in diameter. No lymphoid cells are associated with either of these structures. While it is likely that one or both of these organs represents an abnormal structure derived from the branchial pouches, it has not been proven that either is the counterpart of the normal thymic epithelium.

Neither of these structures is populated by lymphocytes when normal bone marrow cells are injected into nude mice (Wortis *et al.,* 1971), nor do they become lymphoid when grafted to normal mice (Wortis *et al.,* 1971).

Bach *et al.* (1973*a*) have described a material in the sera of normal mice and absent in nudes and thymectomized mice, which they believe is a functional product of the thymus. The assay of this thymic active material is complex. The assay takes advantage of the fact that approximately 0.1% of normal mouse spleen, thymus, and bone marrow cells form rosettes (bind) to sheep red blood cells (Bach and Dardenne, 1972*a*). All thymus cell rosettes and 75% of spleen cell rosettes can be inhibited by either low doses of azathioprine (1 μg/ml) or small amounts of anti-θ serum (Bach and Dardenne, 1972*b*). However, bone marrow cell rosettes and splenic cell rosettes from nude mice or thymectomized animals are insensitive to this treatment. When normal bone marrow or spleen cells from thymectomized mice are incubated *in vitro* with thymus active material, the cells become sensitive to inhibition (Bach *et al.,* 1973*b*). Bach calls this ability to confer sensitivity to inhibition, thymic activity. Material with thymic activity appears to be closely related to thymosin (Bach *et al.,* 1971*a*).

Taken together, these results demonstrate that nude mice lack a thymic dependent hormonelike material normally found in the serum. The biological significance of this observation is not so certain. For instance, it has not been demonstrated that thymosin or material with thymic activity converts stem cells into T cells or changes the function of lymphocytes. We tested this directly by treating nude mice with a preparation of thymosin supplied by Dr. A. L. Goldstein (Goldstein *et al.,* 1970). Neonatal nude mice were given thrice weekly intraperitoneal injections of 500 μg of thymosin or an equivalent amount of a

Table I. Thymus Replacement

Group	Median survival (days)	Mean survival (days)	Weight (g) 40–50 days	Lymphocyte count/mm³ 40–50 days
Untreated	28	-	9.4 (9)	359 ± 152
Thymus grafted	> 60	> 113	14.6 (8)	3290 ± 2578
Thymosin	21 (5)	29	9.4 (4)	2000, 1600, 516, 120
Spleen extract	18 (7)	30	9.0 (3)	2700, 650, 580
Normal littermate	>> 365	>> 365	18.6 (14)	3461 ± 1359

spleen extract prepared in a similar manner. The mice were weighed regularly and white blood cell counts and differential counts made. As can be seen in Table I, there was no difference between groups in survival time, weight gain, or lymphocyte counts. Further, the thymosin treated group did no better than untreated nudes and not nearly as well as mice that had received whole thymus grafts.

Although they involved small numbers of animals, the criteria used as a measure of successful replacement of thymus function were stringent, and the results were negative, I believe that these experiments cast some doubt on the role of thymosin as an inducer of stem to T cell maturation. Rather, they suggest that the many effects of thymosin previously reported (Goldstein et al., 1970; Bach et al., 1971a) might be due to an effect on peripheral differentiated cells (Bach et al., 1971b). These cells might be T cells (Lance et al., 1973), but effects on B cells have not been ruled out. In other words, the thymus plays a dual role, inducing maturation in stem cells which enter it and exercising an effect on peripheral lymphocytes. The peripheral effect could be that of a mitogen or adjuvant.

Thymocyte Precursors

Bone marrow of nude mice can be used to supply precursors to repopulate the thymus of an irradiated but otherwise normal mouse (Wortis et al., 1971; Pritchard and Micklem, 1973). Similarly, a thymus, grafted to a nude, is repopulated by precursors from the nude host (Pritchard and Micklem, 1973). Therefore, there is no evidence of a defect in the lymphocyte stem cell population of nude mice.

Thymus-Derived Lymphocytes

The thymus dependent areas of lymph nodes, Peyer's patches, and spleens of nude mice lack lymphocytes (de Sousa *et al.,* 1969). Circulating lymphocytes are also much reduced (Wortis, 1971). The lymph nodes of nudes are grossly deficient in cells sensitive to cytotoxic anti-θ serum (Raff and Wortis, 1970). Less than 5% of nude lymph node lymphocytes are killed by anti-θ as compared to the 40% of littermate lymphocytes killed by similar treatment. It is not known whether the few apparently θ-positive cells in nude mice are actually cells killed by antibody to non-θ antigens or are truly θ-positive. If the latter proved to be the case, it would suggest that even in the absence of a thymus there is a slow maturation of "thymus-derived" cells.

After thymus grafting, peripheral T cells of nude origin appear. This can be shown by using donor thymus from mice bearing the T6 chromosome. Under these conditions, cells with host (nude) karyotype can be readily identified (Pritchard and Micklem, 1973). Alternatively, thymus from AKR mice can be grafted to nudes known to be genotypically θ^{C3H}. Within a few weeks the spleens of such grafted animals have many cells with θ^{C3H} which are cells of host origin that have matured in an allogeneic thymic milieu (Wortis, 1973).

Thymus Independent Lymphocytes

Primary follicles of lymph nodes, spleen, and Peyer's patches are normal in nude mice (de Sousa *et al.,* 1969; Mitchell *et al.,* 1972*a*). Virtually all their thoracic duct lymphocytes have receptors for antigen-antibody complexes, a presumed B cell property (Basten *et al.,* 1972). In normal mice no more than 20% of thoracic duct lymphocytes bind significant amounts of complex. Readily detectable cell surface immunoglobulin is also characteristic of mouse B cells (Raff, 1970). As many as 94% of nude thoracic duct lymphocytes have this feature, in contrast to the 25% found in normal CBA mice (Bankhurst and Warner, 1972). Over 90% of splenic lymphocytes of nude mice are positive for a newly identified alloantigen limited to B lymphocytes (McKenzie, personal communication). Zeiller *et al.* (1971) reported that normal lymphocytes could be divided into two populations based on electrophoretic mobility. They suggested that the slow-moving population was equivalent to B cells and the rapid to T cells. Sabolovic *et al.* (1972) found that all nude lymphocytes were of slow mobility. Vujanovic *et al.* (1972) reported that they could distinguish by light microscopy B cells from T cells, and that nude lymphocytes were exclusively of B cell type.

Study of the intramembranous fracture plane of lymphocyte membrane obtained by freeze-fracture methods reveals that the inner fracture face contains a variable number of granules. Peripheral lymphocytes can be classed as poly-granular (aggregates of five or more particles) or monogranular (aggregates of less than five particles). In CBA mice the spleen has 30-35% and lymph nodes have 60% polygranular cells. In contrast, the splenic lymphocytes of nudes are less than 30% and lymph node cells are less than 0.5% polygranular (Mandel, 1972). B cells drained from nude thoracic ducts had a life span of five to seven weeks (Sprent and Basten, 1973). As shown by their depletion during prolonged drainage, B cells were found to recirculate slowly. Thus, after 24 hours of drainage of normal mice, the thymus dependent areas of lymph nodes were depleted, but only after a week were the B cell areas depleted (Sprent, 1973). A large proportion of ^{51}Cr labeled B cells injected into either normal or nude mice settled in the spleen within four hours. But, while T cells would then migrate to peripheral nodes, B cells appeared to remain in the spleen (Sprent and Miller, 1972; Sprent, 1973).

RESPONSE TO MITOGENS

Nude mice fail to respond to phytohemagglutinin *in vivo* as measured by local lymph node enlargement (Wortis, 1971). In culture their cells give no mitogenic response to Phytohemagglutinin P (Janossy and Greaves, 1971; Vischer, 1972) or concanavalin A (Andersson *et al.*, 1972*a*; Watson *et al.*, 1973). The data on response to pokeweed mitogen is conflicting. Janossy and Greaves (1971) and Vischer (1972) obtained a mitogenic response, while Watson *et al.* (1973) failed to detect a response. Lipopolysaccharide from *Escherichia coli* (Andersson *et al.*, 1972*a*) and *Salmonella typhosa* (Watson *et al.*, 1973) are strong mitogens for nude spleen cells. These results are in accord with the idea that concanavalin A and phytohemagglutinin are T cell specific mitogens and lipopolysaccharides are B cell specific mitogens. It has also been reported that wheat germ agglutinin and soy bean agglutinin will agglutinate lymphocytes from nudes (Schnebli and Dukor, 1972). It is possible to induce a mitogenic response to concanavalin A by culturing nude spleen cells with the supernate from a 24-hour culture of thymocytes. The supernate is not mitogenic by itself nor does it facilitate the response to lipopolysaccharide (Andersson *et al.*, 1972*b*).

MITOGENIC RESPONSE TO ALLOGENEIC CELLS

Spleen cells of nude mice are reported to proliferate in response to allogeneic spleen cells (Wagner, 1972). The experiments reported lacked controls of syngeneic target cells and controls for the release of nonantigenic mitogenic factors released by T cells from the target spleen. If this result were confirmed, it would contrast with results from other workers who have shown that B cells purified from normal spleens do not respond in mixed lymphocyte cultures (Mosier and Cantor, 1971; Andersson *et al.*, 1973).

MITOGENIC RESPONSES TO ANTIGENS

There are virtually no data available on this important topic. The mitogenic response to lipopolysaccharide noted above under Response to Mitogens should not be construed as an example of antigenic stimulation of mitosis since mice tolerant to lipopolysaccharide can still be stimulated by it (Andersson et al., 1972c). Vischer (1972) has reported that the supernatant fluid of cultures of normal spleen cells and keyhole limpet haemocyanin will induce proliferation of nude spleen cells.

ANTIGEN BINDING

Using ^{125}I labeled antigen and radioautography, Dwyer et al. (1971) demonstrated that the proportion of antigen binding cells per 10^4 splenic lymphocytes is the same for nude mice as for CBA mice. Flagellin from Salmonella adelaide, haemocyanin from Jasus lalandii, dinitrophenylated bovine serum albumin, and the synthetic copolymer Tyr·Glu·Ala·Lys were used as test antigens. In nonimmunized mice, the number of spleen cells capable of forming rosettes with sheep red blood cells is similar in nude mice (1220 ± 140), CBA mice (1440 ± 110), C57BL/6 (1060 ± 120), and Swiss mice (1050 ± 140) (Bach and Dardenne, 1972a). Similar results were obtained by Greaves and Hogg (1971).

Since at least some antigen binding cells must be T cells and since nude mice lack T cells, too much should not be made of the similarity of the numbers of antigen binding cells in nudes and normals as reported above. What these data do indicate is that even in the absence of T cells, B cells with the ability to specifically bind antigen can and do appear. That is, the differentiation from stem cell to antigen specific B cell appears to be independent of T cell (or thymus) mediation. However, while this appears likely, it has not been shown that these cells in nudes make homogeneous antibody of one specificity or that they are genetically committed to the production of antibody of one specificity.

IMMUNOGLOBULIN LEVELS

The serum levels of immunoglobulin in nude mice have been the subject of numerous investigations (Crewther and Warner, 1972; Luzzati and Jacobson, 1972; Manning and Jutila, 1972; Bloemmen and Eyssen, 1973; Pritchard et al., 1973). There is general agreement about the facts which can be summarized. IgM levels of nude mice are equal to those of littermates. IgA and IgG_1 levels are usually less than 10% of control values. IgG_{2a} and IgG_{2b} levels are depressed, but only to about 20% of littermates.

As nude mice mature the difference between their Ig levels and control levels becomes greater. This is because synthesis of IgG_1, IgG_2, and IgA does not begin until several weeks after birth and because maternal immunoglobulin passes to the fetus and neonate (Herzenberg *et al.*, 1967).

These results lead to the conclusion that IgM synthesis and secretion are thymus independent while IgG_1 and IgA are both highly thymus dependent. IgG_2 synthesis is apparently facilitated by the thymus (or T cells), but this is not an absolute requirement. That the low levels of IgA are due to a low synthetic rate rather than a high catabolic rate has been clearly shown by Crewther and Warner (1972).

The low levels of circulating immunoglobulin contrast with the large numbers of B cells found in nude lymphoid tissue. Normally, B cells both secrete immunoglobulin and have a high density of cell surface immunoglobulin (Walters and Wigzell, 1970). In nudes, however, B cells with surface IgM, IgG, and IgA exist (Bankhurst and Warner, 1972), but secrete little IgG or IgA. However, in nudes it appears that the majority of cells have more than one class of Ig on their surfaces, in sharp contrast to the situation in normal mice (Bankhurst and Warner, 1972). This raises the possibility that prior to a thymus (and antigen?) dependent differentiation step, B cells are uncommitted with regard to the class of immunoglobulin that they can synthesize.

RESPONSE TO THYMUS INDEPENDENT ANTIGENS

Antigens which can provoke immune responses in thymectomized animals equivalent to those seen in intact animals are thymus independent antigens (Armstrong *et al.*, 1969). They share the property of having multiple small repeating units and of illiciting a response that is predominantly, if not exclusively, of IgM antibody (Andersson and Blomgren, 1971). Experiments in which nude mice were immunized with some of these antigens are shown in Table II. In all cases the responses of nudes were at least equivalent to those of their phenotypically normal littermates.

Reed and Jutila (1972) showed that nudes can be primed to *E. coli* lipopolysaccharide. That is, memory to a thymus independent antigen occurs in the absence of the thymus. A similar result was obtained by Feldmann (1972) using DNP-flagellin.

There is a growing body of evidence which suggests that thymus-derived cells can suppress the response to thymus independent antigens (Baker *et al.*, 1970*a*). One indication that this may be the case is the paradoxical finding that treatment with antilymphocyte serum augments the responses to pneumococcus SSSIII (Baker *et al.*, 1970*b*) and polyvinylpyrrolidone (Kerbel and Eidinger, 1971). If the mechanism of enhancement depends on the ability of antilymphocyte serum to prevent thymus-derived suppressor cells from functioning, then no

Table II. Thymus Independent Antigens

Antigen	Immunization	Day of assay	Assay[a]	Reference[b]
E. coli 0113 lipopolysaccharide	10 μg i.v.	4	PFC	(1)
"	0.1–100 μg i.v.	4	PFC	(2)
"	10⁹ E. coli	4	PFC	(2)
"	1 μg i.v. day 0 10 μg i.v. day 21	25	PFC	(2)
Pneumococcal poly-saccharide SSSIII	0.5 μg i.v.	5	PFC HA	(1)
In vitro				
Dinitrophenylated polymeric flagellin	100 ng	4	PFC	(3)
E. coli 0113 lipopolysaccharide	4 × 10⁶ E. coli	5	PFC	(4)

[a] PFC; plaque forming cells; HA, hemagglutinating antibody.

[b] (1) Manning *et al.* (1972); (2) Reed *et al.* (1973); (3) Feldmann *et al.* (1972); (4) Aden and Reed (1973).

enhancement should be seen when nude mice are treated with antilymphocyte serum. This prediction was confirmed by Baker *et al.* (1973).

Tolerance can be induced to thymus independent antigens such as pneumococcal polysaccharide and lipopolysaccharides. However, with the establishment of the existence of thymic dependent suppressor cells (Gershon and Kondo, 1971), the question was raised as to whether tolerance was itself a thymic dependent function. That this need not be the case was shown by Nossal *et al.* (1973). The response to dinitrophenol covalently bound to flagellin is thymus independent (Feldmann, 1972). Treatment of intact mice with the dinitrophenylated copolymer D glutamic acid-D lysine render them specifically tolerant to DNP even when the DNP is bound to flagellin (Katz *et al.*, 1972). Nudes can be rendered specifically tolerant to DNP by this procedure (Nossal *et al.*, 1973) proving that tolerance can be achieved in B cells in the absence of T cells. However, this might represent a special case since DNP-D-GL, like other D polymers, is probably not readily metabolized (Katz, personal communication; Gill, 1972).

Nudes should prove to be a fruitful source of information on the nature of the immune response to thymus independent antigens. The relationship of the mitogenic and antigenic properties of substances such as lipopolysaccharide has not been defined. For instance: Are there two separate cell surface sites that can bind lipopolysaccharide, one evoking mitosis and the other antigen specific? Is the increase in antibody forming cells following lipopolysaccharide immunization due to division or recruitment? (Sjöberg *et al.*, 1972). Are the cells that make antibody to thymus independent antigens a subclass of B cells?

RESPONSE TO THYMUS DEPENDENT ANTIGEN

Sheep Red Blood Cells

Sheep red blood cells present a problem. On the one hand, they are very easy to use as an antigen and provoke a response which is easy to quantify by both serological and cellular means. On the other hand, they are not a single antigen—not even a complex molecule with many determinants, but a mixture of many molecules with unknown antigenic, mitogenic, or other characteristics. They have been extensively used in studies of nudes, but until the parts played by the several components of sheep red blood cells are better understood, some caution is necessary in interpretation of results.

IgM

During the first five days after immunization, nude mice have as many plaque forming cells/10^6 spleen cells as do their littermates, but they have far fewer plaque forming cells/spleen (Wortis, 1971; Pantelouris and Flisch, 1972*a;* Pritchard *et al.*, 1973). Thereafter, as first pointed out by Pantelouris and Flisch (1971*b*), nudes do much less well than do controls. The fact that there is a greater discrepancy between nudes and normal splenic plaque forming cells late in the response suggests that either there is both a thymic dependent antigen and a thymic independent antigen in sheep red cells (Playfair and Purves, 1971) or that there are two types (two classes?) of IgM response, one thymus dependent (Plotz *et al.*, 1968).

This difference is more clearly seen if circulating antibody is measured (Kindred, 1971*a;* Pantelouris and Flisch, 1972*a;* Pritchard *et al.*, 1973; Reed and Jutila, 1972).

In normal mice there is a circulation of antibody forming cells (and their precursors) from the spleen to the lymph nodes, thymus, and bone marrow beginning on day four after immunization (Dresser *et al.*, 1972). After that point much of the antibody is produced in the nodes. This suggests that there may be a failure of peripheralization of antibody production in the nudes, that is, the migration of (B?) cells from the spleen to the nodes is thymus dependent. Or, alternatively, that all antibody production in the nodes is thymus dependent. Study of the distribution of antibody forming cells in nudes might answer this question.

Nudes do not produce a secondary response to sheep red blood cells. Rather, they produce a second primary (Kindred, 1971a; Pantelouris and Flisch, 1972a). This again suggests a partial thymic dependence of the IgM response to this antigen.

Most workers report that nude spleen cells in culture can give a meager response to sheep red blood cells (Adams, 1972; Aden et al., 1972; Feldmann and Basten, 1972; Feldmann et al., 1973; Gisler and Dukor, 1972; Sjöberg et al., 1972), but Watson et al. (1973) reported no response at all.

IgG

As measured by indirect plaque forming cells, there is a profound depression (1.2% of normal) of IgG antibody produced in response to sheep red blood cells (Kindred, 1971a; Pantelouris and Flisch, 1972a; Pritchard et al., 1973; Reed and Jutila, 1972; Wortis, 1971). This is reflected in the amount of circulating mercaptoethanol resistant antibody (Pritchard et al., 1973). This result confirms a finding made in thymectomized animals, namely that IgG responses are virtually totally thymus dependent, unlike IgM responses (Taylor and Wortis, 1968; Mitchell et al., 1972b). Since the presence of thymus cells can both augment the IgM response and facilitate the induction of an IgG response (see below) the question is raised as to whether these are accomplished by one or two mechanisms.

Other Antigens

Study of other antigens [streptococcal group A carbohydrate (Braun et al., 1972), chicken red blood cells (Reed and Jutila, 1972), bacteriophage fd (Kolsch et al., 1972), bacteriophage T4 (Kindred, 1971a), and Brucella abortus (Crewther and Warner, 1972)] has confirmed the basic findings obtained with sheep red blood cells: some IgM antibody, no secondary IgM response, and little, if any, IgG response.

In culture systems nude spleen cells show no response to dinitrophenylated fowl gammaglobulin or keyhole limpet haemocyanin (Feldmann and Basten, 1972).

Surprisingly, the ability of nude mice to capture antigen (both thymic dependent and independent) in lymph node follicles is not impaired (Mitchell et al., 1972a). This was demonstrated using ^{125}I labeled antigen and noting the localization of label in radioautographs of lymphoid organs taken from mice sacrificed at various times after immunization.

CONTACT SENSITIVITY

In a carefully controlled study, Pritchard and Micklem (1972) showed that nudes cannot be sensitized by skin painting with oxazalone as measured by ear thickness, weight increase of draining lymph nodes, or uptake of 5 iododeoxyuridine I^{125}.

CELL MEDIATED CYTOTOXICITY

Nude spleens cannot generate cytotoxic or killer cells with specificity for alloantigens. This was shown by Wagner (1972) and Feldmann et al. (1972). Nude spleen cells were cultured with mitomycin treated allogeneic Balb/C ($H-2^d$) spleen cells. After six days in culture the cells were harvested and their ability to kill ^{51}Cr labeled $H-2^d$ mastocytoma assessed. Even at killer/target ratios of 400:1, no killing was observed, whereas 90% of the target cells can be killed by normal sensitized spleen cells at ratios of as little as 10:1.

SKIN GRAFTS

Since the original publication by Rygaard (1969) that rat skin will survive for prolonged periods when grafted to nudes, there have been many reports confirming this observation. Allografts are maintained for the lifetime of the nude (Kindred, 1971; Pantelouris, 1971; Pennycuik, 1971; Wortis, 1971). Xenografts, too, are not rejected, but this can be demonstrated only when care is taken to prevent damage to the graft by scratching or biting. Under these conditions, Manning et al. (1973) were able to show that nudes would accept for their lifetime grafts not only from cats and humans but from chickens, lizards, and tree frogs. The results can be truly spectacular (Fig. 1). From this study it can be concluded that for graft rejection there is an absolute requirement for a thymus. Results from earlier experiments in which chicken skin grafts appeared to be rejected (Shaffer et al., 1973) are now explained as the result of trauma rather than true rejection.

TUMOR GRAFTS

Rouse et al. (1973) demonstrated that nude mice are killed by a transplanted allogeneic plasma cell tumor which regresses when transplanted to a normal syngeneic host.

Rygaard and Povlsen (1969) were able to grow a highly differentiated human adenocarcinoma of the colon in nude mice and to effect a second transfer to more nudes. Subsequently, they reported (Povlsen and Rygaard, 1971) successful transplantation of six out of nine human adenocarcinomas to nudes. Of these, five were serially transplanted. The tumors maintained their

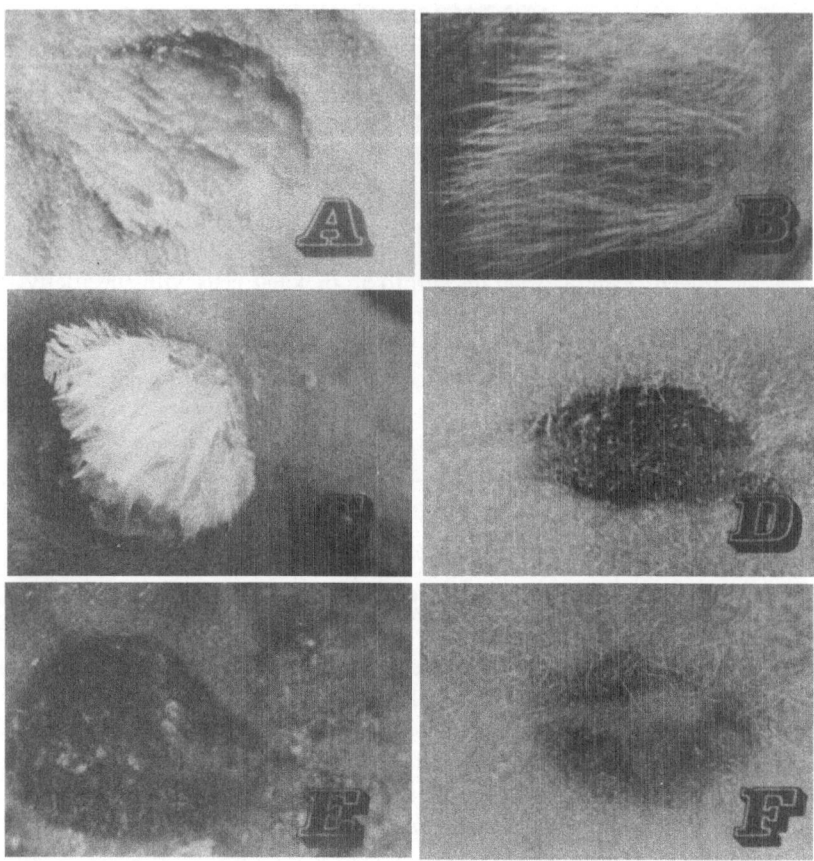

Figure 1. Outward appearance of skin xenografts maintained on nude mice. (A) Human graft at Day 60. (B) Cat graft at Day 51. This graft began hair growth at 20 days and continued growth until death of the recipient at 102 days. (C) Chicken graft at Day 32. This skin was grafted with feathers intact. (D) Chameleon graft at Day 41. (E) Fence lizard graft at Day 28. (F) Tree frog graft at Day 40. The pale central area represents a white stripe on the living frog. (Reprinted with permission from the *Journal of Experimental Medicine,* Vol. 138, No. 2, 1973.)

histological appearance but failed to metastasize. Giovanella *et al.* (1972) have grown a human melanoma in nudes. The tumor was invasive.

SPONTANEOUS TUMORS

Spontaneous malignant tumors have not been seen in untreated nude mice (Wortis, unpublished; Reed and Jutila, personal communication). This is an intriguing observation since it plays havoc with the notion that thymus dependent immunological surveillance (Thomas, 1959; Burnet, 1969) is important in tumor prevention. However, it should be remembered that few nudes raised in a conventional environment live much beyond four months; hence the number of observed mice at risk has been very small.

Still, several additional observations bear on this point. One is that within several months after receiving thymus grafts, nudes do develop tumors (Wortis, unpublished). Reticulum cell sarcoma, thymoma (of the graft), and adeno-carcinoma have been observed. Mammary adenocarcinoma occurs spontaneously in the CBA line to which the nude gene has been introduced (Staats, 1972). Reticulum cell carcinoma can follow chronic graft *vs.* host disease (Andre-Schwartz *et al.,* 1967) and thymoma may occur in thymus grafts (Hays, 1968). It is too soon to say with certainty that thymus grafted nudes are more susceptible to tumor development than their normal littermates.

The evidence at hand suggests the possibility that athymic nudes are resistant to tumor development. This has been directly examined by Johnson *et al.* (unpublished). They have tried to induce tumors by skin painting animals with dimethylbenzanthracene. Under conditions in which their littermates develop papillomas nudes develop no tumors. Since there was a possibility that the abnormality in nudes which blocks normal hair development might also prevent the carcinogenic action of this agent, normal skin was grafted to nudes. This skin, too, failed to develop tumors. This suggests a central "lesion." Further-more, after a thymus graft, nudes do develop tumors when skin painted. Friend virus fails to induce leukemia in nudes unless the recipient has been given a thymus graft (Kouttab *et al.,* unpublished).

There are several alternative explanations for these data, such as: (1) a normal immune mechanism is needed for carcinogenesis; (2) the target cells in these experiments were T cells; and (3) the thymus provides a stimulus (perhaps mitogenic) necessary for tumorogenesis. These are readily verifiable hypotheses, and no doubt we shall soon have some insight into this problem. In the meantime, it remains an intriguing paradox.

EFFECT OF MITOGENS ON ANTIBODY PRODUCTION *IN VITRO*

Lipopolysaccharides, when added in microgram quantities to nude spleen cell cultures, increase the number of plaque forming cells to sheep red blood cells (Sjöberg *et al.,* 1972). When sheep red cells are also included in the culture, the added lipopolysaccharide further augments the plaque forming cell response (Sjöberg *et al.,* 1972; Watson *et al.,* 1973). No IgG plaque forming cells are seen under these conditions (Andersson *et al.,* 1972c). Neither concanavalin A nor pokeweed mitogen has any enhancing effect on nude cultures in contrast to their effect on normal spleen cells which have been depleted of T cells by treatment with anti-θ serum and complement (Watson *et al.,* 1973). Since, at first glance, spleen cells depleted of θ-positive cells and nude cells would appear to be equivalent, this appears to be a paradox; but perhaps enough T cells escaped the anti-θ treatment to interact with B cells, although there were not enough to produce measurable DNA synthesis. This could be directly tested by noting the effect of small numbers of T cells plus concanavalin A on the response of nude cells to sheep red blood cells. Alternatively, the thymus-derived cells which enhanced the immune response could have been θ-negative. It has long been known that θ-positive cells disappear from the lymph nodes of thymectomized mice before the mice become functionally athymic (Schlesinger and Yron, 1970).

It is already known that if the supernate from thymocytes cultured 24 hours is added to a culture of nude spleen cells, the latter become responsive to the mitogenic action of concanavalin A (Andersson et al., 1972b).

Supernates from concanavalin A stimulated thymocytes are more effective than those from nonstimulated cultures, but it is not clear that this is a specific response. It is not known whether such supernates will augment the mitogenic response of nude cultures to phytohemagglutinin, pokeweed, allogeneic cells, or sheep red blood cells, although it was shown that they were not themselves mitogenic and did not augment the response to lipopolysaccharide.

EFFECT OF THYMOCYTES AND THYMUS-DERIVED CELLS ON ANTIBODY PRODUCTION *IN VITRO*

The addition of normal thymocytes to nude spleen cell cultures greatly enhances the plaque forming response to sheep red blood cells (Aden et al., 1972; Cone and Marchalonis, 1972; Feldmann et al., 1972; Bosing-Schneider and Kindred, 1972). This is also seen with peripheral T cells (Adams, 1972) and with cortisone acetate resistant thymocytes (Gisler and Dukor, 1972). But this effect is not readily seen with normal spleen cells which have been T cell-deprived (Hartmann, 1970). The explanation for this apparent discrepancy is that since nudes are not an inbred strain, the addition of thymocytes necessarily means that an allogeneic response is evoked, and it is well known that allogeneically stimulated thymocytes are able to augment antibody production (Haskill et al., 1970; Schimpl and Wecker, 1971).

T cells appear to be able to augment B cell responses by at least two mechanisms: a nonspecific factor evoked by stimuli such as allogeneic cells and an antigen specific factor. Feldmann and Basten (1972) and Feldmann (1972) were able to show that the nonspecific factor augments a variety of thymus independent responses and (in the presence of the antigen specific factor) thymus dependent responses. It could pass through a dialysis membrane and did not require the presence of macrophages. In contrast, the antigen specific factor augmented responses only to the antigen used to stimulate the thymocytes, could pass through nucleopore membrane (but not dialysis membrane), could initiate a response, and unlike the nonspecific factor, it required macrophages.

Whether the thymus produces only two such factors and whether they bear any relation to thymosin or to the materials which permit B cells to respond to concanavalin A and which allow IgG synthesis is unknown.

The ability of T cells to augment nude spleen cell responses to sheep red blood cells is further enhanced by the addition of polymers of polyadenylic and polyuridylic acid (Cone and Marchalonis, 1972). This polymer is a known stimulator of antibody formation (Braun *et al.*, 1968). Since it causes no augmentation in the absence of T cells, it is believed that it has no direct affect on B cells.

THYMUS GRAFTS *IN VIVO*

Thirty days after receiving a thymus graft, nudes can respond normally to sensitization with oxazalone (Pritchard and Micklem, 1972). Ten days after receiving an injection of a thymus cell suspension, nudes can reject allogeneic skin grafts (Pantelouris, 1971). Both thymus grafts and thymus cell suspensions allow nudes to produce normal levels of IgG_1, IgG_{2a}, and IgA (Pritchard *et al.*, 1973).

Thymus cell suspensions enable nudes to respond to sheep red blood cells (Kindred, 1971*b*) and when the donor and recipient differ with respect to the allotypic alleles at the Ig-1 locus [coding for the constant region of the heavy chain of IgG_{2a} subclass (Mishell and Fahey, 1964)], then the antibody produced is of the host (nude) phenotype. This type of restoration was also seen when other lymphoid tissue was used in the injected inoculum (Kindred and Weiler, 1972). There appears to be a requirement for the donor and recipient to share H-2 alleles for this type of restoration to work (Kindred and Shreffler, personal communication), a point established previously with thymectomized mice (Aisenberg, 1970). The situation here where interaction between thymus and host takes place over many weeks should not be confused with the *in vitro* reaction which lasts for only a few days and in which allogeneic combinations work much better than a syngeneic combination (see above). An exception to this observation is the work reported by Kindred (1972) in which thymus cells had the same H-2 specificities but not the same Ig-1 allotype as the recipient nudes. These grafts augmented the immune response to a variety of antigens (including graft rejection) but did not restore the ability of the nude to make antibody to Ig-1[b], the allotype produced by B cells of the donor strain. This suggested that either the thymocytes were inducing tolerance to this antigen or were themselves genetically incapable of recognizing Ig-1[b] molecules. The tolerance theory seems unlikely as nudes which received simultaneous injections of thymocytes from mice of Ig-1^b phenotype and of Ig-1^a phenotypes were able to make anti Ig-1^b antibody.

COMMENTS

Until recently, most studies of the immune response in nudes have confirmed principles previously established in experiments using thymectomized or suppressed mice. Now that colonies have been established in several laboratories, the focus is likely to shift and nudes will supply new rather than confirmatory data. The findings that xenograft rejection requires a thymus, and that IgA is particularly sensitive to a thymic presence are examples of this.

Although it is early, the likelihood is that the development of neoplasia in nudes will be a prime target area. Also the life history of B cells will no doubt be examined more thoroughly with a particular emphasis on their abilities to differentiate when free of thymic influence. All this plus interest in the pathogenesis of nudity itself will continue to make these animals a popular research subject.

ACKNOWLEDGMENTS

This work was supported by a grant from the National Institutes of Health (No. AM-15369-03). The assistance of B. Galgocci and Ms. R. Spitz is gratefully acknowledged.

NOTE ADDED IN PROOF

Strong evidence has been presented that the antigen and mitogenic properties of lipopolysaccharides are attributes of two portions of the molecule, the polysaccharide bearing the antigenic determinants and the lipid A acting as a mitogen and adjuvant (Chiller *et al.*, 1973; Andersson *et al.*, 1973).

A variety of substances, including poly adenylic-uridlyic acid, thymus extracts (and possibly endotoxin and muscle extracts) have been reported as inducing the expression of TL and θ antigen in nude mice (Scheid *et al.*, 1973).

REFERENCES

Adams, P. B., 1972. *In vitro* reconstitution by purified T cells of nude mouse spleen antibody response to SRBC antigen. *Aust. J. Exp. Biol. Med. Sci.* 50:665.
Aden, D. P., and Reed, N. D., 1973. *In vitro* immune response to lipopolysaccharide: Thymus-derived cells not required. *Immunol. Commun.*
Aden, D. P., Reed, N. D., and Jutila, J. W., 1972. Reconstitution of the *in vitro* immune response of congenitally thymusless (nude) mice. *Proc. Soc. Exp. Biol. Med.* 140:548.

Aisenberg, A. C., 1970. Allogeneic thymus grafts and the restoration of immune function in irradiated thymectomized mice. *J. Exp. Med.* **131**:275.

Andersson, B., and Blomgren, H., 1971. Evidence for thymus-independent humoral antibody production in mice against polyvinylpyrrolidone and *E. coli* lipopolysaccharide. *Cell. Immunol* **2**:411.

Andersson, J., Melchers, F., Galanos, C., and Luderitz, O., 1973. The mitogenic effect of lipopolysaccharide on bone marrow-derived mouse lymphocytes. *J. Exp. Med.* **137**: 943.

Andersson, J., Möller, G., and Sjöberg, O., 1972a. Selective induction of DNA synthesis in T and B lymphocytes. *Cell Immunol.* **4**:381.

Andersson, J., Möller, G., and Sjöberg, O., 1972b. B lymphocytes can be stimulated by concanavalin A in the presence of humoral factors released by T cells. *Eur. J. Immunol.* **2**:99.

Andersson, J., Sjöberg, O., and Möller, G., 1972c. Induction of immunoglobulin and antibody synthesis *in vitro* by lipopolysaccharides. *Eur. J. Immunol.* **2**:349.

Andersson, L. C., Nordling, S., and Hayry, P., 1973. Proliferation of B and T cells in mixed lymphocyte cultures. *J. Exp. Med.* **138**:324.

Andre-Schwartz, J., Schwartz, R. S., Mirtl, L., and Beldotti, L., 1967. Neoplastic sequelae of allogeneic disease ii. Electron-microscopic study of a neoplasm (reticuloendo theliosis) in survivors of the graft vs. host reaction. *Am. J. Pathol.* **50**:707.

Armstrong, W. D., Diener, E., and Shellam, G. R., 1969. Antigen-reactive cells in normal, immunized, and tolerant mice. *J. Exp. Med.* **129**:393.

Bach, J. F., and Dardenne, M., 1972a. Antigen recognition by T lymphocytes. I. Thymus and marrow dependence of spontaneous rosette forming cells in the mouse. *Cell. Immunol.* **3**:1.

Bach, J. F., and Dardenne, M., 1972b. Antigen recognition by T lymphocytes II. Similar effects of Azathioprine, antilymphocyte serum, and anti-theta serum on rosette-forming lymphocytes in normal and neonatally thymectomized mice. *Cell. Immunol.* **3**:11.

Bach, J. F., Dardenne, M., and Bach, M. A., 1973a. Detection of a circulating thymic hormone using T-rosette forming cells. In F. Daguillard (ed.), *Proceedings of the Seventh Leucocyte Culture Conference, June 6–11, 1972*, Academic Press, New York, pp. 271–287.

Bach, J. F., Dardenne, M., and Bach, M. A., 1973b. Demonstration of a circulating thymic hormone in mouse and in man. *Transpl. Proc.* **5**:99.

Bach, J. F., Dardenne, M., Goldstein, A. G., Guha, A., and White, A., 1971a. Appearance of T cell markers in bone marrow rosette-forming cells after incubation with thymosin, a thymic hormone. *Proc. Nat. Acad. Sci. U.S.A.* **68**:2734.

Bach, J. F., Dardenne, M., and Davis, A. J. S., 1971b. Early effect of adult thymectomy. *Nature New Biol.* **231**:110.

Baker, P. J., Stashak, P. W., Amsbaugh, D. F., Prescott, B., and Barth, R. F., 1970a. Evidence for the existence of two functionally distinct types of cells which regulate the antibody response to Type III pneumococcal polysaccharide. *J. Immunol.* **105**:1581.

Baker, P. J., Barth, R. F., Stashak, P. W., and Amsbaugh, D. F., 1970b. Enhancement of the antibody response to Type III pneumococcal polysaccharide in mice treated with antilymphocyte serum. *J. Immunol.* **104**:1313.

Baker, P. J., Reed, N. D., Stashak, P. W., Amsbaugh, D. F., and Prescott, B., 1973. Regulation of the antibody response to Type III pneumococcal polysaccharide. I. Nature of regulatory cells, *J. Exp. Med.* **137**:1431.

Bankhurst, A. D., and Warner, N. L., 1972. Surface immunoglobulins on the thoracic duct lymphocytes of the congenitally athymic (nude) mouse. *Aust. J. Exp. Biol. Med. Sci.* **50**:661.

Basten, A., Miller, J. F. A. P., Sprent, J., and Pye, J., 1972. A receptor for antibody on B lymphocytes I. Method of detection and functional significance. *J. Exp. Med.* **135**:610.

Bloemmen, J., and Eyssen, H., 1973. Immunoglobulin levels of sera of genetically thymus-less (nude) mice. *Eur. J. Immunol.* **3**:117.

Bosing-Schneider, R., and Kindred, B., 1972. Stimulation of "nude" spleen cells *in vitro* under the influence of thymus lymphocytes. *Cell. Immunol.* 5:593.

Braun, D. G., Kindred, B., and Jacobson, E. B., 1972. Streptococcal group A carbohydrate antibodies in mice: Evidence for strain differences in magnitude and restriction of the response, and for thymus dependence. *Eur. J. Immunol.* 2:138.

Braun, W., Nakano, M., Jaraskova, L., Yagima, Y., and Jiminez, H., 1968. Stimulation of antibody-forming cells by oligonucleotides of known composition. In O. J. Plescia and W. Braun (eds.), *Nucleic Acids in Immunology*, Springer Verlag, New York, p. 347.

Burnet, F. M., 1969. *Cellular Immunology*, Cambridge University Press, London.

Chiller, J. M., Skidmore, B. J., Morrison, D. C., and Weigle, W. O., 1973. The mitogenic effect of lipopolysaccharide on bone marrow-derived mouse lymphocytes. *J. Exp. Med.* 137:943.

Cone, R. E., and Marchalonis, J. J., 1972. Adjuvant action of poly (A:U) on T cells during the primary immune response *in vitro. Aust. J. Exp. Biol. Med. Sci.* 50:69.

Crewther, P., and Warner, N. L., 1972. Serum immunoglobulins and antibodies in congenitally athymic (nude) mice. *Aust. J. Exp. Biol. Med. Sci.* 50:625.

de Sousa, M. A. B., Parrott, D. M. V., and Pantelouris, E. M., 1969. The lymphoid tissues in mice with congenital aplasia of the thymus. *Clin. Exp. Immunol.* 4:637.

Dresser, D. W., Wortis, H. H., and Andersson, H. R., 1972. The effect of pertussis vaccine on the immune response of mice to sheep red blood cells. *Clin. Exp. Immunol.* 7:817.

Dwyer, J. M., Mason, S., Warner, N. L., and Mackay, I. R., 1971. Antigen binding lymphocytes in congenitally athymic (nude) mice. *Nature New Biol.* 234:252.

Feldmann, M., 1972. Cell interactions in the immune response *in vitro* V. Specific collaboration via complexes of antigen and thymus-derived cell immunoglobulins. *J. Exp. Med.* 136:737.

Feldmann, M., and Basten, A., 1972. Cell interactions in the immune response *in vitro* IV. Comparison of the effects of antigen-specific and allogeneic thymus-derived cell factors. *J. Exp. Med.* 136:722.

Feldmann, M., Wagner, H., Basten, A., and Holmes, M., 1972. Humoral and cell mediated responses *in vitro* of spleen cells from mice with thymic aplasia (nude mice). *Aust. J. Exp. Biol. Med. Sci.* 50:651.

Flanagan, S. P., 1966. "Nude," a new hairless gene with pleiotropic effects in the mouse. *Genet. Res. Camb.* 8:295.

Gershon, R. K., and Kondo, K., 1971. Infectious immunological tolerance. *Immunology* 21:903.

Gill, T. J., III, 1972. The chemistry of antigens and its influence on immunogenicity. In F. Borek (ed.), *Immunogenicity*, North Holland Publishing Company, London, pp. 5–44.

Giovanella, B. C., Yim, S. O., Stehlin, J. S., and Williams, L. J., 1972. Brief Communication: Development of invasive tumors in the "nude" mouse after injection of cultured human melanoma cells. *J. Nat. Cancer Inst.* 48:1531.

Gisler, R. H., and Dukor, P., 1972. A three-cell mosaic culture: *In vitro* immune response by a combination of pure B and T cells with peritoneal macrophages. *Cell. Immunol.* 4:341.

Goldstein, A. L., Asanuma, Y., and White, A., 1970. The thymus as an endocrine gland: Properties of thymosin, a new thymus hormone. In *Recent Progress in Hormone Research*, Vol. 26, Academic Press, New York, pp. 505–538.

Greaves, M. F., and Hogg, N. M., 1971. Immunoglobulin determinants on the surface of antigen binding T and B lymphocytes in mice. In B. Amos (ed.), *Progress in Immunology*, Academic Press, New York, pp. 111–126.

Hartmann, K., 1970. Induction of a hemolysin response *in vitro*. Interaction of cells of bone marrow origin and thymic origin. *J. Exp. Med.* 132:1267.

Haskill, J. S., Byrt, P., and Marbrook, J., 1970. *In vitro* and *in vivo* studies of the immune response to sheep erythrocytes using partially purified cell preparations. *J. Exp. Med.* 131:57.

Hayes, E. F., 1968. The role of thymus epithelial reticular cells in viral leukemogenesis. *Cancer Res.* 28:21.

Herzenberg, L. A., Herzenberg, L. A., Goodlin, R. C., and Rivera, E. C., 1967. Immunoglobulin synthesis in mice. Suppression by anti-allotype antibody. *J. Exp. Med.* 126:701.

Janossy, G., and Greaves, M. F., 1971. Lymphocyte activation I. Response of T and B lymphocytes to phytomitogens. *Clin. Exp. Immunol.* 9:483.

Katz, D. H., Hamaoka, T., and Benacerraf, B., 1972. Immunological tolerance in bone marrow-derived lymphocytes. I. Evidence for an intracellular mechanism of inactivation of hapten-specific precursors of antibody-forming cells. *J. Exp. Med.* 136:1404.

Kerbel, R. S., and Eidinger, D., 1971. Variable effects of antilymphocyte serum on humoral antibody formation: Role of thymus dependency of antigen. *J. Immunol.* 106:917.

Kindred, B., 1971a. Immunological unresponsiveness of genetically thymusless (nude) mice. *Eur. J. Immunol.* 1:59.

Kindred, B., 1971b. Antibody response in genetically thymusless nude mice injected with normal thymus cells. *J. Immunol.* 107:1291.

Kindred, B., 1972. Specificity of antigen recognition by normal thymus cells in nude mice. *Eur. J. Immunol.* 2:383.

Kindred, B., and Weiler, E., 1972. The response to SRBC by nude mice injected with lymphoid cells other than thymus cells. *J. Immunol.* 109:382.

Kolsch, E., Davies, A. J. S., and Leuchars, E., 1972. The immune response to phage fd in normal and thymus-deprived animals of a low responding inbred strain and in genetically thymusless mice. *Eur. J. Immunol.* 2:541.

Lance, E. M., Gillette, S. C., Goldstein, A. L., White, A., and Zatz, M. M., 1973. On the mode of action of thymosin. *Cell. Immunol.* 6:123.

Luzzati, A. L., and Jacobson, E. B., 1972. Serum immunoglobulin levels in nude mice. *Eur. J. Immunol.* 2:473.

Mandel, T. E., 1972. Intramembraneous marker in T lymphocytes. *Nature New Biol.* 239:112.

Manning, D. D., and Jutila, J. W., 1972. Immunosuppression of mice injected with heterologous anti-immunoglobulin heavy chain antisera. *J. Exp. Med.* 135:1316.

Manning, D. D., Reed, N. D., and Shaffer, C. F., 1973. Maintenance of skin xenografts of widely divergent phylogenetic origin on congenitally athymic (nude) mice. *J. Exp. Med.* 138:488.

Manning, J. K., Reed, N. D., and Jutila, J. W., 1972. Antibody response to Escherichia Coli lipopolysaccharide and Type III pneumococcal polysaccharide by congenitally thymusless (nude) mice. *J. Immunol.* 108:1470.

Mishell, R., and Fahey, J. L., 1964. Molecular and submolecular localization of two isoantigen (allotypes) of mouse immunoglobulins. *Science* 143:1440.

Mitchell, J., Pye, J., Holmes, M. C., and Nossal, G. J. V., 1972a. Antigens in immunity. Antigen localization in congenitally athymic "nude" mice. *Aust. J. Exp. Biol. Med. Sci.* 50:637.

Mitchell, G. F., Grumet, F. C., and McDevitt, H. O., 1972b. Genetic control of the immune response. The effect of thymectomy on the primary and secondary antibody response of mice to poly-L (Tyr, Glu)-poly-D, L-Ala-poly-L-Lys. *J. Exp. Med.* 135:126.

Mosier, D., and Cantor, H., 1971. Functional maturation of mouse thymic lymphocytes. *Eur. J. Immunol.* 1:459.

Nossal, G. J. V., Pike, B. L., and Katz, D. H., 1973. Induction of B cell tolerance *in vitro* to 2,4-dinitrophenyl coupled to a copolymer of d-glutamic acid and d-lysine (DNP-d-GL). *J. Exp. Med.* 138:312.

Pantelouris, E. M., 1971. Observation on the immunobiology of "nude" mice. *Immunology* 20:247.

Pantelouris, E. M., 1968. Absence of thymus in a mouse mutant. *Nature* 217:370.

Pantelouris, E. M., and Flisch, P. A., 1972a. Responses of athymic ("nude") mice to sheep red blood cells. *Eur. J. Immunol.* 2:236.

Pantelouris, E. M., and Flisch, P. A., 1972b. Estimation of PFC and serum haemolysin response to SRBC in "nude" mice. *Immunology* 22:159.

Pantelouris, E. M., and Hair, J., 1970. Thymus dysgenesis in nude (nu nu) mice. *J. Embryol. Exp. Morph.* 24:615.

Pennycuik, P. R., 1971. Unresponsiveness of nude mice to skin allografts. *Transplantation* 2:417.

Playfair, J. H. L., and Purves, E. C., 1971. Antibody formation by bone marrow cells in irradiated mice. I. Thymus-dependent and thymus-independent responses to sheep erythrocytes. *Immunology* 21:113.

Plotz, P. H., Colten, H., and Talal, N., 1968. Mouse macroglobulin antibody to sheep erythrocytes: A non-complement-fixing type. *J. Immunol.* 100:752.

Povlsen, C. O., and Rygaard, J., 1971. Heterotransplantation of human adenocarcinomas of the colon and rectum to the mouse mutant nude. A study of nine consecutive transplantations. *Acta Pathol. Microbiol. Scand.* 79:159.

Pritchard, H., and Micklem, H. S., 1973. Haematopoietic stem cells and progenitors of functional T lymphocytes in the bone marrow of "nude" mice. *Clin. Exp. Immunol.*

Pritchard, H., and Micklem, H. S., 1972. Immune responses in congenitally thymusless mice I. Absence of response to oxazolone. *Clin. Exp. Immunol.* 10:151.

Pritchard, H., Riddaway, J., and Micklem, H. S., 1973. Immune responses in congenitally thymusless mice II–Quantitative studies of serum immunoglobulins, the antibody response to sheep erythrocytes, and the effect of thymus allografting. *Clin. Exp. Immunol.* 13:125.

Raff, M. C., 1970. Two distinct populations of peripheral lymphocytes in mice distinguishable by immunofluorescence. *Immunology* 19:637.

Raff, M. C., and Wortis, H. H., 1970. Thymus dependence of θ-bearing cells in the peripheral lymphoid tissues of mice. *Immunology* 18:931.

Reed, N. D., and Jutila, J. W., 1972. Immune response of congenitally thymusless mice to heterologous erythrocytes. *Proc. Soc. Exp. Biol. Med.* 139:1234.

Reed, N. D., Manning, J. K., and Rudbach, J. A., 1973. Immunological responsiveness of mice to LPS from Escherichia coli. *J. Infectious Diseases* (Endotoxin Supplement).

Rouse, B. T., Rollinghoff, M., and Warner, N. L., 1973. Tumor immunity to murine plasma cell tumors II. Essential role of T lymphocytes in immune response. *Eur. J. Immunol.* 3:218.

Rygaard, J., 1969. Immunobiology of the mouse mutant "nude." Preliminary investigations. *Acta Pathol. Microbiol. Scand.* 77:761.

Rygaard, J., and Povlsen, C. O., 1969. Heterotransplantation of a human malignant tumor to "nude" mice. *Acta Pathol. Microbiol. Scand.* 77:758.

Sabolovic, D., Sabolovic, N., and Dumont, F., 1972. Identification of T and B cells in mouse and man. *Lancet* (October 28), p. 927.

Schaible, R. H., and Gowen, J. W., 1961. A new dwarf mouse. *Genetics* 46:896.

Scheid, M. P., Hoffman, M. K., Komuro, K., Hammerling, U., Abbott, J., Boyse, E. A., Cohen, G. H., Hooper, J. A., Schulof, R. S., Goldstein, A. L., 1973. Differentiation of T-cells induced by preparations from thymus and by non-thymic agents. *J. Exp. Med.* 138:1027.

Schimpl, A., and Wecker, E., 1971. Reconstitution of a thymus cell derived immune system by syngeneic and allogeneic thymocytes *in vitro*. *Eur. J. Immunol.* 1:304.

Schlesinger, M., and Yron, I., 1970. Serologic demonstration of a thymus-dependent population of lymph node cells. *J. Immunol.* 104:798.

Schnebli, H. P., and Dukor, P., 1972. Plant agglutinins used to distinguish between different classes of mouse lymphocytes. *Eur. J. Immunol.* 2:607.

Shaffer, C. F., Reed, N. D., and Jutila, J. W., 1973. Comparative survival of skin grafts from several donor species on congenitally athymic mice. *Transpl. Proc.* 5:711.

Sjöberg, O., Andersson, J., and Möller, G., 1972. Lipopolysaccharide can substitute for helper cells in the antibody response *in vitro*. *Eur. J. Immunol.* 2:326.

Sprent, J., 1973. Circulating T and B lymphocytes of the mouse I. Migratory properties. *Cell. Immunol.* 7:10.

Sprent, J., and Basten, A., 1973. Circulating T and B lymphocytes of the mouse II. Lifespan. *Cell. Immunol.* 7:40.

Sprent, J., and Miller, J. F. A. P., 1972. Thoracic duct lymphocytes from nude mice: Migratory properties and lifespan. *Eur. J. Immunol.* 2:384.

Staats, J., 1972. Standardized nomenclature for inbred strains of mice: Fifth listing. *Cancer Res.* **32**:1609.

Taylor, R. B., and Wortis, H. H., 1968. Thymus dependence of antibody response: Variation with dose of antigen and class of antibody. *Nature* **220**:927.

Thomas, L., 1959. In H. S. Lawrence (ed.), *Cellular and Humoral Aspects of the Hypersensitive States,* Cassell, London, p. 529.

Vischer, T. L., 1972. Mitogenic factors produced by lymphocyte activation: Effect on T and B cells. *J. Immunol.* **109**:401.

Vujanovic, N., Kinsky, R. G., and Voisin, G. A., 1972. Premiere demonstration de differences morphologiques entre des lymphocytes appartenant a des populations cellulaires thymo-dependantes et thymo-independantes. *C.R. Acad. Sci. (Paris)* **275**:1933.

Wagner, H., 1972. The correlation between the proliferative and the cytotoxic responses of mouse lymphocytes to allogeneic cells *in vitro. J. Immunol.* **109**:630.

Walters, C. S., and Wigzell, H., 1970. Demonstration of heavy and light chain antigenic determinants on the cell-bound receptor for antigen, similarities between membrane-attached and humoral antibodies produced by the same cell. *J. Exp. Med.* **132**:1233.

Watson, J., Epstein, R., Nakoinz, I., and Ralph, P., 1973. The role of humoral factors in the initiation of *in vitro* primary immune responses ii. Effects of lymphocyte mitogens. *J. Immunol.* **110**:43.

Wortis, H. H., 1973. Pleiotropic effects of the nude mutation in D. Bergsma and R. Good (eds.) *Proceedings of the Second International Workshop on Primary Immunodeficiency Diseases,* in press.

Wortis, H. H., 1971. Immunological responses of "nude" mice. *Clin. Exp. Immunol.* **8**:305.

Wortis, H. H., Nehlsen, S., and Owen, J. J., 1971. Abnormal development of the thymus in "nude" mice. *J. Exp. Med.* **134**:681.

Zeiller, K., Liebich, H. G., and Hannig, K., 1971. Free-flow electrophoretic separation of lymphocytes. Two thoracic duct lymphocyte subpopulations studied after prolonged cannulation and immunization. *Eur. J. Immunol.* **1**:315.

Index